# More Pr[a]
## *The Enlighte[n]*

"Now that the evidence favoring the health value of a plant-based diet is becoming so overwhelming, it is time to provide some straightforward 'how-to' books and recipes. For the sake of your palate, I highly recommend Marie Oser's book!"

— T. COLIN CAMPBELL, PH.D.,
Jacob Gould Schurman Professor Emeritus
of Nutritional Biochemistry, Cornell University

"*The Enlightened Kitchen* will help bring you and your family into the twenty-first century—well informed about the importance of plant-based nutrition, and in excellent health. Marie Oser continues her tradition of bringing you the very best in healthful vegetarian cooking."

— JOHN MCDOUGALL, M.D.,
internist, author, lecturer

"Marie Oser has done it again! Her recipes are to be enjoyed and her message taken to heart: to protect and support your health, begin moving toward a more plant-based diet today. *The Enlightened Kitchen* can help show you the way."

— SUZANNE HAVALA HOBBS, DR.P.H., M.S., R.D.,
author, *Being Vegetarian for Dummies*,
Adjunct Assistant Professor, School of Public Health,
The University of North Carolina at Chapel Hill

"I've heard Marie Oser referred to as the vegan Martha Stewart, and I have to agree: she has indeed turned the meatless kitchen into an extraordinary and delicious experience. Oser knows her stuff."

— GERALD ETTER,
food editor, *Philadelphia Inquirer*

# THE
# ENLIGHTENED
# KITCHEN

# THE ENLIGHTENED KITCHEN

*Eat Your Way to Better Health*

Marie Oser

John Wiley & Sons, Inc.

Published by John Wiley & Sons, Inc., Hoboken, New Jersey
Published simultaneously in Canada

Design and production by Navta Associates, Inc.

For general information about our other products and services, please contact our Customer Care
Department within the United States at (800) 762-2974, outside the United States at (317) 572-3993
or fax (317) 572-4002.

Wiley also publishes its books in a variety of electronic formats. Some content that appears in print may
not be available in electronic books.

ISBN 0-471-08929-X

Printed in the United States of America

10 9 8 7 6 5 4 3 2 1

*To all who would strive to make this world a better place—*
*for people, for the planet, and for our trusting friends, the animals.*
*And, as always, to Justin, my son and my pride and joy.*

# Contents

Foreword    xi

Acknowledgments    xiii

Introduction    1

Good Food, Good Health    5

Have a Heart    5

An Ounce of Prevention . . .    7

Dairy . . . What's Up with That?    10
Got Osteoporosis?    10

Plant Protein    15

Permanent Weight Control    18

Plant-Based Cuisine: The Shift Starts Here    21

Mainstreaming    23

Nature's Pharmacy: The Incredible Edibles    25
Antioxidants    25
Phytochemicals    26

The Enlightened Pantry: What to Have on Hand    31

Notes on Ingredients    36
All about Soyfoods    37
Other Plant-Based Ingredients    41

The Recipes

Enlightened Entertaining    53

Soups, Salads, and Starters    89

Enticing Entrées    111

Contents

ᴄᴡ

x

Savory Sides    161

Self-Sufficient Gourmet    191

Marvelous Muffins and Loaves    223

Sweet Sensations    241

Resource Guide    269

Internet Resources    275

Recommended Reading    279

Bibliography    281

Index    287

# FOREWORD

There was a time when most of us thought that eating healthfully meant depriving ourselves of pleasure. It meant consuming austere diets of brown rice, painstakingly measuring calories, or dutifully combining proteins and laboriously comparing amino acid charts.

Now, though, we are realizing that eating healthfully can be a joyous adventure full of new taste delights and delicious discoveries.

That is, of course, if we know how.

And this is just exactly where Marie Oser's new book, *The Enlightened Kitchen,* comes to our aid. This book—full of healthy, low fat, plant-based recipes made with easy-to-use ingredients—opens a door to a marvelous world of wholesome gourmet meals. If you love to cook, you will find recipe after recipe here to stimulate your creativity and expand your repertoire. If, on the other hand, cooking has always seemed to you to be a necessary evil, prepare to have your horizons expanded and your orientation shifted, because these recipes are fun to create, and even more fun to eat.

Have you ever wondered if a meal was too high in fat, or sodium, and not known how to tell? Each recipe here comes with a comparative analysis, providing you the information you need to be assured that you are preparing food that is in alignment with your health goals.

May you enjoy each and every minute involved in using this book to prepare the food that you and others will eat. It's a good feeling knowing that the meals you bring forth will be both delicious and nutritious.

—John Robbins,
author of *The Food Revolution*
and *Diet for a New America*

# ACKNOWLEDGMENTS

Grateful acknowledgment to:

▶ *My editor, Elizabeth Zack,* for her guidance and skillful editing. Working with Elizabeth is like sharing a favored project with a very good friend. Her ongoing enthusiasm, support, and good humor have made working with her a delight.

▶ *Jeff and Sabrina Nelson of VegSource.* They are the heart that beats within the VegSource Family, an interactive Web site notable as a tremendous resource for health-conscious consumers. The VegSource community includes many prominent professionals with a common goal: to disseminate cutting edge health and nutrition information. I am proud to be a VegSourcer.

▶ *The Physicians Committee for Responsible Medicine,* for the timely research data and health recommendations they provide for professionals and laypeople alike. And for their diligence in confronting institutions and government agencies about policies involving issues of nutrition, preventive medicine, and ethical research practices.

▶ *EarthSave International,* an outstanding organization that promotes healthy food choices for people and for the planet. EarthSave chapters provide education, support, and encouragement to anyone interested in issues of diet.

▶ *John Robbins, Dr. Neal Barnard, Dr. John McDougall, Dr. T. Colin Campbell, and Dr. Dean Ornish,* the most prominent among health professionals and advocates who have laid the groundwork for promoting the plant-based diet. They provide the logical, scientific, and compassionate framework on which I build my "kitchen science." They are my heroes!

▶ *Jerry Etter,* editor of *The Philadelphia Inquirer,* who was the first editor to run my column, "The Enlightened Kitchen." A terrific editor and a wonderful person who has since retired after thirty years of service. God bless you, Jerry.

Acknowledgments

xiv

 *Linda Martinez,* food editor at the Ventura County Star, a Scripps Howard and Food Network affiliate, for her support and encouragement. Linda's assistance has been critical to integrating the various aspects of my work to other media.

 *Ellen Tarantino, Mary Kathleen Benson, and Patricia Jones,* my personal assistants and VegTv crew, who help make it possible for me to accomplish my goals.

 *Sherry Brooks, George Brooks, Patricia and George Jones, Ellen and Paul Tarantino, Judy Rae, Dale Hallcom, and Gail Storch,* who are my tasters.

 *And my dear son, Justin Oser,* who is always there for me. He has been my bridge between the MAC and PC worlds, reformatting documents, relaying emails, and doing whatever he could to help me finish this work within deadline. All without complaint!

# Introduction

Welcome to *The Enlightened Kitchen,* a comprehensive guide for the health-conscious cook interested in delicious, wholesome food. "The Enlightened Kitchen," the newspaper column, made its debut in the Sunday edition of *The Philadelphia Inquirer* on October 10, 1999. The first plant-based column to be syndicated, "The Enlightened Kitchen" has been expanded here for my readers to enjoy in a more permanent collection.

In this book you will find the latest information regarding how to implement healthy plant-based options and the resulting health benefits. You will be introduced to concepts, techniques, and ingredients that can transform heavy traditional fare *delectably!* In *The Enlightened Kitchen* we make traditional meals healthfully, without losing flavor, texture, or eye appeal. These wholesome, richly satisfying dishes, from hearty entrées to lavishly delectable desserts, are enticing and delicious. Each recipe features a complete nutrition analysis of each dish, as well as a comparative analysis of the dish if it were made with animal products. The feature "Notes on Ingredients" not only describes easy-to-use and widely available ingredients, it also tells you where to find them.

Most people try to "eat healthy" these days. Many are cutting back on red meat and adding more fruits and vegetables to their diet. Is this enough to make a difference? Enlightened nutrition experts say "no," and my own personal story supports this recommendation. Let me explain. I became vegetarian in 1971, after reading Frances Moore Lappé's *Diet for a Small Planet.* At the time I became a lacto-ovo vegetarian, which means that eggs and dairy products were still part of my diet. I thought I was eating a healthy diet because I ate no "flesh foods"—beef, pork, chicken, or fish. This was my diet for many years. But in early 1990, I received a startling wake-up call.

In the course of a routine medical exam, it was determined that my blood cholesterol level was 240, much higher than it should have been. I was very surprised since, after all, I walked 15 miles briskly each week. So my decision to "kick" eggs and dairy was immediate. I began exploring plant-based alternatives and started using soyfoods extensively. I continued to make exceptional desserts, and you will note that my baked goods are made without added fat. The techniques developed in *The Enlightened Kitchen* are all the result of my commitment to the plant-based diet. As a result of these further changes to my diet, my blood cholesterol began dropping almost immediately. At the end of six months I had lost 40 pounds and my blood cholesterol was 170. It also helps that I remain fit and active, hiking 3 miles most days and spending an average of 6 hours a week at the gym. My weight has remained stable since 1990, and as I write this, at 5 feet 2 inches, I weigh 107 pounds and wear a size 1.

Making positive lifestyle changes has been cited as the most important step a person can take toward improving health. But just what is the "plant-based" diet, and how do you employ the elements of this much touted regime?

The plant-based diet is one that takes full advantage of legumes, grains, vegetables, and fruits. The health-conscious consumer looks for ways to "lighten" the menu and needs useful information beyond the usual "5 a Day" plan. Most health-conscious cooks are aware that there is a pressing need to reduce, and even eliminate, the high fat, cholesterol-laden ingredients found in traditional Western meals, and to incorporate nutritious, fiber-rich plant foods into every course of every meal. And that is what we do on every page of this book.

It is my belief that making healthful food choices will increase the odds of your being well and staying well. I am supported in this position by a multitude of studies that have been conducted since the early 1970s. There is a health crisis and an epidemic of obesity in America. The scientific evidence is overwhelming. Animal products contribute an extraordinary amount of cholesterol, fat, saturated fat, and protein to the Western diet. The ramifications are devastating! Coronary heart disease, breast cancer, prostate cancer, colon cancer, diabetes, and even Alzheimer's disease have all been linked to diet and lifestyle.

The link between the consumption of fruits, vegetables, and whole grains and disease prevention is clear and convincing. In study after study, components within these foods have demonstrated the ability to protect against—and sometimes even reverse—heart disease and the cancer process! Noted medical professionals, such as Drs. Dean Ornish, John McDougall, Neal Barnard, T. Colin Campbell, and Benjamin Spock are unanimous in recommending a plant-based diet for optimal health.

If you are like most people, you might think healthy eating means that all of your family favorites are suddenly off-limits. Perhaps you believe that it will be difficult to make meals that are good-tasting *and* good for you. But making food choices that lead to optimal health and well-being has never been easier. Enter *The Enlightened Kitchen,* and embark on an adventure in healthy eating as we explore the many wholesome alternatives available to health-conscious consumers. Introducing plant-based ingredients with proven health benefits to your diet, while eliminating unhealthy traditional ingredients, can be the most powerful health choice that you can make. *Adding while subtracting . . . what a concept!* It's so easy when you know how!

# Good Food, Good Health

## Have a Heart

Food is essential to life. And what we choose to eat will affect the way we look, feel, and function. Enlightened medical counsel recommends that Americans adopt a menu that is *low in fat, high in fiber,* and *rich in phytochemicals.* It seems as though a new study is released every day that emphasizes the need to reassess the meat-centered diet that has been the gold standard for most of the last century. Medical and nutrition professionals are saying that the key to good health lies in the plant kingdom, and that a healthy plant-based diet can help protect against heart disease. There are a number of reasons for this.

Plant-based diets are cholesterol-free and lower in total fat, especially saturated fat, than meat-based diets. They are higher in fiber, antioxidants, and phytochemicals. Animal products are the primary source of saturated fats, which cause the liver to produce more cholesterol, raising LDL ("bad" cholesterol) levels dramatically. Saturated fat does not occur in the plant kingdom in any significant amount, except in tropical oils, such as coconut and palm oil, and in cocoa butter. Animal products contain no fiber, whereas a plant-based diet is high in fiber, which carries excess hormones and cholesterol out of the body.

Consuming the conventional American diet over time will cause excess fats and cholesterol to build in the bloodstream, scarring the inner lining of the arteries. These scars collect fat and cholesterol and begin to swell, forming growths called "plaque." Plaque prevents the artery wall from remaining flexible, and as plaque increases in size, it will cause the arteries to narrow, reducing the flow of blood to the heart. This condition, called ischemia, can progress to angina, marked by mild to severe pains in the center of the chest due to diminished blood flow. Over time, this deadly buildup will cause arteries to become more fragile. Any increase in pressure can rupture the arterial wall. Should these plaque deposits break off, a clot can travel into the heart, leading to a heart attack, or to the brain, resulting in a stroke.

Yet when a patient presents with coronary heart disease, the remedy offered by the medical community at large is overwhelmingly either coronary bypass surgery, or angioplasty combined with cholesterol-lowering drugs. This is because Western medicine continues to be more focused on treating the symptoms rather than the cause. Therefore, generally a surgeon is called in to reroute the veins around the blockage (bypass surgery) or inflate a balloon inside the offending arteries (angioplasty) in order to "clear the blockage." And what is the composition of the blockage? The lab results always come back with the same analysis: *cholesterol and saturated fat.*

Bestselling author John Robbins, in his brilliantly provocative book, *The Food Revolution,* points out that in patients who undergo bypass surgery and angioplasty, the likelihood that their arteries will become blocked again within six months, can be as much as 50 percent—*if* they continue to eat a meat-based diet. Additionally, it is best to avoid these kinds of procedures as there is a risk of sustaining permanent brain damage as a result of bypass surgery. And while the risks of complications or death during angioplasty are much less, studies have shown that the number of heart attacks prevented, or lives prolonged by angioplasty, to be *zero.*

Coronary heart disease does not materialize without cause, and the answer does not lie in the surgeon's hand. We have become a nation so caught up in searching for the "magic bullet" that we have forgotten that we are the masters of our fate, and that we ourselves hold the key to good health and longevity!

The Framingham Heart Study, conducted over four decades with thousands of participants, determined that if an individual's cholesterol level remained below 150, the probability of a heart attack was very unlikely. The typical American diet is high in animal products, which contribute to the buildup of dietary cholesterol in the bloodstream. All flesh foods, including beef, pork products, poultry, and seafood, as well as eggs and dairy products, are the *only* source of dietary cholesterol, and the leading source of saturated fat.

Chicken consumption has almost doubled in the past 20 years, with North Americans eating more than 50 pounds of chicken per capita annually. This is due, in part, to a concentrated marketing campaign by the U.S. Department of Agriculture (USDA), which promotes chicken as a low-fat and wholesome food choice.

While the USDA has evolved into a government agency that sets nutrition standards and guidelines, its primary purpose at the outset was to support agriculture and promote farming interests. No matter how you view this agency, promoting the interests of consumers while acting as an advocate for agribusiness produces an obvious conflict of interest. As a result, consumers are often given selective information regarding issues surrounding food choices. For instance, you might be surprised to learn that beef and chicken have the same amount of cholesterol: 25 milligrams per ounce. And that 4 ounces of beef or chicken, half an egg, or 3 cups of milk all contain an equal amount of cholesterol: 100 milligrams. How about the fact that cholesterol is located primarily in the *lean* portion of meat?

Every 100 milligrams of dietary cholesterol increases cholesterol levels in your blood by about 5 points. Conversely, clinical studies have demonstrated that a one-third reduction in the amount of cholesterol in the bloodstream, say from 300 milligrams per deciliter to 200, can reduce the risk of a heart attack by as much as *two-thirds*. Adopting *The Enlightened Kitchen* style of cooking will enable you to eliminate unhealthy foods and help maintain a healthy heart.

# An Ounce of Prevention . . .

One in four individuals in North America will likely die of cancer. It's the second most common cause of death in the United States. Cancers that are most often associated with diet are cancer of the mouth, pharynx, larynx, esophagus, stomach, colon, rectum, liver, pancreas, lung, breast, uterus, and prostate.

There are many risk factors for cancer, and diet seems to account for the dramatic differences in the occurrence of the disease around the world. In fact, scientific evaluation of the typical Western diet strongly suggests a direct correlation between nutrition and disease prevention. Indeed, population studies have provided some of the most compelling evidence establishing the link between nutrition and cancer. The best-known is the highly regarded China-Cornell-Oxford Project, conducted in 1983 by Dr. T. Colin Campbell, the former senior science advisor to the American Institute for Cancer Research.

This landmark study investigated chronic degenerative disease, including a variety of cancers, cardiovascular diseases, and diabetes. It was found that degenerative diseases tended to cluster in the more urbanized, industrialized counties, while communicable diseases were primarily found in the more agricultural counties. The dietary and lifestyle factors chiefly associated with those counties where degenerative diseases were clustered included diets richer in animal products and higher in total fat. In fact, disease patterns suggested strongly that the intake of much larger quantities of animal-based foods was the major dietary factor responsible. Dr. Campbell wrote, at the conclusion of the study, "We found a significant association between the consumption of even small amounts of animal-based foods and the increasing prevalence of heart disease, cancer, and similar diseases."

An important study, released in 1997 was the result of the collaboration of the American Institute for Cancer Research, (AICR) and the World Cancer Research Fund. The resulting 660-page report, called *Food, Nutrition and the Prevention of Cancer: a Global Perspective,* was based on more than 4,500 research studies reviewed by contributors and peer-reviewers from the World Health Organization, the Food and Agriculture Organization of the United Nations, the International Agency on Research in Cancer, and the U.S. National Cancer Institute.

The key message of this comprehensive scientific analysis? *Cancer is a preventable disease,* and as many as 375,000 cases of cancer (at current cancer rates) could be prevented each year in the United States alone through healthy dietary choices. The recommendations include adopting a predominantly plant-based diet, rich in a variety of vegetables, fruits, grains, and legumes, maintaining a healthy weight, and performing at least one hour of vigorous exercise each week. According to the National Cancer Institute, 80 percent of cancers are due to factors that have been identified and can potentially be prevented. Lifestyle choices are the most significant contributor, with 30 percent due to tobacco use, and as much as 50 percent due to food choices.

Let's examine several kinds of cancer that are closely linked to diet. Cancer of the colon is defined as an abnormal and malignant mass of rapidly multiplying cells originating in the inner lining of the large intestine. The colon is the part of the large intestine that extends from the end of the small intestine to the rectum and people have an increasing risk for this type of cancer starting at the age of 40. One of the most striking features of colon cancer is the marked difference in the rate of incidence around the world. In less developed countries, such as parts of Asia, Africa, and Central and South America, this type of cancer is very rare; in developed countries such as Europe and North America, the incidence can be as much as 10 times greater. This has been attributed to, for the most part, differences in diet.

The human intestine is lengthy and is coiled inside the abdomen, so it requires a good deal of fiber to help move things along. The high levels of fat and lack of fiber that characterize all flesh foods foster the growth of bacteria that combine with certain bile acids to form carcinogenic substances. A diet high in fiber and low in fat is believed protective in that it speeds the movement of food through the body, actually reducing the production of carcinogenic substances in the intestine.

Diets high in fat also may have a negative effect on breast cancer survival rates. According to the Physicians Committee for Responsible Medicine, one reason is that foods affect the action of hormones in the body, as well as the strength of the immune system. For instance, several of the more common types of cancer, such as cancer of the breast, ovary, uterus, and prostate, are linked to sex hormones. In large part, the amount of hormones in our bodies and their actions are determined by the foods we eat.

High-fat diets can set you up for an increased risk of breast cancer, because fats increase the amount of estrogen in the blood. Estrogen stimulates breast cells in such a way that cancer is more likely to occur and is more aggressive. Plus, diets high in fatty foods lead to obesity, which also causes higher estrogen levels in the blood. However, if you ask any doctor what you should do in order to prevent breast cancer, the response will most likely be to get an annual mammogram, beginning at age 40 or 50. But mammograms do not prevent cancer . . . they only *find* cancer. Enlightened medical counsel recommend eating a low-fat, plant-based diet to eliminate foods that raise hormones in the blood. Additionally, vegetables and other healthful plant foods are rich in fiber, which helps reduce the risk of breast cancer by naturally decreasing estrogen levels. Add soy to the low-fat, plant-based diet, and you have an opportunity to downgrade the amount of estrogen in the blood even more radically. Soy products contain phytoestrogens. These phytochemicals are very weak plant estrogens that reduce human estrogens' ability to attach to your cells. This results in a marked reduction of estrogen in the blood and less estrogen stimulation of cells.

And what about prostate cancer? A recent study at the University of California at Los Angeles has shown that men who go on a low-fat, high-fiber diet and simultaneously exercise can favorably affect the hormones and serum growth factors that influence prostate cancer growth. The subjects adhered to a diet regimen that contained less than 10 percent of calories from fat, and lots of vegetables, fruits, and whole grains. The exercise component involved walking 30 to 60 minutes, at a quick pace, 4 to 5 days a week. The results suggested that exercise and a low-fat, high-fiber diet significantly reduced the growth of prostate cancer cells.

The scientific evidence is compelling. The recommendations are clear: replacing animal products with vegetables and other health-supporting plant foods and reducing overall fat should be your first line of defense against heart disease and many forms of cancer. As Dr. William Harris, in his classic book, *The Scientific Basis of Vegetarianism,* states, "The vegan (plant-based) diet, extolled by its advocates for at least 150 years as a cancer preventive strategy, is the logical end point of the dietary recommendations, now made by scientific organizations, to reduce animal food consumption."

# Dairy . . . What's Up with That?

### Got Osteoporosis?

If you were to believe the advertising associated with the "Milk Mustache" campaign, you would be concerned if you didn't get three glasses of milk a day. Consumers have been deluged with "Got Milk?" ads for years. This highly successful crusade features well-known celebrities (and even government officials!) sporting milk mustaches. Yet this campaign has been greeted with criticism from many medical and nutrition professionals. Why? Because of misleading information.

In July 2000, the Physicians Committee for Responsible Medicine (PCRM), a nonprofit health advocacy and research organization, filed a petition with the Federal Trade Commission. In September of 2001, the U.S. Department of Agriculture expert panel responded to the complaint with a report largely supporting the physicians' complaints, finding that many of the milk ads make "untruthful health claims."

In fact, a significant amount of scientific research has prompted serious concerns regarding the health risks associated with consuming dairy products. Cow's milk and the majority of products made from it are high in fat (particularly saturated fat) and cholesterol, and contain excess protein and contaminants, from pesticides to drugs. The advertising, sponsored by the National Dairy Council, gives the distinct impression that there is a "calcium emergency," and that we need to drink milk in order to keep our bones strong and healthy. Yet, according to Dr. Walter Willett, in *Eat, Drink, and Be Healthy,* osteoporosis is *not* a problem that should be associated with lack of calcium *intake.* Osteoporosis results from calcium *loss,* with excess dietary protein being a critical factor. He suggests that the substantial amount of protein in milk can result in a 50 percent loss of calcium in the urine! Clinical studies also have established that high protein intake aggravates calcium loss. For example, a 1994 report in the *American Journal of Clinical Nutrition* showed that when animal proteins were eliminated from the diet, calcium losses were cut in half.

The Harvard Nurses' Health Study, which followed more than 75,000 women for 12 years, showed no protective effect from increased milk consumption on fracture risk. What this study also revealed was that increased intake of calcium from dairy products was actually associated with a higher fracture risk. Despite this mounting evidence, the drinking of milk is diligently promoted for preventing osteoporosis. But, if consuming lots of dairy did prevent osteoporosis, Sweden, Finland, the United States, and Great Britain, having the highest rates of dairy consumption, would not enjoy the dubious distinction of also having the highest rates of osteoporosis and hip fractures in the world.

So what *is* in milk? Beyond the overload of fat, saturated fat, cholesterol, and protein, there are pesticides and antibiotics, and a powerful growth hormone, insulin-like growth factor, or IGF-1. According to the Journal of the National Institutes of Health, and many scientific studies, this hormone is linked to the proliferation of breast cancer cells. Prostate cancer is the fourth most common malignancy among men worldwide, with an estimated 400,000 new cases diagnosed annually. Dairy product consumption has also been shown to increase serum concentrations of IGF-I. Case-control studies in diverse populations have shown a strong and consistent association between serum IGF-I concentrations and prostate cancer risk.

A recent study released by the Harvard School of Public Health also has linked the high intake of dairy products to an increased risk of prostate cancer. Initially, researchers suspected that fat might be a factor, since whole milk is a source of excess fat and saturated fat. However, because 83 percent of the subjects in the study drank nonfat or skim milk, the researchers had to turn their attention to other possibilities. Dairy cows are treated with bovine growth hormone (rBGH) in order to boost milk production. This causes the level of IGF-1 to double in the cow's milk. Dr. Neal Barnard of the Physicians Committee for Responsible Medicine, says, "IGF-1 is indeed a growth factor, as the name implies. It causes things to grow. If you mix some of it with prostate cancer cells they grow like crazy. Other research studies have shown that when men (or women, for that matter) drink 2 or 3 glasses of milk a day, the amount of IGF-1 rises by about 10 percent. If you have more of this growth factor in your blood, the belief is that this would increase the likelihood that prostate cancer would arise." Dr. Barnard indicated that there have been a number of similar studies that have shown that men who have more IGF-1 in their blood have more prostate cancer risk. He also said that "even if a person drinks milk from a cow not treated with bovine growth hormone, there still is, we believe, sufficient evidence that IGF-1 levels in a human will rise . . . that the concentrated sugars and animal proteins (in cow's milk) stimulate the production of IGF-1 within the human body."

In *Eat to Beat Cancer,* Dr. Robert Hatherill, a research scientist at the University of California at Santa Barbara, indicates that we can set ourselves up for serious disease by exposing the body to dairy products. Infants with milk allergies make antibodies to fight milk proteins that are linked to destroying cells in the pancreas. In the case of cataracts, milk sugar can build up in the lens of the eye, causing irreversible clouding or cataract. Dr. Hatherill, whose field is environmental toxicology, also points out that cow's milk enhances the uptake of lead, cadmium, mercury, and other metals.

Is it possible for us to get the calcium we need without consuming lots of milk and dairy products? Just how much calcium *do* we need for healthy teeth and bones, and to stave off osteoporosis? In fact, the official recommended dietary allowance (RDA) in the United States is set at a hefty 1,000 milligrams per day for ages 19 to 50, and more for those over fifty and for pregnant and lactating women. But these recommendations are skewed, as they are set higher in order to compensate for the loss of calcium caused by the typical American diet based on animal products. Countries where dietary protein intake is very low set somewhat lower national recommendations. The World Health Organization recommends 500 milligrams of calcium for children and 800 for adults. Consider that elderly South African Bantu women consume a diet of about 50 grams of protein and only 450 milligrams of calcium per day, and do not develop osteoporosis. (In contrast, Eskimos, who consume a very high-protein diet with 250 to 400 grams of protein per day from fish, and a calcium intake of over 2,000 milligrams per day, have the highest rate of osteoporosis in the world!)

Dr. Charles Attwood points out in "Milk, A Catch-22" that adequate amounts of vegetables are *better sources of calcium than milk and cheese.* A cup of broccoli contains about the same amount of calcium as a cup of milk. A 1990 report in the *American Journal of Clinical Nutrition* concluded that greens such as broccoli and kale have high levels of calcium that are absorbed at least as well as that in milk. Excellent calcium balance on a nondairy diet is easily attained because all vegetables and legumes contain calcium, and collectively it's more than adequate. Plus, this calcium stays in the bones, unlike much of that from the high-protein dairy products. In addition, while dairy products may seem to contain an impressive amount of calcium, in order for our bodies to absorb calcium another mineral, magnesium, must be present in comparable amounts. As milk and dairy products contain only small amounts of magnesium, calcium absorption from milk is only about 32 percent. The excess calcium is then utilized by the body in a number of damaging ways. For example, it may be converted by the kidneys into painful stones that block the urinary tract and contribute to arthritis, or even gout. Dr. Neal Pinckney, author and founder of The Healing Heart Foundation, has said, "magnesium . . . is richest in vegetables and whole grains."

So, milk does not offer any nutrients that cannot be found in a far healthier form in other foods. And milk's major selling point—that drinking it will prevent osteoporosis—has been discredited by a mountain of scientific evidence. *A diet with a modest amount of protein and foods rich in calcium, that includes regular exercise is the prescription for protecting your bones.* Listed here are some of the healthful sources of calcium in the plant kingdom.

## PLANT SOURCES OF CALCIUM

| | | |
|---|---|---|
| Apple | 1 medium | 10 mg |
| Almonds | 1 ounce | 26 mg |
| Artichokes | ½ cup | 54 mg |
| Asparagus, cooked | 4 spears | 22 mg |
| Baked beans, vegetarian | 1 cup | 128 mg |

PLANT SOURCES OF CALCIUM *(continued)*

| | | |
|---|---|---|
| Banana | 1 medium | 7 mg |
| Blackstrap molasses | 2 tablespoons | 274 mg |
| Bok choy, cooked | 1 cup | 158 mg |
| Brazil nuts | 1 ounce | 50 mg |
| Broccoli, cooked | 1 cup | 94 mg |
| Brussels sprouts, cooked | 8 pieces | 56 mg |
| Brown rice, cooked | 1 cup | 23 mg |
| Butternut squash, cooked | 1 cup | 84 mg |
| Carrots | 2 medium | 38 mg |
| Cauliflower, cooked | 1 cup | 34 mg |
| Celery, cooked | 1 cup, cooked | 54 mg |
| Corn tortilla | one tortilla | 42 mg |
| Collard greens, cooked | 1 cup | 357 mg |
| Couscous, cooked | 1 cup | 15 mg |
| Cranberry beans, boiled | 1 cup | 88 mg |
| Figs, dried | 1 cup | 286 mg |
| Garbanzo beans, canned | 1 cup | 78 mg |
| Golden raisins, packed | 1 cup | 87 mg |
| Great Northern beans, boiled | 1 cup | 121 mg |
| Green peas | 1 cup | 44 mg |
| Kale, cooked | 1 cup | 94 mg |
| Kidney beans, boiled | 1 cup | 50 mg |
| Lentils, boiled | 1 cup | 37 mg |
| Lima beans | 1 cup | 52 mg |
| Navy beans, boiled | 1 cup | 128 mg |
| Oatmeal, cooked | 1 cup | 20 mg |
| Onions, cooked | 1 cup | 58 mg |
| Orange juice, fortified | 1 cup | 300 mg |
| Orange, navel | 1 medium | 56 mg |
| Pear, bartlett | 1 medium | 19 mg |
| Peanuts | 1 ounce | 15 mg |

| | | |
|---|---|---|
| Pita bread, enriched | one pita | 51 mg |
| Pinto beans, boiled | 1 cup | 82 mg |
| Raspberries | 1 cup | 35 mg |
| Rye bread | 1 slice | 20 mg |
| Soybeans, boiled | 1 cup | 175 mg |
| Soymilk, fortified | 1 cup | 240 mg |
| Sweet potato, boiled | 1 cup | 70 mg |
| Tahini | 2 tablespoons | 128 mg |
| Tempeh | 1 cup | 154 mg |
| Textured Vegetable Protein, dry | ⅝ cup | 160 mg |
| Tofu | ½ cup | 120–392 mg |
| Turnip greens, cooked | 1 cup | 249 mg |
| Turtle beans, boiled | 1 cup | 103 mg |
| Wax beans, canned | 1 cup | 174 mg |
| White beans, small, boiled | 1 cup | 131 mg |
| White potato, baked | 1 cup | 20 mg |
| Whole wheat bread | 1 slice | 20 mg |
| Whole wheat flour | 1 cup | 40 mg |

# Plant Protein

Protein is an important nutrient needed to maintain body tissues and muscle. It is made up of amino acids, the "building blocks" of the body, whose main function is building cells and repairing tissue. Amino acids can be synthesized by plants and micro-organisms, but not by animals. With proper nutrition, our bodies can make most of the different amino acids, but there are eight "essential" amino acids that cannot be synthesized by our bodies and must be obtained from dietary sources. It is a common misconception that essential amino acids are only available in animal products. A variety of legumes, grains, and vegetables can also provide all of the essential amino acids. Besides, when we obtain protein from animal sources such as cows, chickens, and pigs, we are getting these essential nutrients *second-hand*. These animals are naturally vegetarian. In the case of cows, for example, they graze on pasture land nibbling *plants* and eat grain-based feed.

High-protein animal foods provide the framework of the Western diet, but as you already know, they contribute an extraordinary amount of cholesterol and saturated fat. While there has been an overemphasis on high-protein animal products in American culture, quality protein from the plant kingdom has been greatly underestimated. Replacing animal foods with plant foods can be the most important health choice that you make.

In order to calculate your protein requirements, simply multiply your body weight (in pounds) by .36. For example, I weigh 107 pounds, (107 × 0.36 = 38.52). That means my daily protein requirement is 38.5 grams An adult male who weighs 160 pounds (160 × 0.36 = 57.6) needs less than 58 grams of protein a day. Yet the average American consumes about 103 grams of protein daily, 70 grams of which come from animal sources. Even pregnant women—who are eating for two—need only about 75 grams of protein a day.

High-protein diets are unhealthy, in that many respected medical and nutrition professionals link diets high in protein with bone mineral loss, or osteoporosis (see "Got Osteoporosis?" earlier in this chapter). A recent study conducted at the University of California at San Francisco demonstrates a strong link between animal protein consumption and osteoporosis. These findings suggest that a decrease in animal protein and an increase in vegetable protein may decrease bone loss and risk of hip fracture.

According to Dr. John McDougall, author of *The McDougall Program,* "When the protein content in the diet exceeds 15 percent of the calories consumed, the liver and kidneys are burdened with the task of ridding the body of excess protein. Under this strain, these organs enlarge and the physiology of the kidneys changes." He further states that animal protein, unlike vegetable protein, is plentiful in sulphur-containing amino acids, which encourage more calcium loss. Dr. Neal Barnard, in *Food for Life,* also observes, "High protein intakes have been found to contribute to progressive kidney damage." Dr. Robert Kradjian, author of *Save Yourself from Breast Cancer,* says, "There seems to be a consistent and profound association between cancer and large amounts of animal protein."

The adequate amounts of protein needed to maintain body tissue can be easily obtained on a vegetarian diet. Each day include: five or more servings of grains, three or more servings of vegetables, and two to three servings of legumes.

| | | |
|---|---|---|
| Almonds, blanched | 1 ounce | 5.8 gr |
| Barley, cooked | 1 cup | 19.8 gr |
| Broccoli, raw | 1 medium | 4.5 gr |
| Brown rice, cooked | 1 cup | 5 gr |
| Chinese-style tofu | 3 ounces | 9 gr |
| Edamame, boiled | 1 cup | 22.2 gr |
| Garbanzo beans, boiled | 1 cup | 14.5 gr |
| Gimme Lean | 2 ounces | 9 gr |
| Japanese-style tofu | 3 ounces | 6 gr |
| Jumbo veggie hot dogs | each | 16 gr |
| Kidney beans, boiled | 1 cup | 15.4 gr |
| Lentils, cooked | 1 cup | 17.9 gr |
| Lima beans, boiled | 1 cup | 14.7 gr |
| Marinated, baked tofu | 3½ ounces | 18 gr |
| Millet, cooked | 1 cup | 8.4 gr |
| Miso | ½ cup | 6.3 gr |
| Mung beans, boiled | 1 cup | 14.2 gr |
| Navy beans, boiled | 1 cup | 15.8 gr |
| Oatmeal, cooked | 1 cup | 6 gr |
| Peanuts, dry roasted | ¼ cup | 8.65 gr |
| Pinto beans, boiled | 1 cup | 14 gr |
| Pumpkin seeds, roasted | 1 ounce | 9.4 gr |
| Rye flour, dark | 1 cup | 18 gr |
| Sunflower seeds, roasted | 1 ounce | 5.5 gr |
| Sesame seeds, toasted | 1 ounce | 4.8 gr |
| Soybeans, boiled | 1 cup | 28.6 gr |
| Soy flour | 1 cup | 29.4 gr |
| Soynuts | 1 ounce | 13 gr |
| Spinach, raw | 10 ounces | 5.8 gr |
| Split peas, cooked | 1 cup | 16.3 gr |
| Textured Vegetable Protein, cooked | 3.5 ounces | 17.3 gr |

PLANT SOURCES OF PROTEIN *(continued)*

| | | |
|---|---|---|
| Veggie burger | each | 16 gr |
| Veggie ground round | 3 ounces | 10 gr |
| Wheat flour, wh. grain | 1 cup | 16.4 gr |
| Wheat germ, toasted | ¼ cup | 8.23 gr |
| White rice, cooked | 1 cup | 5.5gr |

# Permanent Weight Control

Americans are now among the fattest people on earth. One third of the nation is obese, and between 1980 and 1994, the percentage of obese teenagers doubled. New studies report that 55 percent of American women, 63 percent of men, and 25 percent of children are overweight. Americans' sedentary lifestyle and preference for high-fat, cholesterol-laden meals expose them to numerous health risks. Physicians estimate that 300,000 Americans die annually from obesity-related illnesses, which include heart disease, gall-bladder disease, diabetes, stroke, some cancers, and arthritis. Many doctors are calling obesity an epidemic, especially among the young.

For many people "dieting" is a constant battle. Most believe that to lose weight they have to go on a low-calorie diet, often starving until the diet is no longer tolerable. Then the weight comes right back and then some. Very-low-calorie diets are doomed because they lower the body's metabolic rate, which makes losing weight even more difficult, and can lead to bingeing.

Today the most popular diet plans are based on a high-protein, low-carbohydrate regimen. The focus is on protein-rich meats, poultry, fish, and cheese, and the severe restriction of carbohydrates. In contrast, the plant-based lifestyle I recommend is based on a high-carbohydrate, low-fat, and low-protein intake. Therefore the high-protein "Zone"-type diets are diametrically opposed to every enlightened principle that I support. People who follow these diets run the risk of developing potentially dangerous side effects, because of the excess protein, fat, saturated fat, and cholesterol they consume can lead to an increased risk of heart disease, osteoporosis, kidney stones, and cancer. The weight loss such diets offer is immediate, but cannot be sustained over the long term.

Dr. John McDougall, founder of the highly successful McDougall Plan for Healthy Living, offers a low-fat, plant-based diet that promotes a broad range of dramatic and lasting health benefits, such as weight loss and reversing of serious illness, such as heart disease, all without drugs.

Dr. Dean Ornish, founder and director of the Preventive Medicine Research Institute, is famous for his 17-year study on reversing heart disease through lifestyle changes alone. One interesting result of the study (which uses a plant-based diet, moderate exercise, and meditation) was that the participants who followed his program also lost an average of 22 pounds in the first year, although the focus of the study was not weight loss. Equally significant, the patients who participated in the program were showing even more improvement after four years.

A popular misperception today is that pasta, potatoes, rice, and bread are fattening. Not true. In fact, while making you feel full, carbohydrates contain less than half the calories of fat. Besides, carbohydrates are called "energy foods" because the body readily burns off 23 percent of the calories in carbohydrates. Yet, just 3 percent of the calories in fat are burned in the process of conversion and storage. So a diet high in starchy foods is perfect for permanent weight control.

Fats are the most concentrated source of food energy, contributing 9 calories per gram, which is more than double that of carbohydrates and proteins. So our Enlightened cakes, brownies, muffins, and quickbreads do not make use of added fat. You'll discover throughout *The Enlightened Kitchen* that we keep the use of oil to a minimum. At the start of my characteristic braise, I use only a scant teaspoon or two of olive oil. Olive oil is the only oil that I use, and there are several reasons for that. The flavor is superior to other oils, but more importantly, olive oil is monounsaturated, and monounsaturated fats are thought to lower cholesterol.

On the other hand, even though vegetable oil is of plant origin, it is not a health food. Vegetable oils are fluid and are primarily polyunsaturated fat, whereas fats from animal sources are solid at room temperature, and are the major source of saturated fat. There are also trans-fats which are fashioned from vegetable oils, and are also solid at room temperature, like shortening or margarine. Hydrogenation is the darling of the commercial baking industry, because it extends shelf life considerably. When a label lists "partially hydrogenated oil" as an ingredient, that is hydrogenated oil. With chemically induced hydrogen saturation, the structure of the oil is changed, so that what was once unsaturated is now saturated. This alters the way the body metabolizes these fats, and tends to raise the level of blood cholesterol, thereby increasing the risk of coronary heart disease. In *The Enlightened Kitchen* we

"Just Say No" to saturated fat, trans-fats, and even polyunsaturated oils, opting instead for a very small amount of olive oil.

If you wish to succeed at maintaining weight loss, exercise is critical. It is an essential component to any healthy lifestyle. A combination of workout activities will help you achieve a slimmer, firmer, healthier body. Aerobic exercise speeds up the breakdown of fat in the body, while toning exercises and weight-lifting help firm muscles and increase muscle mass. Find the kinds of activities that you enjoy and that can fit your lifestyle. If you are not sure how to start, simply try walking; you don't need to join a gym to work out and there are many "walking clubs," where a group will meet on a regular basis, perhaps a few times a week.

# Plant-Based Cuisine
## *The Shift Starts Here*

How do we make the necessary changes in diet and lifestyle without sacrificing familiar dishes, flavor, and texture? Does healthy eating mean that all of your family favorites are suddenly off-limits? Can you still have creamy dips, hearty entrées, and outrageous desserts? It is not difficult to make meals that are good tasting and good for you, too—not at all. *Making food choices that lead to optimal health and overall well-being has never been easier.* The key is in using wholesome alternatives that do a great job of standing in for unhealthy traditional ingredients. Is there an easy way to make that transition? Absolutely!

Soyfoods have exploded onto the market. Once popular only among vegetarians, soy is going mainstream. High in quality protein, very low in saturated fat, and with no cholesterol, soy has achieved much recognition recently because of hundreds of exciting clinical studies demonstrating its powerful health benefits. In 1976, the *New England Journal of Medicine* published a landmark study by Dr. James Anderson, which concluded that the addition of soy protein to a low-fat diet reduced cholesterol levels dramatically. Soyfoods have many amazing health benefits, such as significantly reducing the risk of cancer and heart disease, lowering cholesterol and blood pressure, and aiding the body's fight against osteoporosis, kidney disease, and diabetes. The Food and Drug Administration recommends that consumers incorporate at least 25 grams of soy protein each day as part of a low-fat diet, in order to reduce the risk of coronary heart disease. Is it easy to include 25 grams of soy each day? Yes! 8 ounces of soymilk contains 8 grams of soy protein; 1 soy burger, 16 grams; and ¼ cup (1 ounce) of soynuts, 13 grams of soy protein.

Soybeans contain all three of the acronutrients required for good nutrition: complete protein, carbohydrates, and fats, as well as vitamins and minerals, including calcium, folic acid, and iron. The calcium in soy is thought to be better utilized by the body to guard against osteoporosis. Furthermore, *soybeans are the only vegetable that contains complete protein, providing all of the essential amino acids in the amounts needed for human health.* The amino acid pattern of soy is virtually identical to that of meat, milk, and egg products, but without all of the health risks that have been discussed earlier. Additionally, soy protein is the source of phytochemicals that have been credited with many health benefits.

Certainly soy is the "superstar" among legumes. However, a well-balanced plant-based diet need not rely solely on soyfoods for sufficient protein. According to Dr. McDougall, "All the protein needed to grow large muscles is present in vegetable foods. Vegetables provide two to four times the protein anyone would need during any activity." Potatoes provide 11 percent protein; corn, 12 percent; oranges, 8 percent; cauliflower, 4 percent; and legumes, like beans, peas, and lentils, 28 percent.

Plant-based menus are easier than ever! If your daily menu simply includes a balance of foods from the four food groups—vegetables, grains, legumes, and fruit—your nutritional requirements are readily met. For those of us who desire traditional fare but want to eat the plant-based, healthy way, manufacturers have really stepped up to the plate, producing high-quality soy and wheat gluten-based alternatives.

An extensive variety of meat analogs (substitutes) are available not only at health food stores, but at most supermarkets. Look for products like Yves Veggie Canadian Bacon, Veggie Dogs, Ground Round, Veggie Pepperoni, and a variety of deli slices. There are many brands of ground beef alternatives, plant-based "chicken" and "turkey" strips, "chicken" nuggets, soy burgers, and several kinds of sausage. My favorite soy sausages are made by Lightlife Foods. I use their Smart Links Italian to make dishes like Sautéed Polenta with Sweet Italian "Sausage." Also, you can roll "meatballs" right out of the package if you buy Gimme Lean ground beef flavor. Serve the meatballs to family and friends, who will not know that they are eating healthy, plant-based food. These are all made with the goodness of soy!

You can also find many brands of soymilk and styles of tofu that have a number of applications for the health-conscious cook, and you don't have to go out of your way to find them. In fact, you can substitute soymilk for cow's milk, one to one, in any recipe. Most brands feature enriched varieties, with added vitamins, minerals, and calcium. And most are conveniently packaged in aseptic containers. Do they taste good? There are many that are popular with consumers, especially those sold in gable-topped containers in the cold case in supermarkets and health food stores. One even beat cow's milk in a blind taste test on a network television show (White Wave Silk).

Tofu is the best known of all soyfoods, and is widely available in supermarkets and health food stores. If you are looking for a hearty ingredient, try tempeh. Tempeh, a delicious soyfood found in the refrigerator or freezer case at health food stores. Because tempeh is made from the whole bean, it is richer in flavor and nutrients than tofu. Tempeh, a source of vitamin B$_{12}$, has a chewy texture and a distinctive nutty flavor. I make delicious chili and shish kebabs using tempeh.

Is soy that magic bullet we have all been looking for? If soyfoods represent the magic bullet, then it is the enlightened medical community who have pulled the trigger. Soyfoods have an impressive resume and have been well-positioned in the modern marketplace to assume a beneficial role in encouraging health-supporting choices. *Replacing animal products with plant foods can be the most important health choice that you can make. And with soyfoods in the mix, you can enjoy variety, texture, and flavor along with many healthful benefits.*

# Mainstreaming

Vegan (VEE-gan): A person who consumes a plant-based diet, that is, a dietary regimen that avoids animal products of any kind. This lifestyle choice often includes the avoidance of other animal products such as leather and silk.

Adopting a healthier lifestyle is a matter of choice, and home cooks are choosing nonmeat alternatives more often than ever before. They are discovering many advantages that result from substituting with plant foods. New and improved meat alternatives enter the market every day, and in addition to appearing in the usual health food and specialty stores, these innovative products are turning up on the shelves of supermarkets nationwide. Manufacturers, responding to pressure from consumers, are introducing a wide selection of quick-and-easy prep, snack, and prepared food options for busy consumers.

Before you say that the the term "Mainstream Vegan" is an oxymoron, consider that the market for meat alternatives, particularly those that are soy-based, has exploded. Today, soyfood items such as burgers, breakfast sausages, beverages, snack bars, and baked goods have moved out of small, niche health food stores into mainstream supermarkets. According to industry analyst Frost & Sullivan, the meat alternatives market generated $622 million in 2000. Manufacturers' sales of soyfoods alone are projected to top $6.9 billion in 2005, according to a study conducted by Business Communications Co., Inc., of Norwalk, Connecticut.

The people who purchase these products are not all vegetarian. Many are health-conscious, mainstream consumers who are very interested in pursuing a healthier lifestyle. When questioned, these shoppers say they are interested in these alternatives and choose to prepare vegetarian meals at least part of the time because of the health benefits. Home cooks who are looking for ways to embrace healthy eating while making traditional-style meals have discovered that they can use these products without losing flavor, texture, or eye appeal. It is the addition of these new consumers to the plant-based foods market that is fueling the tremendous growth in this sector. And, while consumers have been driven to purchase plant-based products by reports of numerous health benefits associated with animal-free foods, one hidden benefit is the tendency to lose weight when eliminating animal products from the menu—an outcome that tends to hold the interest of many people!

In the past, the term "vegetarian" conjured up images of youthful, activist, hippie types, very much out of the mainstream. However, the overwhelming majority of people for whom plant foods comprise most, if not all of their diet, are just like you and me . . . physicians and nurses, stockbrokers and executives, housewives and career women, teachers and secretaries, writers and programmers, young and old, liberal and conservative. We are at the forefront of a major lifestyle shift, one that will have a positive impact on the quality of life not only for humanity, but for the planet, and for our friends, the animals.

# Nature's Pharmacy:
# The Incredible Edibles

Mom always said, "Eat your fruits and vegetables; they'll help you grow big and strong." There are many studies that verify why, in scientific terms, Mom was right. Numerous studies have demonstrated that people who eat plant-rich diets are healthier and generally live longer. Beyond vitamins and minerals, their investigations revealed that foods of plant origin contain a whole range of protective chemicals that can be profoundly beneficial to our health.

I have already presented a number of compelling reasons for replacing animal products with plant-based foods. Additionally, however vegetables, legumes, grains, and fruits contain certain recognized compounds with health-supporting properties. These protective plant components fall into two categories: antioxidants and phytochemicals.

## Antioxidants

Antioxidants are a class of nutrients with proven disease-fighting abilities. The best-known and most thoroughly studied antioxidants are vitamins C and E, beta-carotene, folic acid, and the mineral selenium. These nutrients have been recognized for their ability to slow the aging process and disable free radicals. What are free radicals? When oxygen is metabolized or burned by the body, cells form byproducts called free radicals. Free radicals result from routine metabolic processes and from breathing. While free radicals can promote beneficial oxidation that produces energy and kills bacterial invaders, in excess they produce harmful oxidation. These unstable oxygen molecules ricochet dangerously inside cells, disrupting the structure of other molecules and resulting in cellular damage.

Many environmental and lifestyle factors encourage the formation of free radicals, such as stress, pollution, injury, smoking, ozone, chemotherapy, radiation, and certain foods. You can take control of this process by *choosing foods rich in antioxidants and avoiding items like deep-fried foods, and rancid fats and oils.* Animal products, which are high in iron, should be avoided, as iron is a known oxidizer. People who eat adequate amounts of fruits and vegetables high in antioxidants have a lower incidence of cardiovascular disease, certain cancers, and cataracts. Antioxidants protect key cell components from damage by neutralizing the free radicals and may block most of the damage. Here's where antioxidants are found most plentifully in the plant-based food supply.

## ANTIOXIDANT VITAMINS IN FOODS

| Source (1 cup serving) | Vitamin C (mg.) | Beta Carotene (mg.) | Vitamin E (mg.) |
|---|---|---|---|
| Apple (1 medium) | 8 | 0.04 | 0.44 |
| Broccoli | 116 | 1.30 | 1.32 |
| Brown rice | 0 | 0.00 | 4.00 |
| Brussels sprouts | 96 | 0.67 | 1.33 |
| Carrot (1 medium) | 7 | 12.00 | .28 |
| Cauliflower | 54 | 0.01 | 0.05 |
| Corn | 10 | 0.22 | 0.15 |
| Garbanzo beans | 2 | 0.02 | 0.57 |
| Grapefruit (½) | 47 | 0.19 | 0.31 |
| Navy beans | 2 | 0.00 | 4.10 |
| Orange, medium | 75 | 0.16 | 0.31 |
| Orange juice | 124 | 0.30 | 0.22 |
| Pineapple | 24 | 0.02 | 0.16 |
| Soybeans | 3 | 0.01 | 3.35 |
| Spinach, fresh | 16 | 2.30 | 0.57 |
| Strawberries | 84 | 0.02 | 0.23 |
| Sweet potato, medium | 28 | 15.00 | 0.32 |

## Phytochemicals

There are thousands of biologically active compounds in plants, called phytochemicals, or plant chemicals (*phyto* is Greek for "plants"). Phytochemicals are non-nutritive, meaning they are neither vitamins nor minerals. Many hundreds of these bioactive plant chemicals are found in dietary sources of fruits, vegetables, legumes, whole grains, nuts, seeds, herbs, and spices.

These compounds have specific medicinal properties that are credited for much of the health-promoting properties of fruits and vegetables, and show promise for preventing a myriad of diseases.

For example plant estrogens, including daidzein, equol, and enterolactone, which are found in soybeans, whole wheat, berries, and flax seed, may help reduce the risk for certain hormone-stimulated cancers, such as breast and prostate, by replacing human estrogen with the benign plant estrogens they contain. They may also inhibit the proliferation of existing cancer cells.

The phytochemicals sulforaphane and isothiocyanates are found in cruciferous vegetables. These may block the effects of carcinogens and suppress tumor growth. While fruits and vegetables, especially brightly colored ones, are especially rich in phytochemicals, so too are whole grains and legumes. Consuming whole grains can reduce the risk of cardiovascular disease and cancer. The phytochemicals in legumes, especially those concentrated in soy, have received a great deal of attention regarding their anticarcinogenic properties and ability to reduce cholesterol levels in the bloodstream.

Flavonoids, found in apples, onions, tea, and red wine, are being investigated for possible anticarcinogenic properties. Some researchers suggest that the protective effect of red wine against cardiovascular disease may be due, in part, to the phytoestrogen resveratrol, which is found in grape skin. Organosulfur compounds that are found in the onion and garlic family may have very potent properties in blocking carcinogenic substances. Some experts advise drinking four cups of green tea daily, as green tea is thought to protect against certain cancers.

All in all, there are numerous phytochemicals that give plants their distinctive pigment, flavor, and aroma. There are almost 2,000 recognized plant pigments in our food, including over 800 flavonoids, 450 carotenoids, and 150 anthocyanins (red pigments found in fruits). Like antioxidants, phytochemicals have powerful disease-preventive properties. Here are some of the more impressive ones known to date.

## PHYTOCHEMICALS OF INTEREST

| Phytochemical | Source | Health Benefit |
| --- | --- | --- |
| Canthaxanthin | Paprika | Antioxidant |
| Capsaicin | Hot peppers | Reduces pain, anti-inflammatory |
| Carotenoids | Red, yellow, and green fruits and vegetables | Antioxidants that reduce plaque formation, and promote cell differentiation |
| Chlorophyll | Most plants | Detoxifies blood, deters tumors |
| Coumarin | Soybeans, whole grains, flax seeds, cruciferous vegetables, squash, melons, green tea | Blood thinning agent, anticarcinogenic |
| Curcumin | Turmeric | Arthritis relief |
| Flavonoids | Most fruits, particularly citrus and apples; vegetables; onions; tea | Antioxidants that block carcinogens, anti-inflammatory |
| Gingerol | Ginger | Antioxidant; arthritis relief, deters ulcers |
| Indoles | Broccoli, cabbage, kale | Block cancer-causing substances |
| Isoflavones | Soyfoods: tofu, tempeh, soymilk, edamame, soynuts | Lower cholesterol, reduces estrogren levels in blood; reduces risk of many cancers |
| Isothiocyanate | Cabbage | Induces protective enzymes, deters lung and other tumors |
| Lignans | Flax seeds, whole grains, berries | Anti-inflammatory; protective against colon cancer and heart disease |

| Lycopene | Tomatoes | Antioxidant; carotenoid; prostate cancer preventive |
|---|---|---|
| Organosulfurs | Garlic, onion, leeks, scallions, shallots, chives | Block cancer-causing agents, boosts immunity, prevents infection |
| Phenolic acid | Most fruits, vegetables, whole grains, berries, especially squash, yams, and citrus fruits | Antioxidant; anti-inflammatory; inhibits carcinogen-induced cell proliferation |
| Protease inhibitors | All plants, soybeans | Antiviral, and anti-bacterial; slows tumor growth, blocks cancer-causing enzymes |
| Quercetin | Citrus fruits | flavonoid; antihistamine and anti-inflammatory activity |
| Rosmarinic acid | Rosemary | Deters tumors |
| Saponins | Soybeans, legumes, garlic, ginseng, sunflower seeds | Lowers level of fats in the bloodstream; inhibits tumors |
| Sulforaphane | Cruciferous vegetables | Suppresses tumor growth. |
| Terpenes | Grapefruit, oranges, and lemons | Induce protective enzymes; interfere with carcinogens; prevent dental decay |

# The Enlightened Pantry
## *What to Have on Hand*

Whether a plant-based lifestyle is your ultimate goal or you just want to have a greater variety of healthy ingredients at hand, you can use this guide to stock up on items that make creating healthy meals a snap. Listed here are products and ingredients that I use in my kitchen. You needn't go out and buy them all at once: purchase what you need for a particular recipe, and each time you are at the store, pick up a few more items suggested here. Let's look at some of these food choices in detail first:

You can cook **dried beans** from scratch—a pressure cooker will cut the cooking time considerably—or you can choose canned beans. While canned ingredients can be very convenient, sodium is an issue, as are additives and preservatives. When choosing canned beans, look for good quality beans without additives, organic if possible. I like to use Eden brand canned products; they are far lower in sodium than other brands, are flavored with sea vegetables, and are organic.

Keeping **canned tomatoes** on hand is not only convenient, but more healthful: canned tomatoes are a better source of lycopene than fresh. Lycopene is the phytochemical that has been credited with reducing the risk for prostate cancer. Still, it is important to read the labels of canned tomatoes. For example, when purchasing tomato paste, avoid flavored types, such as

"Italian Tomato Paste," as they invariably contain cheese. (This is not generally an issue with stewed tomatoes.)

Another time-saving ingredient in recipes are **prepared soups.** They help make terrific entrées and side dishes easy and delicious. The new Mori Nu soups come in 32-ounce and 11-ounce (single serve) aseptic packages. They are made with tofu purée, and I have used them as a base for sauces, casseroles, and other fabulous dishes.

**Broth powders** are invaluable flavorings in any kitchen. In *The Enlightened Kitchen* I use wholesome broth powders to rehydrate **textured vegetable protein (TVP),** and to flavor dips and sauces. Textured vegetable protein is *The Enlightened Kitchen's* version of fast food! Rehydrated with boiling broth, this shelf-stable soyfood is ready to incorporate into any dish in minutes. *(Note: DDC is the acronym I use throughout this book for any ingredient from the Dixie Diners Club product line, such as broth powder.)* **Imagine No-Chicken Broth**—organic and ready-to-use this is a very convenient item to use in place of Chicken-Flavored Vegetarian broth powder.

When purchasing **whole grains** and **flour,** it's best not to buy more than a 3-month supply, and it's also a good idea to refrigerate flour during the summer. This will reduce the likelihood of infestation or rancidity. For **oat flour,** I place rolled oats in the food processor (you may also use a blender) and process into flour in less than a minute. Rolled oats are a staple with many uses, but I don't generally use enough oat flour to warrant keeping it on hand.

Keep a variety of **herbs** and **spices** available. As herbs and spices lose flavor and pungency over time, it's best to purchase smaller size jars and store them in a cool, dark place. I've listed below those that I use most, such as the crushed red pepper, (also labeled as: red chile pepper or red pepper flakes). Whole chile peppers, whether fresh or dried, need special handling and some take extra time to prepare. I have used crushed chile to "perfume the oil" at the beginning of my sauté for many years, and find it to be a convenient and very effective way to add depth of flavor to most dishes. Granulated spices are stronger and more flavorful than ground spices, and I always prefer them.

**Nutritional yeast** is a must for every plant-based kitchen. Not only nutritious, nutritional yeast is downright delicious, adding a rich, cheeselike flavor and a creaminess to any dish. These versatile flakes are very high in protein and B vitamins. Do not confuse with brewer's yeast, which has a bitter taste. I recommend Red Star Nutritional Yeast, and KAL Nutritional Yeast. They are both labeled Vegetarian Support Formula, are consistant in quality, and contain Vitamin $B_{12}$.

I use only **fruit-sweetened ketchup** and **barbecue sauce.** Muir Glen (my favorite) is also organic. Bragg Liquid Aminos is a wholesome and delicious, all-purpose, **soy seasoning.** Vegenaise, my "hands-down" favorite eggless mayonnaise, is made by Follow Your Heart. The **salsas** listed work well as a flavorful ingredient in many dishes.

I have several **sweeteners** of choice. One is Sucanat, an unrefined cane sugar made by Wholesome Sweeteners. Any recipe calling for Sucanat is referring to this dark brown granular sugar that is used to replace brown sugar in any recipe. Evaporated cane sugar is a slightly refined sugar. Light tan in color, it is available from Wholesome Sweeteners and Florida Crystals. Liquid Fruitsource is made from grapes and grains and is safe for type 1 and type 2 diabetics, who can use it as a fruit or a grain exchange. This wholesome sweetener is used just like honey or rice syrup.

A pantry stocked with these wholesome ingredients will help you make healthy and delicious meals without having to make lots of special trips. We all lead such busy lives, and having ready-to-use, wholesome ingredients handy is the first step in making health-supporting meals nearly effortless. The following list includes ingredients that I feel are essential to have on hand to ensure flexibility in meal preparation. (Note: This list doesn't include perishable soy-foods, or fruits and vegetables, which you should purchase as you need them.)

## Canned and Jarred Goods

### Beans

Black beans
Black-eyed peas
Garbanzo beans
Great Northern beans
Kidney beans (red)
Pinto beans
White beans, small
White kidney beans (cannellini)

### Vegetables, canned and jarred

*Canned:*
Artichoke hearts, quartered
Coconut milk, lite
Water chestnuts, sliced
Bamboo shoots

Mexican-style stewed tomatoes
Italian-style stewed tomatoes
Peeled and diced tomatoes
Tomato paste

*Jarred:*
Melissa's Fire Roasted Whole Red and Green Chiles
Thai green chile paste
Capers

## Soups

Mori Nu Soups: Tomato, Garden Pea, Butternut Squash, and Corn

### *Vegetarian Broth Powders:*

DDC (Dixie Diners Club) Official Broth Powder, Official Onion Flavor
    Broth Powder, and Crème of Mushroom Soup, Sauce and Gravy Mix
Harvest Direct Vegetarian Chicken Broth Powder
Imagine No-Chicken Broth

## Dry Goods

Laura Beans soybeans
Tosteds soynuts
Melissa's soynuts
Brown rice, short grain
Basmati rice, white
Barley, quick-cooking
Quinoa
Couscous, whole wheat
Couscous, roasted garlic
San Gennaro Foods polenta (cellophane "chubs")
Brown lentils

## Pasta

Fettuccini
Linguine
Spaghetti
Penne
Penette (or other small salad pasta)
Orzo
Barilla No-Cook Lasagna Noodles

## Flours, Cereals, and Baking Needs:

Whole wheat flour
Whole wheat pastry flour
Unbleached white flour
Whole grain yellow cornmeal
Soy flour
Rolled oats
Celtic sea salt
Rumford nonaluminum baking powder
EnerG egg replacer powder
Dixie Diners Club Egg Not!
Dixie Diners Club Crème It!
Barbara's mashed potato flakes
Applesauce, unsweetened
Solo prune puree
Chocolate chips, dairy-free
Vanilla extract, pure
Rosewater
Orange blossom water

## Sweeteners

Sucanat unrefined sugar
Evaporated cane sugar
Liquid Fruitsource
Maple syrup, pure

## Miscellaneous

Red Star nutritional yeast, Vegetarian Support Formula
Tofu Hero dehydrated vegetable and spice blends: Eggless Salad, Italian
    Herb Medley, Shanghai Stir Fry, Garden Scramble
Shelf-stable tofu: Mori Nu Lite Silken Tofu, Mori Nu Silken Tofu
    (regular)
Dried mushrooms: Melissa's Dried Mushroom Medley, Melissa's Dried
    Shitake Mushrooms
Sea vegetables: kombu, wakame, agar, nigari,
Potatoes: russet, Yukon Gold, red, fingerling, etc.
Yams
Onions, yellow and red

Garlic, fresh

Shallots

Melissa's Roasted Sweet Corn

Pine nuts

Walnuts

Dried fruit: currants, blueberries, cranberries, cherries, pineapple chunks, peaches

Herbs and spices: crushed red pepper, granulated garlic, granulated onion, dried basil, dried thyme, dried marjoram, dried Mexican oregano, ground cinnamon, ground nutmeg, ground ginger, curry powder, turmeric, paprika, ground cloves, ground cumin, coarse black pepper, lemon pepper

Thickeners: arrowroot, cornstarch

Oils: extra virgin olive oil, mild olive oil, dark sesame oil

Vinegars: balsamic vinegar, red wine vinegar, rice vinegar

## Prepared Sauces and Condiments

Fat-free tomato sauce

Basil and tomato sauce

Roasted red pepper tomato sauce

Tamari (regular and lite)

Bragg Liquid Aminos

Vegetarian Worcestershire sauce (Robbies or The Wizard)

Tabasco sauce

Vegenaise Dressing and Sandwich Spread

Salad dressings by Follow Your Heart (note: not all are dairy-free)

Salad dressings by Nasoya

Salad dressings by Simply Delicious

Fire-roasted chile salsa

Pineapple salsa

Mango salsa

Artichoke salsa

# Notes on Ingredients

Presented here are health-supporting ingredients that play an essential role in creating enlightened meals. These healthy options are easy to use and widely available, and have a number of applications. Most are available in health food stores, and many can now be found in supermarkets. For information regarding a particular product or manufacturer, see the Resource Guide (page 000).

## All about Soyfoods

**Baked tofu**   Marinated, precooked, and ready-to-eat, baked tofu can be sliced and added to salads and sandwiches right from the package. Baked tofu is available in many flavors, including Savory, Five Spice, Hickory Smoked, Teriyaki, Italian, Mexican, Thai, Oriental, and more. These products have a flavor reminiscent of smoked meats or roast duck and have many applications. I like to use baked tofu as a quick high-protein addition to stir-fry and baked dishes. Among the brands of baked tofu available at health food stores are The Soy Deli, White Wave, Wildwood Foods, and Tree Of Life.

**Beef Not!**   DDC analog: unflavored strips, chunks, and ground beef. See TVP (Textured Vegetable Protein).

**Bragg Liquid Aminos**   This tasty liquid seasoning is used in the same way as soy sauce. A highly concentrated source of minerals and soy protein (420 milligrams per ½ teaspoon), Bragg Aminos is not fermented and is available from Live Food Products.

**Broth powder**   DDC Official Broth powder, made from soybeans, is used in *The Enlightened Kitchen* to rehydrate Beef Not! and Chicken Not! and in many other dishes.

**Chicken Not!**   DDC analog: unflavored strips, chunks, and ground poultry.

**Chick'n Strips**   Lightlife Foods analog. See Smart Chick'n Strips.

**Crème It!**   DDC powdered tofu product with a variety of uses. Adds a rich-tasting creaminess to dishes.

**Edamame**   Green vegetable soybeans are available in the pod, usually frozen. Harvested when about 80 percent mature, green vegetable soybeans are delicious and have none of the stronger "beany" taste associated with mature beans. Use as a nutritious snack or a delicious addition to an appetizer buffet.

**Egg Not!**   From DDC, this very effective egg replacer powder is made from soy lecithin.

**Fairview Farms soybeans**   See Laura Beans, and Tosteds.

**Firm nigari tofu**   A very firmly pressed tofu with a dense texture that is lower in fat (3 grams per 4 ounces) than traditional water-packed tofu. Sold in vacuum packaging, it will keep, unopened, in the refrigerator for up to two months. Once opened, it should be used in a few days. Made from organic soybeans from The Soy Deli, this tofu has a subtle sweetness and handles well because of its firm texture.

**Gimme Lean**   Made by Lightlife, this wholesome meat alternative is a favorite in *The Enlightened Kitchen,* because of its authentic flavor, texture, appearance, and aroma. It is available in sausage and ground beef style. Because of the excellent cohesive quality of this product, you can roll delicious "meatballs" or fashion "hamburgers" right out of the package. Look for it in the cold case and freezer section.

**Ground beef alternatives**   These "ready to use" soy products are fat free: Yves Ground Round, Lightlife Smart Ground, and Boca Burger Crumbles. Ready Ground Tofu contains 4 grams of fat per 3 ounce serving. They are all available preseasoned. This type of "ground beef" can be used in any "loose meat" application.

**Laura Beans**   This is the soybean of choice in *The Enlightened Kitchen.* The Laura Bean is non-GMO (not genetically modified), has a pleasant flavor, and is excellent for making soymilk (page 203) and tofu (page 204). Order Laura Beans from Fairview Farms.

**Miso**   A savory, smooth paste with a consistency much like peanut butter. Miso is a fermented food made from soybeans, a grain such as rice or barley, salt, and a mold culture. It is aged in cedar vats for up to three years. Miso should be stored in the refrigerator, where it will keep for several months. Easily digested and highly nutritious, miso adds depth of flavor to soups, sauces, marinades, dips, salad dressings, pâté, and main dishes. It is available from Cold Mountain and Westbrae Foods, among others. I use mellow white miso extensively, but barley miso can be used in its place.

*Barley miso and country barley miso*   Medium tan in color, with a chunky texture and rich flavor.

*Mellow white miso*   This is a highly versatile miso that I use extensively in soups, sauces, fillings, dips, and dressings. It has a rich, creamy texture, and sweet fragrance. Mellow barley miso is similar in color but not as creamy.

**Mori Nu soups**   Really versatile and aseptically packaged, these soups are made with tofu purée. Available in four flavors: Tomato, Garden Pea, Corn, and Butternut Squash.

**Nayonaise**   This popular mayonnaise, made with silken tofu, is much lower in fat and calories than traditional mayonnaise. Made by Nasoya, this wholesome alternative contains no eggs and therefore no cholesterol, and little saturated fat.

**Okara**   Okara is the by-product of soymilk making (see Homemade Soymilk (page 203). It is the fiber left behind after the liquid is extracted from the soybeans. Okara is a hearty and nutritious ingredient that adds protein, fiber, and the goodness of soy to any dish.

**Okara, dry roasted**   Drain okara and spread on a baking pan. Bake in a preheated 300° oven for 20 minutes. This will produce a fluffier okara and increase its shelf life.

**Roasted Chicken Not!**   A mix, complete with sauce from the DDC catalog. Quite authentic in flavor, texture, and appearance. Just add water, and proceed with recipe (see Roasted "Chicken" and Vegetables, page 126).

**Salad dressings**   There are some terrific salad dressings that are made using tofu, miso, or shoyu. My favorites are made by Nasoya and Simply Delicious. They are available in health food stores.

**Shoyu**   A naturally brewed, high-quality soy sauce. Processed in the traditional Japanese way, it is aged two to three years without coloring, additives, or preservatives.

**Silken tofu**   A low-fat (1.5 grams of fat per 3 ounces), Japanese-style tofu that, unlike Chinese-style tofu, has a smooth and "silky" texture. It is widely available in aseptic packages from Mori Nu.

*Lite silken tofu*   Used extensively in *The Enlightened Kitchen,* this very low-fat tofu (.5 gram of fat per 3 ounces) has a rich-tasting, smooth, creamy texture and a custardlike consistency. Its creamy versatility makes it an excellent substitute for eggs and dairy products in baked goods and cream sauces. Because of its aseptic packaging, lite silken tofu is a time-saving ingredient when making dips, spreads, and dressings, because it need not be precooked. Measure for volume by spooning tofu into a liquid measuring cup and stirring down with a fork. Widely available from Morinaga Nutritional Foods, Inc.

**Smart Links Italian Sausage**   Low-fat vegetarian Italian-style sausage links from Lightlife Foods that successfully simulate the appearance, flavor, and texture of Italian sausage. Before they are cooked, these links are fragile, so it is important to handle them gingerly, and brown them first. However, once cooked, they are firm and handle well.

**Smart Chick'n Strips**   Precut and lightly seasoned, this poultry alternative from Lightlife Foods is fat-free and very authentic in flavor, texture, and appearance.

**Smart Steak-Style Strips**   Precut and lightly seasoned, like the Chick'n Strips, this meat analog from Lightlife Foods is also fat-free.

**Soy flour**   Finely ground from roasted soybeans, low in carbohydrates, and very high in protein (35 percent, twice that of wheat flour), soy flour contains no gluten and is combined with other flours in baking. Replace no more than ⅓ of the amount of flour called for in a recipe with soy flour. Available in packages from Bob's Red Mill, and Arrowhead Mills in health food stores and some supermarkets. Also available from the DDC catalog.

**Soy grits**   Sometimes called soya granules, soy grits are whole soybeans that have been lightly toasted and cracked into small pieces. Great for boosting nutrition and adding texture as in gratin toppings. DDC soy grits are available through the catalog, and Red Mill soy grits and Fearn soya granules are available in health food stores.

**Soymage Parmesan cheese alternative**   Sold in shaker packages, this grated soy cheese is low in fat, cholesterol-free, all natural and 100 percent dairy-free.

**Soymilk**   A nondairy beverage made by extracting the liquid from cooked soybeans. Soymilk is a dairy-free and cholesterol-free alternative to cow's milk, and is substituted one-for-one in any recipe. Widely available, it is sold plain, flavored, 1% fat, and fortified. It can be found in shelf-stable aseptic packages and gable-top containers in the dairy case.

**Soynuts**   These roasted, crunchy snacks are similar to peanuts and are widely available. Melissa's makes them: many flavors.

**Soyrizo vegetarian chorizo**   Plant-based version of the highly seasoned pork sausage widely used in Mexican and Spanish cooking. Remove the casing and crumble before browning in a small amount of olive oil.

**Tamari**   A wheat-free, natural soy sauce, tamari has a darker, richer flavor than soy sauce.

**Tempeh**   A traditional Indonesian food, tempeh (tem-pay) is a rich, chewy soyfood with a distinctive nutty flavor. Tempeh is fermented from whole soybeans, and sometimes mixed with another grain such as rice or with sea vegetables. Because tempeh is made from the whole bean, it is richer in flavor and nutrients than tofu. Tempeh is steamed before incorporating into any recipe, and can be can be marinated before adding to a recipe. Tempeh is available from Turtle Island Foods, White Wave, Pacific Foods, Lightlife, and Soy Power, among others, in the refrigerator or freezer section of health food stores.

**Textured vegetable protein (TVP)**   Made from defatted soy flour, TVP is extremely economical, high in protein, and a very credible meat substitute, once rehydrated. Available in a variety of styles including ground, chunk, and strip beef or poultry styles as Beef Not! and Chicken Not! from the DDC catalog. Because of its very low fat content, unprepared TVP has an extended shelf life. TVP is also available through the The Mail Order Catalog. As a rule, the TVP sold in health food stores only in the *flavored* ground-beef style is not used in *The Enlightened Kitchen*.

**Tofu**   Soybean curd that is made from coagulating soymilk with nigari (seaweed) or calcium chloride, in much the same way cheese is made from milk. It is high in protein, very low in saturated fat, and cholesterol-free. Tofu's blandness and ability to absorb flavors make it a very versatile ingredient. Chinese-style tofu has a firm and spongy texture, and is packed in water-filled tubs or clear vacuum packages. Japanese-style is comparatively soft. The majority of silken tofu is aseptically packaged, though it can be found packed in water. Most styles and types of tofu are widely available.

**Tosteds**   Whole roasted soynuts available from Fairview Farms. Use these delicious soynuts as a topping for ice cream or cereal and to replace peanuts in any recipe. (See Kung Pao "Chicken," page 115).

**Yves Veggie Canadian Bacon**   A very authentic, wholesome alternative, very close to Canadian bacon or ham in appearance, aroma, and flavor. Made with soy protein and wheat gluten, this tasty meat analog can be enjoyed right out of the package in sandwiches or salads, or as a delicious addition to stir-fry and baked dishes.

**Yves Veggie Pepperoni**   Presliced soy pepperoni, a very popular meat analog with an authentic appearance and taste. It is perfect for pizza.

## Other Plant-Based Alternatives

This section includes plant-based ingredients that, while not soy based, will also serve to replace unhealthy traditional products and contribute beneficial nutrients, subnutrients, vitamins, and minerals. Combine these wholesome ingredients with soyfoods for a well-balanced plant-based regimen.

**Active dry yeast**   Used to leaven dough, this type of yeast is sold in packages and jars. Quick-rising yeast takes a third to half the time required for regular yeast. Make sure to store yeast in a cool, dry place.

**Applesauce**   In all recipes that call for applesauce as a fat replacer, use *unsweetened* applesauce.

**Arrowroot**   This powder can replace tapioca flour or cornstarch for thickening.

**Artichoke hearts**   Quartered artichoke hearts are available canned from several manufacturers. Or whole canned artichoke hearts can be quartered for any recipe.

**Assorted greens**   Assemble using a variety of greens with a mixture of colors, tastes, and textures. Prepackaged salad greens are conveniently washed and ready to use. Blends can include: baby spinach, arugula, baby romaine, radicchio, sorrel, oak- and red-leaf lettuces, and many other gourmet greens.

**Avocado**   Rich-tasting, pear-shaped fruit with either smooth or textured skin and light green flesh. Hass avocados, with thick, dark green, bumpy skin and buttery flesh are considered to be the superior variety. Select avocados that yield to gentle pressure and store in the refrigerator for several days. In order to hasten ripening, keep at room temperature or in a closed brown paper bag.

**Baby-cut carrots**   These are mature carrots that have been peeled and cut into small carrot shapes, not the delicate baby carrots with feathery leaves attached that are used by chefs for eye appeal. Baby-cut carrots are widely available.

**Baking powder**   Nonaluminum, double-acting baking powder is widely available. Rumford, Featherweight, and Cellu baking powders are all nonaluminum.

**Balsamic vinegar**   Slightly sweet and fragrant with a distinctive depth of flavor, genuine balsamic vinegar is aged for a minimum of six years and produced in Modena, Italy. Most balsamic vinegars made in America are not aged. While these vinegars lack the body and flavor of the well-aged balsamic vinegars, they still possess a fair sweet-and-sour balance of flavor not found in any other vinegars.

**Barbara's Mashed Potato Flakes**   A wholesome product made from whole, unpeeled Idaho potatoes. Distributed by Barbara's Bakery.

**Barilla lasagna noodles**   I use these noodles for my all of my baked lasagna dishes. They do not have to be precooked before baking, and are widely available.

**Basmati rice**   Considered by many cooks as the world's finest, this aromatic, long-grain rice has a faintly nutlike flavor and aroma. In *The Enlightened Kitchen,* white basmati rice is used, as brown basmati takes twice the time to cook.

**Capers**   Sold in jars, capers are flower buds pickled in vinegar brine. The pungent flavor of capers adds a piquant quality to sauces and vegetable medleys.

**Celtic sea salt**   Naturally harvested in Brittany, France, Celtic sea salt is produced using a 2,000-year-old Celtic tradition. This highly superior sea salt has minerals that are naturally balanced and also has an "energy" that is very compatible to the body. You can "feel" it!

**Chile beans with chipotle peppers**   Santa Fe–style pinto beans seasoned with chipotle peppers and spices. Available from S & W Foods at supermarkets.

**Cornstarch**   A fine-textured, powdery flour ground from the white heart of the corn kernel. Cornstarch is used as a neutral-flavored thickening agent in sauces and fillings and to give baked goods a delicate texture. It is sometimes called corn flour.

**Couscous**   Couscous are tiny pellets of semolina, the ground endosperm of durum wheat. A staple in Mediterranean cuisines, where grains, vegetables, fruits, and legumes are the foundation of a healthy diet, couscous is common throughout North Africa, especially in Morocco and Tunisia. Preparation takes 5 minutes.

**Curry powder**   A prepared spice blend used to flavor East Indian–style dishes. Curry powder traditionally includes ground dried chile, cumin, coriander, fenugreek, turmeric, and cloves. Blends labeled "Madras" are often hotter than other commercial products.

**Dairy-free chocolate chips**   Delicious, dairy-free chocolate chips are available in a variety of flavors, including espresso, peanut butter, and semisweet, from Tropical Source, Cloud Nine, or Sunspire.

**Diced tomatoes**   Canned peeled and diced tomatoes are available in plain and flavored styles.

**Dijon mustard**   This distinctive mustard is made from brown or black mustard seeds.

**Dried Fruit**   Wonderful as snacks, dried fruits add special flavor to many dishes.

*Date pieces*    Chopped dates rolled in oat flour rather than sugar.

*Dried apricots*    Pitted whole or halved dried fruits, dried apricots have an intense flavor and moist, chewy texture. They can be eaten out of hand or used as an ingredient in sweet and savory dishes, and in baking.

*Dried blueberries*    These whole blueberries have been kiln-dried to preserve their deep blue-black color and distinctive flavor. In shape and texture, they resemble raisins.

*Dried cranberries*    These also resemble raisins in shape and texture. Lightly sweetened and available year-round, they can be eaten out of hand or used in baking and in sauces and chutneys.

*Dried currants*    The type of currants used in cooking and baking are the small, dark, dried Zante grape. If they are unavailable, substitute raisins.

*Dried peaches*    Sweet and slightly tangy, dried peaches are available halved or quartered.

*Dried pineapple chunks*    These are available in specialty stores and some supermarkets.

**Dried minced garlic**    Widely available on the spice aisle at supermarkets and health food stores. Look for roasted dried minced garlic at specialty stores.

**Dried Mushroom Medley**    A mix of exotic mushrooms from Melissa's, among others. Steep in boiling water for 15 minutes before proceeding with the recipe.

**EnerG egg replacer powder**    A combination of tapioca starch and leavenings. This powder is available in health food stores and through the EnerG catalog.

**Evaporated cane sugar**    This unbleached and minimally processed alternative sweetener is light tan and granulated. It can be substituted on a one-for-one basis for refined white sugar. Available from Wholesome Sweeteners and Florida Crystals.

**Fillo pastry shells**    These wholesome, shelf-stable pastry shells are very low in fat. From Fillo Factory, they are available in the DDC catalog and health food stores.

**Flour**    The finely ground and sifted meal of any edible grain.

*Oat bran*    A fiber-rich bran derived from oats that adds a distinctive hearty flavor to baked goods.

*Oat flour*    This flour may be purchased at health food or specialty stores. However it only takes a few seconds to make fresh oat flour. Simply place rolled oats in a food processor or blender and process into flour.

*Whole grain yellow cornmeal*   I like to include a small amount of yellow cornmeal in many baked goods, as it promotes a wonderful light brown crust. Only whole grain yellow cornmeal is used in *The Enlightened Kitchen.*

*Whole Wheat Flour*   A whole grain flour that contains the wheat germ and has the highest nutritional, fiber, and fat content.

*Whole wheat pastry flour*   This finely milled flour made from soft wheat is the best choice for baked goods such as cakes and quickbreads. It has a low gluten content and is not used in yeast breads. Whole wheat pastry flour is available from Bob's Red Mill and Arrowhead Mills, among others.

**Florida Crystals evaporated cane juice**   Minimally processed cane sugar that is unbleached and light tan in color. Available in convential and organic varieties.

**Food Merchants polenta (San Gennaro)**   A precooked, shelf-stable, and ready-to-use polenta, sold shrink-wrapped in clear cellophane. This conven-ient, time-saving ingredient is available in a variety of flavors. Fat-free and gluten-free, polenta is made from cornmeal and can require 30 minutes or more of preparation before proceeding with the dish.

**Fruitsource**   This wholesome sweetener made from grapes and grains is available in both liquid and granulated forms. However you will find only *liquid Fruitsource* listed in *The Enlightened Kitchen.* Fruitsource also functions as a fat replacer, to some degree, in baked goods because it contains fruit pectins. You may substitute brown rice syrup for Liquid Fruitsource.

**Fruit-sweetened ketchup**   Traditional ketchup is loaded with refined sugar. Delicious fruit-sweetened ketchup is available from Muir Glen and Westbrae.

**Garbanzo beans**   Also called chick peas, or ceci beans, these legumes are buff colored and irregularly shaped, with a firm texture and a mild, nutlike fla-vor. The main ingredient in hummus, garbanzo beans are used extensively in Mediterranean, Indian, and Middle Eastern cuisine.

**Granny Smith apples**   Tart, green-skinned apples, mostly imported from New Zealand and Australia, but also produced in California and Arizona. This all-purpose juicy, crisp apple is excellent for cooking or eating out of hand. Pippin apples are a good substitute.

**Granulated garlic**   Textured into grains like sugar or salt, garlic in this form is far superior to garlic powder in flavor and aroma.

**Great Northern beans**   I love the rich, creamy flavor of these white beans. If unavailable, substitute small white (navy) beans.

**Gingerroot**   This knobby root with an aromatic, spicy ginger flavor is found in the produce department. Fresh gingerroot is generally peeled and grated before adding to the recipes.

**Japanese eggplant**   A small, narrow variety of eggplant with solid purple or variegated skin. Japanese eggplant has tender and slightly sweet flesh, without the characteristic bitterness of the the larger, more common eggplant.

**Kale**   A member of the cabbage family, kale has deep green frilly leaves, sometimes tinged with purple. High in calcium, folic acid, and iron, kale also provides ample amounts of vitamin C and vitamin K.

**Lighter Bake**   A blend of prune purée and applesauce used to replace fat in baking. Made by Sunsweet.

**Lite coconut milk**   This product is much lower in fat and calories than regular coconut milk. Available from Thai Kitchen.

**Mirin**   Lower in alcohol than Japanese sake, mirin is a sweet rice wine used in cooking.

**Mushrooms**   A low-calorie, fat-free way to add meaty texture to many dishes.

*Button mushrooms*   Mild-flavored cultivated white mushrooms in their smallest form. Select firm, plump mushrooms that are not bruised or slimy. Store in the refrigerator unwashed and lightly wrapped.

*Cremini mushrooms*   Similar in size and shape to common cultivated white mushrooms, they are sometimes called Italian or brown mushrooms. They have a more assertive flavor than white mushroom, and a rich brown skin concealing creamy tan flesh.

*Wild mushrooms*   Morrel, chanterelle, oyster, shitake, enoki, Chinese black, wood ear, and porcini (sometimes called cèpe) are some examples of wild mushrooms.

*Shitake mushrooms*   Available both fresh and dried, these distinctive mushrooms are used in stir-fry dishes, soups, and salads.

*Baby portobellos*   Sometimes called stuffing portobellos, this smaller variety of portobello mushrooms provides a reasonable cavity to hold a savory filling. They can also be sliced and added to many dishes. If not available, simply stuff the larger portobello and then divide into portions, or use the largest cremini mushrooms.

**Mushroom broth powder**   DDC Crème of Mushroom Soup, Sauce and Gravy Mix adds the rich flavor of mushrooms to sauces, soups, and gravies.

**Nutmeats**   A number of my recipes, particularly baked goods, use nuts for added crunch and flavor. Nuts are a good source of protein (almonds have 30 grams per cup), but are also high in fat. Usually ⅓ cup of nuts can add just the right crunch and add plenty of flavor.

**Nutritional yeast**   Available at health food stores, these delicious flakes are very high in protein and B vitamins. Not to be confused with Brewers Yeast, which has a characteristically bitter taste, nutritional yeast adds a rich, cheesy flavor, and creaminess.

*Vegetarian Support Formula*   This type of nutritional yeast is available from Red Star, DDC, and KAL brands. The Vegetarian Support Formula classification indicates yeast containing Vitamin $B_{12}$. In health food stores and mail order catalogs.

**Olive oil cooking spray**   Use this widely available cooking spray to grease baking and cooking pans.

**Onions**   Pungent underground bulb essential to cuisines the world over.

*Scallions*   Sometimes called spring onions or green onions, scallions are perfect for stir-fries, salads, and soups. Slice crosswise and include 2 inches of the green with the bulb.

*Shallots*   Shaped more like garlic than onions, shallots are composed of a head with multiple cloves, covered with a papery skin. Used extensively in French cuisine, this mild member of the onion family combines the flavor of onions and garlic.

*Sweet onions*   The sweetest are grown in Vidalia, Georgia; California; Maui, Hawaii; and Texas.

*Yellow onions*   These all-purpose onions are the most pungent. Use in frying, main dishes, stews, and soups.

*White onions*   These all-purpose onions can be as big as the yellows in size, but their flavor is a good deal milder.

*Red onions*   Mild and sweet, red onions perform equally well raw in salads, sandwiches, and antipasto, or cooked in fajitas, medleys, focaccia, or pizza.

*Spanish and Bermuda onions*   Sweeter than yellow or white onions, these onions are not as sweet or as fragile as the Vidalia variety.

*Leeks*   Leeks look like giant scallions. They are used in soups and stir-fries. Wash them carefully.

**Orange blossom water**   The distilled essence of orange blossoms used to perfume sweets in eastern Mediterranean cuisine. It is used sparingly, and when used in baking, fills the house with the fragrance of orange blossoms.

**Orzo**   A light and delicious rice-shaped pasta that is perfect in soups or salads.

**Pearl barley, quick cooking**   Pearl barley has had the bran removed, and has been steamed and polished. Quick-cooking barley takes 10 minutes to prepare.

**Prune purée**   Puréed prunes are a very effective fat replacer in baked goods. Prepared prune purée, sometimes called prune butter or prune filling, can be found in supermarkets with the kosher foods or on the baking aisle under the brand names Solo Lekvar, Baker, and Sokol.

*Homemade prune purée*   Simply place 2 cups of pitted prunes in a food processor or blender with ¾ cup of cold water and 4 teaspoons of pure vanilla extract. Pulse, then blend until smooth, cover, and refrigerate. Because prune purée is very high in sorbitols, a natural preservative, it will keep in the refrigerator for more than two weeks.

**Pure vanilla extract**   Pure vanilla extract is a brown liquid that is clear and richly fragrant. Pure vanilla extract is about twice as expensive as imitation vanilla; however, the flavor, intensity, and quality will allow you to use about half as much.

**Quinoa**   Although new to North Americans, quinoa (pronounced keen'wa) has been cultivated in the South American Andes since 3,000 B.C. High in protein, calcium, and iron, quinoa is exceptionally high in lysine, an amino acid not overly abundant in vegetables.

**Roasted sweet corn**   Dried, roasted corn kernels sold in 3-ounce packages, from Melissa's in the produce section.

**Rose water**   The distilled essence of rose petals is used to perfume sweets in eastern Mediterranean cuisine. Like orange blossom water, it is used sparingly and when used in baking, perfumes the house. Try adding a teaspoon of rose water to hot tea.

**Saffron**   The most expensive spice in the world, the yellow-orange stigmas of the crocus plant must be hand picked and then dried. This pungent, aromatic spice is an exotic flavoring that also adds a lovely hue to Mediterranean dishes. Fortunately, a little goes a long way.

**Sea salt**   Salt derived from evaporated seawater. It retains some natural trace minerals and contains no additives.

**Seitan**   Also called wheat gluten, this meat alternative is available packed in broth or shrink-wrapped in the refrigerated case at health food stores from White Wave and Lightlife, among others. A 1-pound package of seitan packed in broth will yield eight ounces of product and eight ounces of broth.

**Stewed tomatoes**   Flavored stewed tomatoes are used in a number of savory dishes. Mexican-style and Italian-style stewed tomatoes add spice and flavor conveniently. Widely available in supermarkets, from S & W Foods.

**Sucanat Evaporated Cane Sugar**   This is a slightly refined sugar that is substituted for refined granulated white sugar in any recipe one-for-one.

**Sucanat**   Unrefined cane sugar. Made from unrefined cane juice, this alternative sweetener is a whole food and therefore retains the vitamins and minerals found in nature. From Wholesome Sweeteners, it replaces brown sugar one-for-one in any recipe.

**Sun-dried tomatoes**   Ripe tomato halves that have been oven dried, giving them a uniquely intense flavor. I use only the dry variety, which is reconstituted in boiling water, and never those which have been packed in oil. Store unused dry-packed tomatoes airtight at room temperature for up to one year. Organic sun-dried tomatoes are available from Sonoma Foods.

**Tofu Hero (formerly Tofu Helper)**   A wholesome mix of dehydrated vegetables and spices that turn a box of silken tofu into a meal in minutes. You need add only boiling water, or mayonnaise (depending on the variety) to mashed or cubed tofu. Available in four varieties, this product has been incorporated into a number of dishes in *The Enlightened Kitchen,* adding depth of flavor. In some instances, the directions will sometimes differ from those indicated on the package. Use the dry mix only without added water unless otherwise indicated in the recipe instructions.

**Vegenaise**   This eggless alternative dressing tastes just like traditional mayonnaise. It is available in Original, Expeller Pressed, Grapeseed Oil, and Organic, in the refrigerated case in health food stores from Follow Your Heart.

**Vegetarian chicken- and beef-flavored broth powder**   These useful products are used in recipes for some soups, sauces, and gravies.

**Vegetarian Worcestershire sauce**   A condiment with all of the zest and flavor of the traditional, without anchovies or artificial ingredients. Available from The Wizard, Robbie's Foods, and Angostura.

**Vital wheat gluten**   Vital wheat gluten occurs naturally in all wheat flours. Vital wheat gluten helps improve the rise and texture of bread. It is highly rec-

Pantry

ommended that you add vital wheat gluten to the flour in recipes for whole grain breads. Please note: Vital wheat gluten is not the same as gluten flour, which is a combination of flour and vital wheat gluten.

**Whole wheat tortillas**  Most tortillas contain hydrogenated fat but generally, whole wheat tortillas do not. If whole wheat is not available, tortillas made with unbleached flour are fine, as long as the ingredients do not list "partially hydrogenated oil" of any kind.

# The
# Recipes

# Enlightened Entertaining

While it is possible to turn almost any meal into a special occasion, this section offers dishes that lend themselves easily to larger gatherings. Whether planning a festive holiday party or an impromptu gathering of friends, it's best to do as much advance preparation as possible.

This collection includes easy-to-assemble dips and pâtés, and several types of marinated edamame that develop added flavor overnight. It also offers real time-savers—you can cook up a batch of crepes, or make the filling for dishes such as Potato Quesadillas or Sun-Dried Tomato Quiche Bites a day or two ahead of time. Dishes like these are best made a day in advance, so you can easily fit hosting responsibilities into your busy life.

Traditional party fare is loaded with unhealthy ingredients. Take a rich, creamy dip, a classic party favorite. A quick read of ingredients for the standard dip might include such artery-clogging ingredients as sour cream, mayonnaise, grated cheese, and/or cream cheese. All this is too high in fat and cholesterol for today's health-conscious cook.

Does this mean that these enduring favorites are off limits when maintaining a healthy diet? Certainly not! In *The Enlightened Kitchen*, we create creamy, dairy-free dishes using wholesome alternative ingredients that mimic the texture and preserve the character of the traditional dish. For example, you can have a really fun fondue party, a terrific way to bring guests together. Our

Enlightened "Cheesy" Fondue Pot and Richly Chocolate Fondue are richly flavorful, creamy, and delectable without fatty cheese or dairy chocolate.

So, make an outstanding impression. Entertain the *Enlightened Kitchen* way. Arrange the flowers, light the candles, and introduce your guests to delicious, wholesome food.

# Recipes

Potato Quesadillas

Sun-Dried Tomato Quiche Bites

"Cheesy" Fondue Pot

Shelled Edamame and Mushrooms in Spring Onion Marinade

Shelled Edamame in Sesame Marinade

Shelled Edamame in Balsamic Marinade

Creamy "Cheese" Bites

Paella

Spinach-Stuffed Shells

Savory "Sausage" Lasagna

Individual Broccoli Quiche

Hearty Tortilla Wraps

Spinach-Artichoke Dip

"Bacon" and Chive Dip

Garlic and Thyme Pita Crisps

"Sausage" in a Blanket

"Sausage" Turnovers

Festive Holiday Roast

Stuffed Grape Leaves

Tempeh Chili

Mushroom-Okara Pâté

Hoppin' John

Light and Lovely Crepes

Just Peachy Dessert Crepes

Richly Chocolate Fondue

Tosteds Trail Mix

# Potato Quesadillas

*Quesadillas are traditionally high in fat, because they are thick with cheese. These aren't! And they're even better the next day, when reheated under the broiler for few minutes.*

*10 Servings*

olive oil cooking spray
4 medium Yukon Gold potatoes, cut
   to ¼-inch slices
1½ teaspoons olive oil
¼ teaspoon crushed red pepper
4 cloves garlic, minced
1 medium yellow onion, chopped
2 Melissa's fire roasted chiles, one red,
   one green, chopped (about ½ cup)

1 cup enriched 1% fat soymilk
½ cup nutritional yeast
2 teaspoons Bragg Liquid Aminos
2 tablespoons lime juice
1 teaspoon dried cilantro
1 teaspoon dried marjoram
10 flour tortillas, nonhydrogenated

Preheat oven to 375°. Spray two baking pans with olive oil.

Place potatoes in a medium saucepan and cover with salted water. Bring to a boil, reduce heat, and cook for 20 minutes, or until tender. Set aside. In a 10-inch frying pan, heat oil and crushed pepper over medium-high heat for 1 minute. Add garlic, onion, and chopped chiles. Cook for 3 minutes.

Using a slotted spoon, remove potatoes from cooking water and add to the frying pan. Cook mixture, stirring frequently, for 3 minutes. Combine soymilk and yeast. Stir to blend, then add liquid aminos. Add soymilk mixture to the frying pan along with lime juice, cilantro, and marjoram.

Place a tortilla on a prepared baking pan. Spread filling to within 1 inch of the edge. Top with a second tortilla. Repeat until 5 quesadillas are completed. Lightly spray tortilla tops with olive oil and bake for 10 minutes. Turn, using a flat spatula, and bake for 10 more minutes. Cut each quesadilla into quarters, and serve with additional Melissa's fire roasted chiles or salsa on the side.

NUTRITION ANALYSIS: PER 2 QUARTER PORTIONS (1/2 QUESADILLA)

**Enlightened Quesadillas**
Protein 8 g, carbohydrate 63 g, fiber 6 g, fat 2g,
saturated fat 0 g, cholesterol 0 mg,
calcium 55 mg, sodium 227 mg.
Calories 191: from protein 11%,
from carbohydrate 83%, from fat 6%

**Traditional Quesadillas**
Protein 11g, carbohydrate 40 g, fiber 3 g, fat 19 g,
saturated fat 8 g, cholesterol 33 mg,
calcium 225 mg, sodium 489 mg
Calories 370: from protein 11%,
from carbohydrate 43%, from fat 46%

# Sun-Dried Tomato Quiche Bites

*Very easy to assemble, these delicious appetizers can be made in advance and frozen. To reheat, place frozen pastries in a preheated 350° oven for 10 minutes, or until hot. Microwave: wrap up to 8 pastries in (white) paper towel; microwave at 50% power for 60 seconds.*

olive oil cooking spray
1 cup sun-dried tomatoes (about half a 3-ounce package)
1 cup boiling water
2 teaspoons olive oil
⅛ teaspoon crushed red pepper
3 cloves garlic, minced
1 large shallot, minced (about ⅓ cup)
⅓ cup sliced scallions
⅓ cup chopped red bell pepper
1 12.3-ounce package lite silken tofu

3 tablespoons mellow white miso
⅓ cup dry sherry
⅓ cup mashed potato flakes
½ cup nutritional yeast
¼ teaspoon turmeric
1 teaspoon dried basil
½ cup enriched 1% fat soymilk
2 tablespoons lemon juice
60 Fillo Factory shelf-stable mini pastry shells
dried basil for garnish

Preheat oven to 375°. Lightly spray two baking pans with olive oil.

Combine sun-dried tomatoes and boiling water in a small bowl and set aside for at least 15 minutes. In a 10-inch frying pan, heat oil and crushed pepper over medium-high heat for 1 minute. Add garlic, shallots, scallions, and bell pepper. Sauté for 3 minutes. Add reconstituted dried tomatoes, reserving soaking liquid. Lower heat and cook for 8 minutes. Add ½ cup tomato-soaking liquid and return heat to medium high. Cook for 5 minutes, stirring frequently, or until liquid is absorbed. Remove from heat and set aside.

Place tofu in food processor and blend until smooth. Place miso in a small bowl; add sherry and blend with a fork until smooth. Add to the tofu and blend. Add potato flakes, yeast, turmeric, basil, soymilk, and lemon juice. Process thoroughly. Add the sun-dried tomato mixture to the soymilk mixture,

**Sun-Dried Tomato Quiche Bites** *(continued)*

and pulse carefully to chop tomatoes. Press the pulse button lightly—do not
purée. Spoon about 2 tablespoons of filling into each phyllo cup, sprinkle with
additional basil, and bake in prepared pans on middle rack of oven for 15 minutes or until filling is cooked through and firm. Let sit 10 minutes before
serving.

---

NUTRITION ANALYSIS: PER SERVING (3 APPETIZERS)

| Enlightened Quiche Bites | Traditional Quiche Bites |
|---|---|
| Protein 4 g, carbohydrate 10 g, fiber 1 g, fat 3 g, | Protein 5 g, carbohydrate 14 g, fiber 1 g, fat 12 g, |
| saturated fat 0 g, cholesterol 0 mg, | saturated fat 5 g, cholesterol 65 mg, |
| calcium 21 mg, sodium 78 mg | calcium 62 mg, sodium 230 mg |
| Calories 76: from protein 18%, | Calories 184: from protein 11%, |
| from carbohydrate 51%, from fat 31% | from carbohydrate 30%, from fat 59% |

# "Cheesy" Fondue Pot

*Your guests will not believe that there are no dairy products in this fabulous fondue. You can also serve "Sausage" in a Blanket (page 75) with this "cheese" sauce. Very yummy!*

1 cup enriched 1% fat soymilk
2 teaspoons lemon juice
1 12.3-ounce package lite silken tofu
1 12.3-ounce package regular silken tofu
¼ cup sliced scallions
3 cloves garlic, peeled

2 teaspoons vegetarian Worcestershire sauce
1 teaspoon Dijon mustard
1 tablespoon DDC onion broth powder
1 cup nutritional yeast
2 tablespoons mellow white miso
2 tablespoons dry sherry

Combine soymilk and lemon juice in a medium glass measuring cup and set aside. Place tofu in food processor and process to blend. Add scallions, garlic, Worcestershire sauce, mustard, broth powder, and yeast. Blend. In a small bowl, blend miso and sherry, "creaming" to form a thick paste. Add to the tofu mixture along with the soymilk mixture. Blend until smooth. Warm sauce in the microwave or on stovetop before pouring into fondue pot.

DIPPING SUGGESTIONS: cubed crusty whole grain bread, boiled new potatoes, blanched asparagus, broccoli, cauliflower florets

---

## NUTRITION ANALYSIS: PER ½-CUP SERVING

**Enlightened "Cheesy" Fondue**
Protein 8 g, carbohydrate 5 g, fiber 1 g, fat 1 g, saturated fat 0 g, cholesterol 0 mg, calcium 52 mg, sodium 125 mg
Calories 57: from protein 50%, from carbohydrate 35%, from fat 15%

**Traditional Cheese Fondue**
Protein 8 g, carbohydrate 9 g, fiber 0 g, fat 13 g, saturated fat 8 g, cholesterol 43 mg, calcium 242 mg, sodium 293 mg
Calories 189: from protein 17%, from carbohydrate 20%, from fat 63%

# Shelled Edamame and Mushrooms in Spring Onion Marinade

*Serve edamame and sliced cremini mushrooms
in this light marinade as a side dish.*

*12
Servings*

16 to 20 ounces shelled edamame
1 recipe of Spring Onion Marinade
 (page 219)
1 6-ounce package sliced cremini
 mushrooms

½ red onion, thinly sliced and cut in
 half
1 large red bell pepper, chopped

LOOK FOR CONVENIENT,
9- or 10-ounce packages of
ready-to-eat shelled edamame
in the produce section of
supermarkets and health food
stores.

If frozen, cook edamame according to package directions and drain well. Combine marinade ingredients in a medium glass measuring cup. Place edamame in a nonreactive bowl (preferably glass) and combine with marinade. Add mushrooms, onion, and bell pepper and mix thoroughly. Cover and refrigerate at least 4 hours, or overnight for optimal flavor.

---

NUTRITION ANALYSIS: PER ¹/2-CUP SERVING

**Enlightened Marinated Edamame**
Protein 6 g, carbohydrate 8 g, fiber 3 g, fat 3 g,
saturated fat 0 g, cholesterol 0 mg,
calcium 42 mg, sodium 230 mg
Calories 90: from protein 28%,
from carbohydrate 37%, from fat 35%*

**Traditional Marinated Beans and Mushrooms**
Protein 3 g, carbohydrate 12 g, fiber 2 g, fat 19 g,
saturated fat 3 g, cholesterol 0mg,
calcium 24 mg, sodium 506 mg
Calories 227: from protein 5%,
from carbohydrate 25%, from fat 70%

\* The percentage of calories from fat seems high only because the calories are so low.

# Shelled Edamame in Sesame Marinade

*Delivering 6 grams of soy protein in just a third of a cup,
this dish is a healthy and delicious addition
to the buffet table.*

16 to 20 ounces shelled edamame
1 recipe of Savory Sesame Marinade
  (page 218)

½ cup thinly sliced scallions
1 large red bell pepper, chopped

If frozen, cook edamame according to package directions and drain well. Combine marinade ingredients in a medium glass measuring cup. Place edamame in a nonreactive bowl (preferably glass) and combine with marinade. Add scallions and pepper and mix thoroughly. Cover and refrigerate at least 4 hours or overnight for optimal flavor.

NUTRITION ANALYSIS: PER ⅓-CUP SERVING

**Enlightened Marinated Edamame**
Protein 6 g, carbohydrate 7 g, fiber 3 g, fat 7 g,
saturated fat 1 g, cholesterol 0 mg,
calcium 39 mg, sodium 269 mg
Calories 119: from protein 20%,
from carbohydrate 24%, from fat 56%*

**Traditional Marinated Beans**
Protein 3 g, carbohydrate 8 g, fiber 2 g, fat 11 g,
saturated fat 2 g, cholesterol 1 mg,
calcium 26 mg, sodium 771 mg
Calories 137: from protein 8%,
from carbohydrate 25%, from fat 67%

* Percentage of calories from fat seems high only because the calories are so low.

# Shelled Edamame in Balsamic Marinade

*Exquisite balsamic flavor notes add a new dimension*
*to edamame, especially when marinated overnight.*

*12*
*Servings*

16 to 20 ounces shelled edamame
1 recipe of Balsamic Marinade
   (page 209)

½ cup thinly sliced scallions
1 large red bell pepper, chopped

If frozen, cook edamame according to package directions and drain well. Combine marinade ingredients in a medium glass measuring cup. Place edamame in a nonreactive bowl (preferably glass) and combine with marinade. Add scallions and pepper, and mix thoroughly. Cover and refrigerate at least 4 hours, or overnight for optimal flavor.

NUTRITION ANALYSIS: PER ⅓-CUP SERVING

**Enlightened Marinated Edamame**
Protein 6 g, carbohydrate 8 g, fiber 3 g, fat 2 g,
saturated fat 0 g, cholesterol 0 mg,
calcium 46 mg, sodium 118 mg
Calories 82: from protein 30%,
from carbohydrate 43%, from fat 27%*

**Traditional Marinated Beans**
Protein 3 g, carbohydrate 8 g, fiber 2 g, fat 11 g,
saturated fat 2 g, cholesterol 1 mg,
calcium 26 mg, sodium 771 mg
Calories 137: from protein 8%,
from carbohydrate 25%, from fat 67%

* Percentage of calories from fat seems high only because the calories are so low.

# Creamy "Cheese" Bites

*Quick and easy, these delicious appetizers can be made in advance and frozen. To reheat: place frozen pastries in a preheated 350° oven for 10 minutes, or until warm. Or, if using a microwave, wrap up to six pastries in (white) paper towel. Microwave on 50% power for 30 seconds.*

olive oil cooking spray
1 recipe Homemade Dairy-Free
　　"Cheese" (page 202)

45 Fillo Factory shelf-stable mini
　　pastry shells
paprika for garnish

Preheat oven to 375°. Lightly spray two baking pans with olive oil.

Make the "cheese" filling. Fill each pastry shell with a rounded tablespoon of filling. Sprinkle with paprika. Bake 15 minutes or until brown.

---

NUTRITION ANALYSIS: PER SERVING (3 APPETIZERS)

### Enlightened "Cheese" Bites
Protein 6 g, carbohydrate 10 g, fiber 1 g, fat 3 g,
saturated fat 0, cholesterol 0 mg,
calcium 28 mg, sodium 79 mg
Calories 81: from protein 27%,
from carbohydrate 46%, from fat 27%

### Traditional Cheese Bites
Protein 6 g, carbohydrate 12 g, fiber 0 g, fat 14 g,
saturated fat 8 g, cholesterol 68 mg,
calcium 98 mg, sodium 194 mg
Calories 198: from protein 11%,
from carbohydrate 25%, from fat 63%

*8
Servings*

# Paella

*This classic Spanish dish can be the centerpiece
for easy, elegant entertaining.*

1 teaspoon saffron threads
4 cups chicken-flavored vegetarian
   broth, boiling
olive oil cooking spray
½ 12-ounce package Soyrizo
   (6 ounces)
3 cloves garlic, minced
1 cup sliced scallions
1 cup chopped red bell pepper

2 6-ounce packages Smart Chick'n
   Strips
1 15-ounce can cannellini beans
   (white kidney beans)
⅓ cup dry sherry
1 cup raw white rice
1 13¾-ounce can quartered
   artichoke hearts, drained
2 plum tomatoes, diced

THIS ROBUST dish takes its name from the shallow, two-handled metal pan in which it is traditionally cooked.

Stir saffron into broth and set aside.

Spray a Dutch oven or electric frying pan with olive oil and warm over medium-high heat. Squeeze Soyrizo into the pan, discarding the casing. Break Soyrizo into pieces with a fork while cooking for 8 minutes, or until crisp and brown. Remove Soyrizo from the pan and set aside. Spray pan with olive oil, add garlic, scallions, and bell pepper and cook for 3 minutes. Add Chick'n Strips and sauté mixture for 3 minutes. Add the beans and sherry and cook for 2 minutes. Add rice and cook mixture for 3 minutes, stirring frequently. Stir in broth along with artichoke hearts. Reduce heat and simmer for 20 minutes, or until liquid is absorbed. Add cooked Soyrizo. Serve hot or at room temperature.

NUTRITION ANALYSIS: PER 2-CUP SERVING

| Enlightened Paella | Traditional Paella |
|---|---|
| Protein 15 g, carbohydrate 37 g, fiber 7 g, fat 4 g, saturated fat 0 g, cholesterol 0 mg, calcium 75 mg, sodium 581 mg Calories 245: from protein 24%, from carbohydrate 62%, from fat 14% | Protein 30 g, carbohydrate 25 g, fiber 1 g, fat 28 g, saturated fat 9 g, cholesterol 130 mg, calcium 50 mg, sodium 1058 mg Calories 497: from protein 26%, from carbohydrate 21%, from fat 53% |

# Spinach-Stuffed Shells

*A great choice for entertaining, Spinach-Stuffed Shells are
best made in advance and reheated before serving.*

---

1 10-ounce package frozen spinach,
   thawed
1 12-ounce package jumbo shells
3 12.3-ounce packages lite silken tofu
3 cloves garlic, minced
⅓ cup chopped scallions
1 tablespoon DDC onion broth
   powder

⅓ cup nutritional yeast
⅓ cup soy Parmesan cheese
1 teaspoon dried thyme
½ teaspoon granulated garlic
2 28-ounce jars tomato sauce
additional soy Parmesan cheese

Preheat oven to 350°.

Set thawed spinach aside in wire mesh colander to drain. Cook shells according to package directions. Drain and set aside in a colander suspended in a bowl of ice water, keeping the pasta shells hydrated, and rinsing from time to time to avoid sticking.

Place tofu in a large bowl and mash with a potato masher. Add the minced garlic, scallions, and broth powder. Add the spinach, yeast, soy Parmesan, thyme, and granulated garlic. Mix thoroughly and set aside.

*Assembly:* Spread a layer of tomato sauce evenly along the bottom of one 9- by -13-inch and one 8- by 8-inch baking pan. Cupping a cooked shell in the palm of your hand, stuff shell with about 2 tablespoons of filling and set in baking pan. Repeat. This dish freezes well, if that is more than you will need. Top shells with remaining tomato sauce, then sprinkle with soy Parmesan cheese. Cover with foil and bake for 45 minutes. (May be made a day in advance and

**Spinach-Stuffed Shells** *(continued)*

set aside in the refrigerator, at this point). Remove foil and bake for an additional 15 minutes. Let shells sit for 15 minutes before serving. Reheats very well.

---

NUTRITION ANALYSIS: PER SERVING (3 SHELLS)

| Enlightened Spinach-Stuffed Shells | Traditional Spinach-Stuffed Shells |
|---|---|
| Protein 13 g, carbohydrate 26 g, fiber 4 g, fat 1 g, saturated fat 0 g, cholesterol 0 mg, calcium 81 mg, sodium 408 mg | Protein 20 g, carbohydrate 26 g, fiber 1 g, fat 20 g, saturated fat 11 g, cholesterol 90 mg, calcium 426 mg, sodium 1111 mg |
| Calories 146: from protein 31%, from carbohydrate 61%, from fat 8% | Calories 356: from protein 23%, from carbohydrate 28%, from fat 49% |

# Savory "Sausage" Lasagna

*You will love this easy and really delicious dish that tastes even
better the next day. Gimme Lean "sausage" enriches this dish,
imparting great flavor, texture, and the goodness of soy!*

*Savory "Sausage" Tomato Sauce*

1½ teaspoons olive oil
1 tablespoon dried minced garlic
½ cup sliced scallions
1 14-ounce package Gimme Lean
   sausage style

1 28-ounce can Italian Recipe diced
   tomatoes
½ teaspoon dried thyme

*Tofu Layer*

3 12.3-ounce packages lite silken tofu
3 cloves garlic, minced
1 26-gram package Tofu Hero Italian
   Herb Medley
½ cup coarsely shredded carrots
½ cup chopped red onion

⅓ cup nutritional yeast
¼ cup soy Parmesan cheese
1 25-ounce jar fat-free tomato sauce
1 9-ounce package Barilla no-cook
   lasagna noodles
additional soy Parmesan Cheese

Preheat oven to 350°.

*For the sauce:* Warm oil in a medium saucepan over medium-high heat for 1 minute. Add the garlic and scallions and cook for 2 minutes. Add the Gimme Lean and cook the mixture for 5 minutes, stirring frequently and breaking sausage into pieces with a large spoon. Add tomatoes and reduce heat to low. Simmer for 5 minutes, add thyme and set aside.

*For the tofu layer:* Place tofu in a large bowl and mash with a potato masher. Add the garlic, Tofu Hero, carrots, onion, yeast, and soy Parmesan. Mix well and set aside.

*Assembly:* Spread a layer of tomato sauce evenly in the bottom of a 9- by 13-inch baking pan. Top with a layer of noodles. Add any broken noodle pieces around edges to make an even fit. Top with the tofu filling

WHEN ENTERTAINING family and friends, I usually choose Italian-style dishes. They are hearty, flavorful dishes that always lend themselves well to advance preparation— as does this lasagna.

**Savory "Sausage" Lasagne** *(continued)*

followed by a layer of noodles, and cover with sauce. Break remaining noodles into uneven pieces and sprinkle lightly over sauce. Sprinkle with soy Parmesan. Cover casserole with foil and bake for 45 minutes. (May be made a day in advance and set aside in the refrigerator, at this point.) Remove foil and bake for an additional 15 minutes. Let lasagna sit for 15 minutes before serving. Reheats very well.

---

NUTRITION ANALYSIS: PER 1½-CUP SERVING

Enlightened Savory Sausage Lasagna
Protein 18 g, carbohydrate 29 g, fiber 4 g, fat 2 g,
saturated fat 0 g, cholesterol 0 mg,
calcium 47 mg, sodium 574 mg
Calories 193: from protein 35%,
from carbohydrate 57%, from fat 8%

Traditional Sausage Lasagna
Protein 23 g, carbohydrate 18g, fiber 2 g, fat 26 g,
saturated fat 12 g, cholesterol 90 mg,
calcium 300 mg, sodium 792 mg
Calories 398: from protein 23%,
from carbohydrate 19%, from fat 58%

# Individual Broccoli Quiche

*Rich tasting and flavorful, the filling for this delicious dish is made with
wholesome, plant-based alternatives that mimic the flavor and character
of classic quiche. The pastry relies on pectins from liquid
Fruitsource and just one tablespoon of olive oil for elasticity.*

6 Individual
Quiches

### Crust

1 cup rolled oats
1 cup whole wheat flour
¼ teaspoon salt
⅓ cup lite silken tofu

1 tablespoon olive oil
1 tablespoon liquid Fruitsource
¼ cup ice water

### Filling

1 teaspoon olive oil
3 cloves garlic, minced
⅓ cup chopped red onion
¼ cup chopped green bell pepper
2 cups broccoli florets, cut to bite size
1 12.3-ounce package lite silken tofu
⅓ cup dry sherry

3 tablespoons mellow white miso
⅓ cup mashed potato flakes
⅓ cup nutritional yeast
¼ teaspoon turmeric
½ cup enriched 1% fat soymilk
1 tablespoon lemon juice

Preheat oven to 400°.

*For the crust:* Place oats, flour, and salt in food processor
and blend to mix. Add tofu and process. Add oil and Fruitsource and pulse to blend. With the machine running, drizzle
in ice water until the dough begins to form a ball. Turn dough
onto a clean flat surface dusted with flour. Knead the dough a
few times and shape into a ball. Divide the pastry into 6 equal
pieces and roll out to between ⅛ and ¼ inch thick. Press each
into a 4⅝-inch diameter tart pan and set aside.

A GOOD CHOICE FOR a
luncheon or brunch, Individual
Broccoli Quiche will freeze
well. Place frozen quiche in
preheated 350° oven for 20
minutes or until heated
through.

**Individual Broccoli Quiches** *(continued)*

*For the filling:* Heat oil in a 10-inch frying pan over medium-high heat for 1 minute. Add garlic, onion, and pepper. Sauté for 3 minutes. Add broccoli and cook for 4 minutes. Remove from heat and set aside.

Place tofu in food processor and blend until smooth. In a small bowl, blend sherry and miso with a fork until smooth. Add to the tofu with potato flakes, yeast, turmeric, soymilk, and lemon juice. Process thoroughly. Fold tofu mixture into the broccoli and spoon into each pastry-lined pan. Place the pans on a baking sheet and bake on the center rack of the oven for 30 minutes. Serve warm.

---

NUTRITION ANALYSIS: PER INDIVIDUAL QUICHE

| Enlightened Broccoli Quiche | Traditional Broccoli Quiche |
|---|---|
| Protein 17 g, carbohydrate 39 g, fiber 5 g, | Protein 15 g, carbohydrate 35 g, fiber 2 g, |
| fat 6 g, saturated fat 1 g, cholesterol 0 mg, | fat 31 g, saturated fat 18 g, cholesterol 220 mg, |
| calcium 56 mg, sodium 223 mg | calcium 212 mg, sodium 535 mg |
| Calories 267: from protein 24%, | Calories 476: from protein 12%, |
| from carbohydrate 57%, from fat 19% | from carbohydrate 30%, from fat 58% |

# Hearty Tortilla Wraps

*Made in advance, this dish can be a fun picnic item. Simply pack the filling
separately in a covered plastic container, and wrap the tortillas
in foil. Bring along a colorful salad and a bottle of chilled Chardonnay—
and you are ready for an evening dining al fresco!*

3⅓ cups boiling water, divided
2 tablespoons DDC original broth
   powder
2 cups DDC Beef Not! Strips
1½ tablespoons DDC Crème of
   Mushroom soup mix
1½ teaspoons olive oil
¼ teaspoon crushed red pepper
2 cloves garlic, minced

1 medium red onion, chopped
1 stalk celery, sliced
1½ cups shredded carrots
½ cup dry sherry
1 cup frozen corn, thawed
¼ cup nutritional yeast
2 teaspoons dried marjoram
8 whole wheat tortillas

Over medium-high heat, combine 2 cups boiling water, broth powder, and
"beef" strips in a medium saucepan. Bring mixture to a second boil, reduce
heat to medium low, and simmer for 15 minutes, stirring occasionally. Set
aside.

In a medium glass measuring cup, combine 1⅓ cups boiling water and
mushroom soup mix and set aside. In a Dutch oven or electric frying pan, heat oil and crushed pepper over medium-high heat for 1
minute. Add garlic, onion, celery, and carrots. Cook mixture for 5
minutes, stirring occasionally. Add sherry, corn, yeast, and marjoram. Reduce heat to low and simmer for 10 minutes. Warm tortillas in oven at 300° for 5 minutes or microwave (a few at a time)
at 50% power for 30 to 60 seconds.

PITA POCKETS ARE an
easy alternative choice for
tortillas here.

---

### NUTRITION ANALYSIS: PER 2-CUP SERVING

| Enlightened Tortilla Wraps | Traditional Tortilla Wraps |
|---|---|
| Protein 16 g, carbohydrate 37 g, fiber 8 g, fat 2 g, | Protein 17 g, carbohydrate 33 g, fiber 3 g, fat 22 g, |
| saturated fat 0 g, cholesterol 0 mg, | saturated fat 9 g, cholesterol 58 mg, |
| calcium 73 mg, sodium 303 mg | calcium 120 mg, sodium 554 mg |
| Calories 203: from protein 28%, | Calories 404: from protein 17%, |
| from carbohydrate 64%, from fat 8% | from carbohydrate 33%, from fat 50% |

# Spinach-Artichoke Dip

*A delightfully creamy dip
with a light Parmesan flavor.*

1 10-ounce package chopped frozen
    spinach, thawed
1 12.3-ounce package lite silken tofu
1 tablespoon lemon juice
¼ cup eggless mayonnaise
1 tablespoon DDC onion broth
    powder

4 cloves garlic, peeled
⅔ cup chopped red onion
¼ cup chopped shallots
1 13½-ounce can artichoke hearts
⅓ cup soy Parmesan cheese
¼ cup nutritional yeast

Set spinach aside in a wire mesh colander to drain. Place tofu in food processor and blend until smooth. Add the lemon juice, mayonnaise, broth powder, garlic, onion, and shallots; blend. Add spinach and pulse to mix. Add artichoke hearts and pulse to mix. Add soy Parmesan and yeast. Process to blend. Cover and refrigerate for several hours or, optimally, overnight.

SERVE WITH torn pita pockets or pita crisps, and crudités like baby carrots, celery, and broccoli.

---

NUTRITION ANALYSIS: PER ½-CUP SERVING

**Enlightened Spinach-Artichoke Dip**
Protein 6 g, carbohydrate 7 g, fiber 2 g, fat 2 g,
saturated fat 0 g, cholesterol 0 mg,
calcium 54 mg, sodium 228 mg
Calories 55: from protein 35%,
from carbohydrate 40%, from fat 25%

**Traditional Spinach-Artichoke Dip**
Protein 6 g, carbohydrate 7 g, fiber 1 g, fat 19 g,
saturated fat 9 g, cholesterol 36 mg,
calcium 166 mg, sodium 341 mg
Calories 212: from protein 10%,
from carbohydrate 13%, from fat 77%

# "Bacon" and Chive Dip

*Serve this tasty dip with pita crisps or
as a delicious sandwich spread.*

8
*Servings*

½ cup enriched 1% fat soymilk
1 teaspoon lemon juice
1 12.3-ounce package lite silken tofu
3 cloves garlic, peeled
⅓ cup sliced scallions
1 tablespoon Dijon mustard
1 tablespoon liquid Fruitsource
1 teaspoon vegetarian Worcestershire
    sauce

1 tablespoon DDC onion broth
    powder
⅓ cup nutritional yeast
1 6-ounce package veggie Canadian
    bacon, diced
¼ cup chopped fresh chives

Combine soymilk and lemon juice in a medium glass measuring cup and set
aside. Place tofu in food processor and process until smooth. Add garlic, scallions, mustard, Fruitsource, Worcestershire sauce, and soymilk mixture. Blend.
Add onion broth powder and nutritional yeast. Blend until smooth. Add diced
veggie bacon and and chives; process to mix well. Do not purée—the veggie
bacon should remain in very small chunks.

---

NUTRITION ANALYSIS: PER ⅔-CUP SERVING

| Enlightened "Bacon" and Chive Dip | Traditional Bacon and Chive Dip |
|---|---|
| Protein 12 g, carbohydrate 7 g, fiber 1 g, fat 1 g, | Protein 13 g, carbohydrate 11 g, fiber 0 g, fat 19 g, |
| saturated fat 0 g, cholesterol 0 mg, | saturated fat 11 g, cholesterol 62 mg, |
| calcium 42 mg, sodium 314 mg | calcium 92 mg, sodium 772 mg |
| Calories 79: from protein 56%, | Calories 260: from protein 19%, |
| from carbohydrate 35%, from fat 9% | from carbohydrate 18%, from fat 63% |

# Garlic and Thyme Pita Crisps

*Homemade pita crisps can be spiced with just granulated garlic or with
your favorite blend of herbs and spices. Serve with "Bacon" and
Chive Dip (page 73) and Spinach-Artichoke Dip (page 72).*

*24
Servings*

olive oil cooking spray
24 whole wheat pita pockets
1 tablespoon granulated garlic

1 teaspoon granulated onion
1 teaspoon dried thyme
¼ teaspoon lemon pepper

Pita Crisps are a
wholesome alternative
to commercial chips
and crackers, which are
routinely loaded with
hydrogenated fats.

Preheat oven to 400°. Line a baking pan with foil and spray foil with
oil.

Cut pita pockets into eighths and place on prepared baking pan.
Lightly oil spray top side of pita. Mix together herbs and spices, and
sprinkle on top of pita. Bake 10 minutes, or until lightly browned. Set
aside to cool.

NUTRITION ANALYSIS: PER SERVING (8 PITA CRISPS)

| Enlightened Garlic and Thyme Pita Crisps | Traditional Savory Crackers |
|---|---|
| Protein 5 g, carbohydrate 25 g, fiber 3 g, fat 1 g, | Protein 4 g, carbohydrate 29 g, fiber 0 g, fat 11 g, |
| saturated fat 0 g, cholesterol 0 mg, | saturated fat 4 g, cholesterol 0 mg, |
| calcium 8 mg, sodium 239 mg | calcium 13 mg, sodium 521 mg |
| Calories 123: from protein 14%, | Calories 236: from protein 6%, |
| from carbohydrate 77%, from fat 9% | from carbohydrate 51%, from fat 43% |

# "Sausage" in a Blanket

*This appetizer is always a hit. Savory "sausage" is encased in a
light pastry. A dipping sauce such as "Cheesy" Fonduee (page 59)
or tomato sauce makes a nice accompaniment.*

olive oil cooking spray

1 14-ounce package Gimme Lean,
   sausage style

*Pastry*
2 cups unbleached flour
1 teaspoon nonaluminum baking
   powder
½ teaspoon sea salt

⅓ cup lite silken tofu
1 tablespoon olive oil
⅓ cup ice water

Preheat oven to 400°. Spray a baking pan pan with olive oil.

Roll sausage directly from package into 40 small balls. Bake on prepared pan
for 10 to 15 minutes, or until lightly browned. Set aside to cool, but leave oven
on.

*For the pastry:* Place flour, baking powder, and salt in a food processor and
pulse to mix. Add tofu and process. While machine is running, add oil and ice
water through feeding tube. Ingredients will form into a dough ball. Stop
machine and turn dough onto a clean, flat surface. Sprinkle lightly with no
more than a tablespoon of flour, and knead dough for a minute. Using thumb
and forefingers, shape a tablespoon or so of dough around each "sausage" ball.
It will press easily. Spray a clean baking pan with olive oil and bake dough-
wrapped "sausage" balls for 15 minutes or until browned. Serve hot.

---

NUTRITION ANALYSIS: PER SERVING (5 "SAUSAGE" BALLS)

Enlightened "Sausage" in a Blanket
Protein 6 g, carbohydrate 10 g, fiber 1 g, fat 2,
saturated fat 0 g, cholesterol 0 mg,
calcium 23 mg, sodium 287 mg
Calories 76: from protein 33%,
from carbohydrate 53%, from fat 14%

Traditional Sausage in a Blanket
Protein 9 g, carbohydrate 17 g, fiber 1 g, fat 21 g,
saturated fat 10 g, cholesterol 44 mg,
calcium 95 mg, sodium 601 mg
Calories 291: from protein 13%,
from carbohydrate 22%, from fat 65%

# "Sausage" Turnovers

*You can make these easy and delicious turnovers a day in advance.
Reheat at 325° for 20 minutes.*

*40
Appetizers*

olive oil cooking spray
1 10-ounce package DDC Soysage
    Pattie Mix

2¼ cups cold water

*Pastry*

1 cup rolled oats
2 cups whole wheat pastry flour
1 tablespoon EnerG egg replacer
    powder
1 teaspoon nonaluminum baking
    powder
½ teaspoon sea salt

¾ cup lite silken tofu
2 tablespoons olive oil
2 tablespoons liquid Fruitsource
¼ cup ice water
½ cup barbecue sauce or tomato
    sauce

SERVE WITH barbecue
sauce, Dijon mustard, or
tomato sauce on the side.

Preheat oven to 400°. Spray a baking pan with olive oil.

In a large bowl, combine sausage mix with water and set aside
for 15 minutes. *For the pastry:* Place oats in food processor and
process to flour, for less than 30 seconds. Add pastry flour, egg
replacer powder, baking powder, and salt. Process to mix. Measure
out tofu by stirring down in a liquid measuring cup with a fork.
Add tofu to flour and process. While machine is running add oil, Fruitsource,
and water through feeding tube. Ingredients will form a moist dough ball. Stop
machine and turn dough onto a clean, flat surface dusted with pastry flour.
Sprinkle dough with pastry flour, and knead for 5 minutes, adding up to a cup
of flour, until dough is no longer sticky and is smooth and elastic. Cover dough
with a clean towel for 10 minutes.

Divide dough ball in half, keeping reserved half covered with towel. Roll dough to about 11-by-17-inches. Using a round glass or pastry tool about 3½ inches in diameter, cut disks from the dough. Cupping a dough disk in the palm of the hand, place a rounded tablespoon of the sausage filling onto the dough and top filling with a scant teaspoon of barbecue or tomato sauce. Place filled pastry on the pastry board, and press the edges closed with the tines of a fork. Repeat until all dough is used. Any remaining filling can be formed into patties and baked.

Bake for 15 minutes or until brown. Serve hot.

---

## NUTRITION ANALYSIS: PER SERVING (2 TURNOVERS)

| Enlightened "Sausage" Turnovers | Traditional Sausage Turnovers |
|---|---|
| Protein 5 g, carbohydrate 15 g, fiber 2 g, fat 2 g, saturated fat 0 g, cholesterol 0 mg, calcium 38 mg, sodium 137 mg | Protein 8 g, carbohydrate 15 g, fiber 1 g, fat 16 g, saturated fat 6 g, cholesterol 41 mg, calcium 62 mg, sodium 203 mg |
| Calories 98: from protein 21%, from carbohydrate 60%, from fat 19% | Calories 399: from protein 13%, from carbohydrate 26%, from fat 61% |

# Festive Holiday Roast

*You can enjoy a delectably healthy holiday feast and all the fixings with less than 1 gram of saturated fat per serving. (All nutrition analyses are rounded to above or below the .5 g level. The actual saturated fat is .7 g.) Create a bountiful, meatless Thanksgiving celebration that is easy to prepare, as delicious as the traditional meal, and extremely cost-effective.*

*12 Generous Servings*

5 16-ounce packages firm, water-packed tofu

### Stuffing

1½ teaspoons olive oil
4 cloves garlic, minced
1 medium yellow onion, chopped
1 stalk celery, chopped, with leaves
¼ cup chopped red bell pepper
2 ounces portobello mushrooms, diced

1 10-ounce package cubed herb stuffing mix
1 cup chicken-flavor vegetarian broth, boiling
⅔ cup dried cranberries
½ teaspoon dried sage

### Basting Mixture

2 tablespoons mellow white miso
⅓ cup dry sherry
½ cup tamari
⅔ cup fresh orange juice

1 cup chicken-flavor vegetarian broth
1 teaspoon Dijon mustard
1 teaspoon granulated garlic

### Brown Gravy

2 tablespoon olive oil
3 tablespoons whole wheat flour
1½ cups chicken-flavor vegetarian broth, boiling

½ cup nutritional yeast
1 teaspoon granulated garlic

THE DAY BEFORE: Drape a cheesecloth over a 12-inch colander, allowing the sides to overlap, and set over a larger bowl. Set aside. Mash tofu thoroughly, crumble into prepared colander, and fold cheesecloth over the top. Position a deep bowl inside the colander over cheesecloth-covered tofu, and weigh it down with something that weighs at least 5 pounds. Place in refrigerator overnight.

FOLLOWING DAY:

*For the stuffing:* Heat oil in a large saucepan over medium-high heat. Add garlic, onion, celery, bell pepper, and mushrooms. Cook mixture for 5 minutes, then add stuffing mix, broth, cranberries, and sage. Stir to moisten, remove from heat, and set aside.

*For the basting mixture:* Blend miso with sherry in a liquid measuring cup. Add tamari, juice, broth, mustard, and garlic. Blend, and set aside.

Preheat oven to 400°.

Oil spray baking pan lined with foil. Remove tofu from refrigerator and remove 5-pound weight from top bowl. Open the cheesecloth cover. Scoop out a portion of the tofu leaving a 1-inch wide shell. Fill the hollowed shell with stuffing, reserving extra stuffing to cook separately. Cover with remaining tofu and pat down firmly. Place the prepared baking pan over the colander, face-down. Invert, turning the stuffed tofu onto baking pan, flat side down. Baste with a third of the basting mixture, cover roast with foil, and bake for 1 hour. Remove foil, baste with half of remaining mixture. Bake, uncovered, for one more hour, basting again halfway through. (Cook extra stuffing on stovetop for 20 minutes.)

THIS PRODUCES a fabulous holiday meal! The crumbling and pressing technique, coupled with a flavorful basting mixture and delicious stuffing, yield a delectable roast with all the flavor and texture you expect from a holiday entrée. You will need two large bowls and a large colander, of graduating sizes, that can be stacked with the colander fitting in the middle. A large cheesecloth and heavy weight are also necessary.

*For the gravy:* Heat oil in a medium saucepan for 1 minute over medium-high heat. Add flour and stir to form a paste. Lower heat and gradually add broth, stirring constantly. Add nutritional yeast and garlic, and simmer for 5 minutes, stirring occasionally.

Remove roast from oven and set aside for 10 minutes. Garnish with fresh herbs at the center (sage leaves are nice). Slice into wedges and serve with gravy and additional dressing.

---

NUTRITION ANALYSIS: PER $2^1/4$-CUP SERVING WITH STUFFING AND GRAVY

**Enlightened Holiday Roast**
Protein 25 g, carbohydrate 37 g, fiber 4 g, fat 11 g,
saturated fat 1 g, cholesterol 0 mg,
calcium 195 mg, sodium 990 mg
Calories 335: from protein 29%,
from carbohydrate 43%, from fat 28%

**Traditional Roast Turkey**
Protein 58 g, carbohydrate 24 g, fiber 1 g, fat 32 g,
saturated fat 11g, cholesterol 177 mg,
calcium 84 mg, sodium 1098 mg
Calories 631: from protein 38%,
from carbohydrate 15%, from fat 47%

*12
Servings*

# Stuffed Grape Leaves

*A popular Middle Eastern dish, rice-filled grape leaves are usually served at room temperature with lemon wedges and dipping sauce.*

### Filling

1 cup white basmati rice
⅓ cup pine nuts
2 teaspoons olive oil
10 cloves garlic, minced, divided
½ cup thinly sliced scallions
1 12-ounce package vegetarian ground beef alternative
1 14½-ounce can Mexican-style stewed tomatoes, coarsely chopped

⅓ cup golden raisins
1 teaspoon ground cinnamon
½ teaspoon ground allspice
½ cup chopped flat-leaf parsley
½ cup boiling water
1 16-ounce jar grape leaves
juice of 2 fresh lemons
2 cups boiling water
lemon wedges

### Dipping Sauce

1 12.3-ounce package lite silken tofu
3 cloves garlic, peeled
1 tablespoon olive oil
½ teaspoon tamari lite

3 tablespoons mellow white miso
¼ cup dry sherry
juice of 1 lemon
4 teaspoons nutritional yeast

*For the filling:* Rinse rice thoroughly and place in a bowl. Cover with cold water and set aside for 30 minutes.

Place pine nuts in a dry medium pan and toast over medium heat for 3 to 5 minutes, shaking pan vigorously, until nuts are fragrant and lightly browned. Set aside.

Heat oil in a medium saucepan over medium-high heat for 1 minute. Add 4 cloves minced garlic and scallions, and sauté for 3 minutes. Add vegetarian beef and cook mixture for 5 minutes, stirring occasionally. Drain rice and add to the pan. Pulse chopped tomatoes in food processor and add to the pan with the raisins, cinnamon, allspice, parsley, and boiling water. Cook for 10 minutes, or until most of the liquid is absorbed and the rice is softening but not fully cooked. Stir in the toasted pine nuts and set aside to cool.

Ned and Rose Marie Skaff, friends from Wood Ranch, California, showed me how to make this Lebanese appetizer with the unique molded presentation.

*For the dipping sauce:* Place tofu in food processor and process until smooth. Add garlic, olive oil, and tamari. Blend. Place miso in a small bowl, "cream" with sherry, and add to the tofu mixture with the lemon juice and nutritional yeast. Cover and keep refrigerated until ready to use.

Rinse grape leaves in cool water over a colander and remove stems with a sharp knife. Work in batches, laying the leaves flat on a work surface, shiny side down. Place a tablespoonful of filling closer to the stem end of the leaf and roll up, folding the sides in as you go. Do not roll tightly, as the rice will expand during cooking.

Line a medium saucepan with additional grape leaves, overlapping them and draping them over the edges of the pan. Place the filled leaves in the pan, seam side down, arranged in a circular pattern. Drizzle with some of the lemon juice, and sprinkle generously with some of the remaining minced garlic. Top with a second layer of filled grape leaves, arranged in an opposite pattern. Top with lemon and garlic as before, and repeat layering until all of the filled leaves are in the pan. Fold the leaves overlapping the edges of the pan in over the top layer, and cover with additional grape leaves, tucking them down inside the pan with a spatula. Pour the boiling water over all, and top with a heavy plate. Simmer gently over low heat for 45 minutes or until rice is cooked and leaves are tender. Remove plate and set aside to cool. After leaves are cool, invert the pan onto a plate. The stuffed leaves should remain in a perfect mold. Serve at room temperature with dipping sauce and lemon wedges.

---

### NUTRITION ANALYSIS: PER SERVING (3 STUFFED LEAVES)

| Enlightened Stuffed Grape Leaves | Traditional Stuffed Grape Leaves |
|---|---|
| Protein 15 g, carbohydrate 27g, fiber 7 g, fat 1 g, saturated fat 0 g, cholesterol 0 mg, calcium 67 mg, sodium 515 mg Calories 181: from protein 33%, from carbohydrate 61%, from fat 6% | Protein 13 g, carbohydrate 28 g, fiber 2 g, fat 17 g, saturated fat 5 g, cholesterol 31 mg, calcium 334 mg, sodium 235 mg Calories 305: from protein 16%, from carbohydrate 35%, from fat 49% |

# Tempeh Chili

Chili con carne *means "peppers with meat." It is traditionally made with beef, and slow cooked with chile peppers and other spices. Not in* The Enlightened Kitchen! *Here, heart-healthy, chewy tempeh replaces the unhealthy ingredient typically used in this popular dish.*

*8
Servings*

2 8-ounce packages tempeh, cubed
2 teaspoons olive oil
¼ teaspoon crushed red pepper
4 cloves garlic, minced
1 medium red onion, chopped
1 red bell pepper, chopped
6 ounces portobello mushroom, diced

2 14½-ounce cans Mexican-style stewed tomatoes, diced
2 15-ounce cans chile beans with chipotle peppers
2 tablespoons chile powder
1 teaspoon dried basil
½ tablespoon dried Mexican oregano

GREAT DISH FOR a Super Bowl party: Whip up a batch of Tempeh Chili and a few of our dips in advance for an Enlightened gathering.

Steam tempeh over boiling water for 20 minutes and set aside.

In a 5-quart saucepan, heat olive oil and crushed pepper over medium-high heat for 1 minute. Add garlic, onion, and bell pepper, and sauté for 3 minutes, stirring frequently. Crumble steamed tempeh into the pan and add the diced mushrooms. Cook for 5 minutes, stirring occasionally. Add stewed tomatoes, chile beans, chile powder, basil, and oregano. Reduce heat and simmer for 15 minutes.

---

NUTRITION ANALYSIS: PER 1½-CUP SERVING

**Enlightened Tempeh Chili**
Protein 20 g, carbohydrate 33 g, fiber 8 g, fat 5 g, saturated fat 1 g, cholesterol 0 mg, calcium 173 mg, sodium 722 mg
Calories 227: from protein 32%, from carbohydrate 52%, from fat 16%

**Traditional Chili**
Protein 17 g, carbohydrate 27 g, fiber 5 g, fat 22 g, saturated fat 7 g, cholesterol 0 mg, calcium 95 mg, sodium 982 mg
Calories 359: from protein 18%, from carbohydrate 28%, from fat 54%

# Mushroom-Okara Pâté

*This delicious spread for pita crisps or crackers
can be made a day in advance.*

olive oil cooking spray
2 teaspoons olive oil
2 cloves garlic, minced
⅓ cup minced shallots
1 cup chopped red onion
½ cup chopped red bell pepper
6 ounces portobello mushrooms,
  chopped
6 ounces button mushrooms,
  chopped

1¾ cups okara
½ cup dry sherry
2 tablespoons mellow white miso
⅓ cup hot chicken-flavor vegetarian
  broth
¼ cup tomato paste
⅓ cup Barbara's mashed potato flakes
1 26-gram package Tofu Hero Italian
  Herb Medley

Preheat oven to 375°. Spray a 9- by 5-inch loaf pan with olive oil.

Heat oil over medium-high heat in a 10-inch frying pan for 1 minute. Add garlic, shallots, onion, and pepper, and sauté for 3 minutes. Add mushrooms and cook for 5 minutes, stirring frequently. Add okara and sherry, and cook mixture for 3 minutes, stirring occasionally. Pour mixture into food processor and pulse briefly. In a small bowl or liquid measuring cup, blend the miso and hot broth, then add to the mushroom mixture. Add tomato paste, potato flakes, and Italian Herb Medley and process to mix thoroughly. Pour into prepared loaf pan. Bake, uncovered, for 30 minutes. Set aside to cool on wire rack. Cover and refrigerate overnight.

Just before serving, invert onto a serving plate and remove pan. Pâté should be formed into an oblong mold. Serve with pita crisps and crudites.

OKARA, THE pulp that is left behind after soymilk is extracted from soybeans, contains protein and fiber. Those of us who make soymilk and tofu at home produce prodigious amounts of okara, and are *always* looking for good ways to use it.

---

NUTRITION ANALYSIS: PER ½-CUP SERVING

**Mushroom Okara-Pâté**
Protein 3 g, carbohydrate 11 g, fiber 2 g, fat 2 g,
saturated fat 0 g, cholesterol 0 mg,
calcium 27 mg, sodium 223 mg
Calories 68: from protein15%,
from carbohydrate 65%, from fat 20%

**Traditional Pâté**
Protein 6 g, carbohydrate 6 g, fiber 1 g, fat 16 g,
saturated fat 10 g, cholesterol 159 mg,
calcium 29 mg, sodium 288 mg
Calories 209: from protein 13%,
from carbohydrate 13%, from fat 74%

# Hoppin' John

*The Enlightened Kitchen gives a healthy twist to a famous dish
that's traditionally loaded with smoked meat such as ham and sausage.
This updated version uses heart-healthy veggie Canadian bacon,
to add the goodness of soy to this delightful dish.*

*6
Servings*

1½ teaspoons olive oil
2 serrano chiles, seeded and minced
6 cloves garlic, minced
1 medium yellow onion, chopped
½ medium red bell pepper, chopped
1 stalk celery, thinly sliced
1 cup sliced baby-cut carrots

1 6-ounce package veggie Canadian bacon, diced
1 15-ounce can black-eyed peas
2 cups cooked brown rice
1 14½-ounce can Mexican-style stewed tomatoes
2 bay leaves
1 teaspoon dried thyme

POPULAR IN THE southern United States and the Caribbean, Hoppin' John is said to bring good luck when eaten on New Year's Day.

In a medium saucepan, heat oil over medium-high heat and add the chiles, garlic, onion, bell pepper, celery, and carrots. Cook for 3 minutes, then add diced veggie bacon. Cook mixture for 5 minutes, stirring frequently. Add black-eyed peas and rice, mixing thoroughly. Add tomatoes, bay leaves, and thyme, and reduce heat to low. Simmer for 15 minutes, or until ready to serve, stirring occasionally. Remove bay leaves before serving.

---

NUTRITION ANALYSIS: PER 1½-CUP SERVING

**Enlightened Hoppin' John**
Protein 13 g, carbohydrate 38 g, fiber 6g, fat 2 g,
saturated fat 0 g, cholesterol 0 mg,
calcium 112 mg, sodium 411 mg
Calories 222: from protein 23%,
from carbohydrate 68%, from fat 9%

**Traditional Hoppin' John**
Protein 13 g, carbohydrate 33 g, fiber 5 g, fat 16 g,
saturated fat 4 g, cholesterol 23 mg,
calcium 111 mg, sodium 925 mg
Calories 323: from protein 16%,
from carbohydrate 40%, from fat 44%

# Light and Lovely Crepes

*Egg-free, dairy-free, and with just a touch of olive oil, these crepes
are easy to make, delicious, and healthy. Choose Dilled Asparagus and
Wild Mushrooms (page 165) for an elegant savory filling, or Just Peachy
Dessert Crepes (recipe follows) for a delectable dessert.*

*18
Crepes*

2 cups enriched 1% fat soymilk
1 tablespoon lemon juice
¾ cup unbleached white flour
½ cup whole wheat pastry flour
1 teaspoon nonaluminum baking
   powder

½ teaspoon sea salt
⅓ cup lite silken tofu
1 tablespoon prune purée
1 tablespoon olive oil
olive oil cooking spray

Combine soymilk and lemon juice in a medium glass measuring
cup and set aside.

In a large bowl, mix together the unbleached flour, pastry flour,
baking powder, and salt. Set aside.

Place tofu, prune purée, and soymilk mixture in a food processor, and blend. Add oil through feeding tube while processing, and
blend thoroughly. Make a well in the center of the dry ingredients,
and pour in tofu mixture. Mix thoroughly. Set batter aside to rest
for 20 minutes.

Spray a heavy 6-inch skillet with olive oil. Warm over medium
heat and pour a scant ¼ cup of batter into the pan. Lift pan above
heat; tip and swirl pan to distribute batter evenly, covering the bottom of skillet. Cover pan and cook, shaking pan frequently, until underside is golden,
about 3 minutes. Flip crepe over and and cook until edges are lightly browned.
Repeat with remaining batter.

LIGHT AND LOVELY
Crepes may be made up to
two days in advance. Stack
crepes with waxed paper in
between and refrigerate in
a tightly covered container.
Microwave on 50% power
or reheat in a warm oven.

---

NUTRITION ANALYSIS: PER SERVING (2 CREPES)

| Enlightened Light and Lovely Crepes | Traditional Crepes |
| --- | --- |
| Protein 3 g, carbohydrate 12 g, fiber 1 g, fat 2 g, | Protein 4 g, carbohydrate 8 g, fiber 0 g, fat 9 g, |
| saturated fat 0 g, cholesterol 0 mg, | saturated fat 4 g, cholesterol 69 mg, |
| calcium 89 mg, sodium 176 mg | calcium 72 mg, sodium 273 mg |
| Calories 78: from protein 14%, | Calories 123: from protein 12%, |
| from carbohydrate 61%, from fat 25% | from carbohydrate 26%, from fat 62% |

# Just Peachy Dessert Crepes

*Crepes are an elegant choice for entertaining,*
*and making this filling is a snap.*

*18*
*Crepes*

1 recipe Light and Lovely Crepes
   (page 85)
⅔ cup evaporated cane sugar
¼ cup water

4 medium peaches, peeled and diced
1 cup dried cherries
⅓ cup kirsch brandy

MAKE THE CREPES in advance, and store in a tightly covered container in the refrigerator. Stack crepes with waxed paper in between. Microwave on 50% power or reheat in warm oven.

Make Light and Lovely Crepes and set aside.

Place sugar in dry heavy 12-inch skillet and warm for 3 minutes over medium heat, stirring occasionally. Stir in water and cook for 1 minute. Add peaches and cherries and cook, stirring often, for 3 minutes. Add kirsch and reduce heat to medium low. Allow mixture to simmer, covered, for 5 minutes, stirring occasionally. Fill crepes and serve.

---

NUTRITION ANALYSIS: PER SERVING (2 FILLED CREPES)

**Enlightened Peach Dessert Crepes**
Protein 4 g, carbohydrate 40 g, fiber 3 g, fat 3 g,
saturated fat 0 g, cholesterol 0 mg,
calcium 103 mg, sodium 199 mg
Calories 214: from protein 13%,
from carbohydrate 76%, from fat 11%

**Traditional Peach Dessert Crepes**
Protein 8 g, carbohydrate 60 g, fiber 2 g, fat 12 g,
saturated fat 4 g, cholesterol 0 mg,
calcium 80 mg, sodium 228 mg
Calories 398: from protein 8%,
from carbohydrate 64%, from fat 28%

# Richly Chocolate Fondue

*Serve this fondue with fresh strawberries, pineapple cubes, tart apples, peaches, or nectarines—whatever you like! Most anything tastes better dipped in rich, silky chocolate!*

---

2 12.3-ounce packages lite silken tofu
1 cup enriched 1% fat soymilk
½ cup cocoa powder

¾ cup liquid Fruitsource
1 tablespoon vanilla
freshly ground nutmeg for garnish

*12
Servings*

Place tofu in food processor and process until smooth. Add soymilk and blend. Place cocoa in a small bowl and set aside. Heat Fruitsource in microwave on 100% power for 30 seconds or in a pan on the stove over low heat for 2 minutes. Add hot Fruitsource to the cocoa, and using a small wire whisk or fork, blend to form a smooth syrup. Add to the tofu with the vanilla and blend until smooth. Pour into the fondue pot and sprinkle with nutmeg.

FONDUE IS MAKING a comeback—gathering around the fondue pot is a delightful way to bring guests together. Save time by warming the sauce in the microwave before placing in the fondue pot to serve.

---

NUTRITION ANALYSIS: PER ½-CUP SERVING

**Enlightened Chocolate Fondue**
Protein 5 g, carbohydrate 15 g, fiber 1 g, fat 1 g,
saturated fat 0 g, cholesterol 0 mg,
calcium 50 mg, sodium 50 mg
Calories 85: from protein 23%,
from carbohydrate 65%, from fat 12%

**Traditional Chocolate Fondue**
Protein 3 g, carbohydrate 31 g, fiber 2 g, fat 21 g,
saturated fat 13 g, cholesterol 54 mg,
calcium 68 mg, sodium 69 mg
Calories 301: from protein 4%,
from carbohydrate 39%, from fat 57%

*12
Servings*

# Tosteds Trail Mix

*Fairview Farms Tosteds are my favorite choice for trail mix.
They are light, not too salty, and non-GMO (not genetically modified) too!*

2 cups Tosteds soynuts
½ cup golden raisins
½ cup chopped dried pineapple

⅓ cup chopped dried apricots
½ cup dairy-free chocolate chips
½ cup whole grain Chex cereal

Combine all ingredients in a large bowl. Mix thoroughly and store in a covered container or zip-top plastic bag.

NUTRITION ANALYSIS: PER ⅓-CUP-SERVING

**Enlightened Trail Mix**
Protein 8 g, carbohydrate 21 g, fiber 5 g, fat 5 g,
saturated fat 2 g, cholesterol 0 mg,
calcium 41 mg, sodium 39 mg
Calories 158: from protein 20%,
from carbohydrate 52%, from fat 28%

**Traditional Trail Mix**
Protein 8 g, carbohydrate 21 g, fiber 3 g, fat 14 g,
saturated fat 3g, cholesterol 2 mg,
calcium 40 mg, sodium 97 mg
Calories 227: from protein 12%,
from carbohydrate 34%, from fat 54%

# Soups, Salads, and Starters

Steamy soups, terrific salads, and delicious starters are waiting for you in *The Enlightened Kitchen*. Set out a "souper" lunch for friends: after all what could be more welcoming than a warming bowl of soup and a loaf of bread that has been freshly baked or warmed in the oven? Choose the exquisite Gingered Acorn Squash Soup or the delightfully easy "Cream" of Broccoli Soup. Add a colorful salad, and you have a wonderful, healthy luncheon.

Do you prefer a hearty main-dish salad? California Chef's Salad showcases the wonderful contrast of rich, creamy avocado, marinated "chicken" strips, tender baby spinach leaves, and tart fresh strawberries. Another alternative is a chilled salad like Caribbean Pasta Salad, which offers marinated tempeh and orzo pasta in a rich tasting dressing.

Cold, refreshing salads are perfect summertime meals and also travel well in an insulated cooler. Hearty Summer Rice Salad is a great choice for a picnic or barbecue, and really easy to assemble in advance, freeing the cook to enjoy outdoor activities with everyone else. Or arrange chilled asparagus on a serving platter with Creamy Dilled Dressing drizzled over the top for a lovely, light start to most any meal. Cold Sesame Noodles, a personal favorite, are made low-fat and delicious with an intriguing blend of wholesome ingredients. Leftover soup? Offer it with one of these delightful salads, or whip up a quick starter, and you will have a very satisfying meal.

# Recipes

Black Bean Cakes with Creamy Dijon Sauce
Chilled Asparagus with Creamy Dill Dressing
California Chef's Salad with Creamy Italian Dressing
Creamy Italian Dressing
Caribbean Pasta Salad
Chilled Pasta Salad with Edamame
Easy Edamame Salad
Hearty Summer Rice Salad
"Cream" of Broccoli Soup
"Chicken" and Barley Soup
Chunky Vegetable "Beef" Soup
Easy and Delicious Miso Soup
Gingered Acorn Squash Soup
Tomato Vegetable Soup with Garbanzos
Cold Sesame Noodles

# Black Bean Cakes
## with Creamy Dijon Sauce

*Black Bean Cakes are a delicious starter, especially when served with
creamy mustard and salsa. Or add a salad to make a light lunch.*

1 recipe Creamy Dijon Sauce
   (page 199)
2 15-ounce cans black beans,
   drained
3 cloves garlic, peeled
1 small yellow onion, coarsely
   chopped
¾ cup coarsely shredded carrots
⅓ cup nutritional yeast
¼ cup Barbara's mashed potato
   flakes

¼ cup chopped fresh cilantro
2 tablespoons whole wheat bread
   crumbs
2 rounded tablespoons fruity salsa,
   such as pineapple or mango
3 drops hot pepper sauce, or
   to taste
½ cup whole grain yellow
   cornmeal
2 tablespoons olive oil
1 tablespoon chopped fresh cilantro

Prepare Creamy Dijon Sauce. Set aside and keep warm.
Place black beans in food processor with garlic, onion, carrots, yeast, mashed potato flakes, cilantro, bread crumbs,
salsa, and hot pepper sauce. Pulse to mix, and process to
blend. Place cornmeal in a small bowl and set aside. Fill a
small ice cream scoop with black bean mixture and drop
mixture into cornmeal. Using a tablespoon, flip mixture
over and coat second side with cornmeal. Toss between
hands a few times to diminish excess cornmeal. Set aside,
and continue the process with the remaining black bean
mixture. *Note:* Patty will be delicate.

IT IS BEST to make these tasty
starters in advance, then warm them
up in a 300° oven for 10 minutes
before serving. They are delicate
when first cooked, and firm up after
being set aside for about 20 minutes.

**Black Bean Cakes with Creamy Dijon Sauce** *(continued)*

Heat oil in an electric frying pan or 10-inch frying pan for 1 minute. Place black bean cakes into hot pan. Cook on first side for 5 minutes, then gently turn over and cook on second side for 4 minutes, or until brown. Set browned cakes aside on a platter until batter is depleted.

---

NUTRITION ANALYSIS: PER SERVING
(2 BLACK BEAN CAKES WITH ABOUT 3 1/2 TABLESPOONS SAUCE)

Enlightened Black Bean Cakes
with Creamy Dijon Sauce
Protein 9 g, carbohydrate 28 g, fiber 5 g, fat 4 g,
saturated fat 1 g, cholesterol 0 mg,
calcium 61 mg, sodium 150 mg
Calories 163: from protein 20%,
from carbohydrate 61%, from fat 19%

Traditional Black Bean Cakes
with Creamy Dijon Sauce
Protein 12 g, carbohydrate 26 g, fiber 5 g, fat 22 g,
saturated fat 12 g, cholesterol 66 mg,
calcium 108 mg, sodium 312 mg
Calories 305: from protein 14%,
from carbohydrate 30%, from fat 56%

# Chilled Asparagus
## with Creamy Dill Dressing

*For an elegant presentation, arrange chilled asparagus on serving plates, drizzle with dressing, and garnish with sprigs of fresh dill.*

6
*Servings*

1 pound asparagus, trimmed
½ 12.3-ounce package lite silken tofu
1 clove garlic, peeled
1 scallion, sliced, including 2 inches of green
¼ cup eggless mayonnaise
⅓ cup enriched 1% fat soymilk

1 teaspoon rice vinegar
2 teaspoons Dijon mustard
2 tablespoons nutritional yeast
¼ cup chopped fresh dill
½ teaspoon dried dillweed
¼ teaspoon sea salt
⅛ teaspoon coarse black pepper

Steam asparagus for 5 minutes, then plunge immediately into a bowl of ice water. Set aside.

Place tofu in food processor and process. Add remaining ingredients. Process until smooth, but with bits of dill remaining, scraping down once, halfway. Refrigerate at least 1 hour before serving.

Serve Creamy Dill Dressing with salads, or as a delicious dip for crudités.

NUTRITION ANALYSIS: PER SERVING (ASPARAGUS WITH 3½ TABLESPOONS DRESSING)

| Enlightened Chilled Asparagus with Creamy Dill Dressing | Traditional Chilled Asparagus with Creamy Dill Dressing |
|---|---|
| Protein 4 g, carbohydrate 6 g, fiber 2 g, fat 5 g, saturated fat 1 g, cholesterol 0 mg, calcium 38 mg, sodium 130 mg | Protein 3 g, carbohydrate 5 g, fiber 1 g, fat 26 g, saturated fat 6 g, cholesterol 25 mg, calcium 41 mg, sodium 438 mg |
| Calories 81: from protein 20%, from carbohydrate 26%, from fat 54%* | Calories 253: from protein 4%, from carbohydrate 8%, from fat 88% |

\* The percentage of calories from fat seems high only because the calories are so low.

# California Chef's Salad with Creamy Italian Dressing

*This salad showcases wonderful contrasts: rich, creamy avocado; tasty marinated seitan; tender of leaves baby spinach; and tart, fresh strawberries.*

*6
Servings*

2 16-ounce packages seitan, drained
1 recipe Lively Marinade (page 212)
olive oil cooking spray
2 ounces portobello mushrooms, sliced
1 medium avocado, peeled, pitted, and sliced

juice of 1 lime
1 6-ounce package baby spinach
½ medium red onion, thinly sliced
6 large fresh strawberries, sliced
¼ cup chopped fresh cilantro
1 recipe Creamy Italian Dressing (recipe follows)

THIS RECIPE calls for 16 ounces of seitan. One 16-ounce package of seitan, packed in broth, will render about 8 ounces of seitan and 8 ounces of broth.

Tear seitan into bite-size pieces, place in a medium bowl, and combine with marinade. Cover and refrigerate for at least 1 hour. Spray a 10-inch frying pan with olive oil cooking spray, and heat over medium heat for 1 minute. Remove seitan from the marinade with a slotted spoon, reserving about 3 tablespoons of marinade, and add seitan to the pan. Cook for 5 minutes or until lightly browned. Push seitan to one side, spray pan lightly with oil if necessary, add mushrooms, and cook for 3 minutes. Spoon 3 tablespoons of the marinade over the mushrooms and reduce heat to simmer. Keep warm while assembling the salad.

Put sliced avocado on a plate and drizzle with lime juice; set aside. Place spinach in a large salad bowl. Arrange onion, avocado, and strawberries around the perimeter, and mound the seitan and mushrooms in the center and sprinkle with cilantro. Serve with dressing on the side.

NUTRITION ANALYSIS: PER SERVING (1¼ CUPS SALAD PLUS ¼ CUP DRESSING)

| Enlightened California Chef's Salad with Creamy Italian Dressing | Traditional Chef's Salad with Traditional Creamy Italian Dressing |
|---|---|
| Protein 17 g, carbohydrate 21 g, fiber 9 g, fat 5 g, saturated fat 1 g, cholesterol 0 mg, calcium 118 mg, sodium 548 mg Calories 185: from protein 34%, from carbohydrate 42%, from fat 24% | Protein 22 g, carbohydrate 9 g, fiber 2 g, fat 48 g, saturated fat 13 g, cholesterol 79 mg, calcium 134 mg, sodium 1522 mg Calories 550: from protein 16%, from carbohydrate 6%, from fat 78% |

# Creamy Italian Dressing

*This creamy dressing is actually fat-free!*

*Makes
about
3 Cups*

1 12.3-ounce package lite silken tofu,
   drained
2 cloves garlic, peeled
1 large shallot, peeled and quartered
¼ cup sliced scallions

⅔ cup enriched 1% fat soymilk
3½ tablespoons red wine vinegar
1 26-gram package Tofu Hero Italian
   Herb Medley (dry mix only)
1½ teaspoons tamari lite

Place tofu in food processor and process to blend. Add garlic, shallot, and scallions, and blend. Add soymilk, vinegar, Italian Herb Medley, and tamari. Blend
thoroughly. Refrigerate for at least an hour.

---

## NUTRITION ANALYSIS: PER 2-TABLESPOON SERVING

**Enlightened Creamy Italian Dressing**
Protein 3 g, carbohydrate 4 g, fiber 0 g, fat 0 g,
saturated fat 0 g, cholesterol 0 mg,
calcium 31 mg, sodium 136 mg
Calories 28: from protein 38%,
from carbohydrate 50%, from fat 12%

**Traditional Creamy Italian Dressing**
Protein 0 g, carbohydrate 2 g, fiber 0 g, fat 16 g,
saturated fat 2 g, cholesterol 1 mg,
calcium 4 mg, sodium 346 mg
Calories 143: from protein 0%,
from carbohydrate 4%, from fat 96%

# Caribbean Pasta Salad

*This dish is so very creamy, you won't believe it is dairy free!*

1 8-ounce package tempeh, cut into small cubes and steamed

1 recipe Pacific Blend Marinade (page 214)

### Dressing

1 12.3-ounce package lite silken tofu
2 cloves garlic, peeled
⅓ cup eggless mayonnaise
½ cup enriched 1% fat soymilk

2 tablespoons Dijon mustard
juice of 1 lime
½ cup reserved marinade
4 to 5 drops hot pepper sauce

### Salad

1¾ cups orzo pasta
⅓ cup sliced scallions
½ cup chopped red bell pepper
1 stalk celery, chopped
½ cup dried currants

1 medium plum tomato, sliced, for garnish
½ teaspoon dried cilantro, for garnish

MARINATED TEMPEH adds meaty flavor, texture, and heartiness to this cold salad. You may steam tempeh up to 3 days in advance, and set up the marinade the night before making this dish. Always store tempeh in a covered container in the refrigerator.

Combine steamed tempeh with marinade in a nonreactive bowl. Cover and refrigerate for up to 24 hours.

*For the dressing:* Using a slotted spoon, remove the marinated tempeh to a large bowl, reserving ½ cup of the marinade, and set aside. Place tofu in food processor and blend until smooth. Add garlic and mayonnaise; blend, and scrape down. Add soymilk, mustard, lime juice, reserved marinade, and hot pepper sauce. Process to mix thoroughly, and set aside.

*For the salad:* Cook orzo according to package directions; drain. Add cooked orzo to the tempeh. Add scallions, bell pepper, celery, and currants, stirring after each addition. Add dressing and mix thoroughly. Garnish with tomato slices and sprinkle with cilantro. Cover and refrigerate until ready to serve.

---

NUTRITION ANALYSIS: PER 1 ½-CUP SERVING

**Enlightened Caribbean Pasta Salad**
Protein 9 g, carbohydrate 44 g, fiber 4 g, fat 5 g,
saturated fat 0 g, cholesterol 0 mg,
calcium 109 mg, sodium 208 mg
Calories 277: from protein 13%,
from carbohydrate 63%, from fat 24%

**Traditional Caribbean Pasta Salad**
Protein 9 g, carbohydrate 36 g, fiber 2 g, fat 24 g,
saturated fat 8 g, cholesterol 43 mg,
calcium 77 mg, sodium 807 mg
Calories 406: from protein 9%,
from carbohydrate 37%, from fat 54%

# Chilled Pasta Salad with Edamame

*This colorful pasta salad is rich in flavor and and texture.*

1 12-ounce package panette pasta
1½ cups shelled edamame
1 12.3-ounce package lite silken tofu
3 cloves garlic, peeled
⅓ cup eggless mayonnaise
1 26-gram package Tofu Hero
    Italian Herb Medley
¼ cup nutritional yeast

2 tablespoons red wine vinegar
2 tablespoon Dijon mustard
1 cup enriched 1% fat soymilk
2 teaspoons Bragg Liquid Aminos
1 medium onion, chopped
1 medium red bell pepper, chopped
1 cup baby carrots, cut julienne style
1 teaspoon dried marjoram

Cook pasta and edamame (if frozen) according to package directions, and set aside to drain. Rinse pasta occasionally with cold water to keep it from sticking.

Place tofu in food processor and blend until smooth. Add garlic, mayonnaise, herb medley, nutritional yeast, vinegar, and mustard. Process to mix, add soymilk and aminos, and blend until smooth. Set aside. Place drained pasta in a large bowl and add onion, bell pepper, and carrots. Combine pasta mixture with tofu dressing and add edamame. Sprinkle with marjoram and chill thoroughly before serving.

PANETTE PASTA ARE a very small version of the tubular penne pasta. Any small pasta shape can be substituted.

---

NUTRITION ANALYSIS: PER 1-CUP SERVING

**Enlightened Chilled Pasta Salad with Edamame**
Protein 14 g, carbohydrate 48 g, fiber 4 g, fat 5 g,
saturated fat 0 g, cholesterol 0 mg,
calcium 114 mg, sodium 181mg
Calories 215: from protein 19%,
from carbohydrate 66%, from fat 15%

**Traditional Pasta Salad with Ham**
Protein 11 g, carbohydrate 34 g, fiber 3 g, fat 26 g,
saturated fat 7 g, cholesterol 33 mg,
calcium 107 mg, sodium 677 mg
Calories 402: from protein 11%,
from carbohydrate 33%, from fat 56%

*8
Servings*

# Easy Edamame Salad

*Marinating shelled edamame adds a
new dimension to this delicious soyfood.*

1 recipe of Savory Sesame Marinade,
   (page 218)
1 10-ounce package shelled, ready-
   to-eat edamame, or frozen
   edamame
½ medium red onion, thinly sliced
1 medium yellow bell pepper, cut
   into 3-inch strips
1 medium red bell pepper, cut into
   3-inch strips

1 stalk celery with leaves, thinly
   sliced
2 medium plum tomatoes, cut in half
   vertically and cut crosswise into
   thin slices
2 tablespoons capers, rinsed
1 10-ounce package baby spinach, or
   gourmet salad greens

Prepare marinade and set aside. If using ready-to-eat edamame, place in nonreactive bowl (preferably glass) and cover with marinade. If frozen, cook
according to package directions, drain, and pat dry. Then place in nonreactive
bowl and cover with marinade. Refrigerate several hours or overnight.

Mix vegetables with the marinated edamame and serve with greens.

NUTRITION ANALYSIS: PER 1-CUP SERVING

**Enlightened Edamame Salad**
Protein 7 g, carbohydrate 12 g, fiber 9 g, fat 7 g,
saturated fat 1 g, cholesterol 0 mg,
calcium 84 mg, sodium 394 mg
Calories 132: from protein 19%,
from carbohydrate 34%, from fat 47%*

**Traditional Bean Salad**
Protein 6 g, carbohydrate 20 g, fiber 5 g, fat 17 g,
saturated fat 2 g, cholesterol 1 mg,
calcium 99 mg, sodium 883 mg
Calories 239: from protein 9%,
from carbohydrate 31%, from fat 60%

* The percentage of calories from fat seems high only because the calories are so low.

# Hearty Summer Rice Salad

*Cool, casual, and elegant, this chilled salad is easy
to assemble and can be made in advance.*

1 ½ cups short-grain brown rice
3 cups vegetarian chicken broth
1 cup coarsely shredded carrots
½ cup chopped red bell pepper
⅓ cup chopped dried apricots

1 6-ounce package savory baked tofu,
   sliced on an angle
⅓ cup sliced scallions
⅓ cup chopped almonds (optional)

### Dressing

1 12.3-ounce package lite silken tofu
¼ cup eggless mayonnaise
1 26-gram package Tofu Hero
   Italian Herb Medley

1 large shallot, peeled and quartered
2 cloves garlic, peeled
2 tablespoons fresh lemon juice
2 tablespoon nutritional yeast

If using an electric rice cooker, combine the rice with the broth and press "On." On the stovetop, bring the broth to a boil and add rice, reduce heat to low, cover, and simmer for 40 minutes, or until liquid is absorbed.

Place cooked rice in a large bowl and add the carrots, peppers, and apricots. Add the baked tofu, scallions, and almonds to the rice, and set aside.

*For the dressing:* Place silken tofu in the food processor and blend until smooth. Add the mayonnaise, Italian Herb Medley, shallots, and garlic, and process. Add the lemon juice and yeast and blend until smooth. Fold the dressing into the rice mixture, cover, and refrigerate for several hours.

RICH IN FIBER, brown rice has an interesting chewy texture and a longer cooking time because the outer bran layers act as a barrier to heat and moisture. This dish calls for short-grain brown rice, which is a little softer than medium- or long-grain brown rice.

NUTRITION ANALYSIS: PER 1 ½-CUP SERVING

**Enlightened Summer Rice Salad**
Protein 13 g, carbohydrate 42 g, fiber 4 g, fat 4 g,
saturated fat 0 g, cholesterol 0 mg,
calcium 50 mg, sodium 368 mg
Calories 252: from protein 21%,
from carbohydrate 67%, from fat 12%

**Traditional Summer Rice Salad**
Protein 12 g, carbohydrate 39 g, fiber 2 g, fat 28 g,
saturated fat 6 g, cholesterol 24 mg,
calcium 85 mg, sodium 848 mg
Calories 459: from protein 11%,
from carbohydrate 33%, from fat 56%

# "Cream" of Broccoli Soup

*This rich-tasting, creamy soup is easy and delicious.*

4 cups chicken-flavor vegetarian
  broth
1 small yellow onion, chopped
⅓ cup chopped green bell pepper
4 cups sliced broccoli florets
1 12.3-ounce package lite silken tofu
3 cloves garlic, peeled
1 large shallot, chopped
1 cup nutritional yeast

2 tablespoons Barbara's mashed
  potato flakes
1 cup frozen corn, thawed
2 tablespoons cornstarch
2 tablespoons cold water
2 tablespoons tamari lite
1 teaspoon Bragg Liquid Aminos
2 tablespoons chopped Italian
  flat-leaf parsley

Mashed potato flakes add a distinctive texture to this soup.

Combine broth, onion, pepper, and broccoli in a 6-quart saucepan. Bring to a boil, reduce heat, and simmer for 5 minutes. Place tofu in food processor and blend. Add garlic, shallot, yeast, and mashed potato flakes, and process. With a slotted spoon, remove solids from broth and add to the tofu mixture. Process to blend. Spoon into the hot broth, stirring after each addition. Add corn to the soup. In a small bowl, blend cornstarch with cold water and add to the soup with tamari, aminos, and chopped parsley. Simmer for 12 minutes, stirring occasionally.

NUTRITION ANALYSIS: PER 2-CUP SERVING

**Enlightened "Cream" of Broccoli Soup**
Protein 13 g, carbohydrate 38 g, fiber 5 g, fat 1 g,
saturated fat 0 g, cholesterol 0 mg,
calcium 77 mg, sodium 385 mg
Calories 132: from protein 25%,
from carbohydrate 70%, from fat 5%

**Traditional Cream of Broccoli Soup**
Protein 11 g, carbohydrate 21 g, fiber 3 g, fat 15 g,
saturated fat 9 g, cholesterol 40 mg,
calcium 175 mg, sodium 796 mg
Calories 250: from protein 17%,
from carbohydrate 33%, from fat 50%

# "Chicken" and Barley Soup

*This chunky soup is a meal in itself.*
*When reheating, refresh with additional boiling broth.*

1 cup DDC Chicken Not! Strips
1 cup boiling water
1 tablespoon DDC original broth powder
1 piece kombu, rinsed
6 cups cold water
5 cloves garlic, minced
1 large yellow onion, chopped
1 medium yellow bell pepper, chopped
1 tablespoon grated fresh gingerroot
1 medium parsnip, peeled and diced
1 cup sliced baby-cut carrots

3 cups vegetarian chicken broth, boiling
½ cup quick-cooking pearl barley
1 6-ounce can tomato paste
1 14½-ounce can Mexican-style stewed tomatoes
⅓ cup chopped Italian flat-leaf parsley
1 cup frozen peas, thawed
⅔ cup mellow white miso
¾ cup dry vermouth
1 teaspoon granulated garlic
1 teaspoon dried basil
⅛ teaspoon coarse black pepper

Combine Chicken Not! with boiling water and broth powder in a medium saucepan, bring to a boil, and simmer for 8 minutes. Set aside. Place kombu in a large soup pot with the 6 cups of water, and set aside for 15 minutes. To the kombu stock, add the minced garlic, onion, bell pepper, gingerroot, parsnip, and carrots. Bring mixture to a boil, reduce heat to medium, and cook for 10 minutes, stirring occasionally. Add boiling broth and barley and cook for 5 minutes. Cut the reconstituted "chicken" into smaller pieces, and add to the soup. Reduce heat to low, and spoon the tomato

KOMBU, A DARK green sea vegetable, is steeped in water to produce an enriching, flavorful soup broth the Japanese call *dashi.*

## "Chicken" and Barley Soup *(continued)*

paste into the soup. Place the stewed tomatoes in food processor, pulse to chop coarsely, and add to soup with parsley and peas. Combine miso and vermouth in a small bowl, and blend with a fork until smooth. Add to the soup with the granulated garlic, basil, and and black pepper. Remove kombu and set aside for another use. Simmer soup gently for 5 minutes, stirring occasionally. Do not boil.

---

### NUTRITION ANALYSIS: PER 2-CUP SERVING

| Enlightened "Chicken" and Barley Soup | Traditional Chicken and Barley Soup |
|---|---|
| Protein 8 g, carbohydrate 29 g, fiber 7 g, fat 1 g, saturated fat 0 g, cholesterol 0 mg, calcium 66 mg, sodium 608 mg Calories 164: from protein 20%, from carbohydrate 74%, from fat 6% | Protein 16 g, carbohydrate 24 g, fiber 5 g, fat 9 g, saturated fat 5 g, cholesterol 52 mg, calcium 73 mg, sodium 758 mg Calories 236: from protein 27%, from carbohydrate 40%, from fat 33% |

# Chunky Vegetable "Beef" Soup

*Bursting with chunky vegetables, Vegetable "Beef" Soup
is hearty, wholesome, and delicious.*

1 piece kombu, rinsed
2 quarts cold water
5 cloves garlic, minced
1 medium yellow onion, chopped
½ cup chopped red bell pepper
1 stalk celery, with leaves, chopped
1 tablespoon grated fresh gingerroot
2 cups green beans, cut into 2-inch
  pieces
2 cups thinly sliced zucchini
⅔ cup DDC Beef Not!, ground

2 cups boiling water
2 tablespoons DDC original broth
  powder
1 6-ounce can tomato paste
⅔ cup mellow white miso
⅔ cup white wine or vegetable broth
2 teaspoons granulated garlic
1 teaspoon ground ginger
2 teaspoons dried basil
1½ teaspoons dried thyme

In a large soup pot, combine kombu and cold water and set aside for 15 minutes. To the kombu stock, add minced garlic, onion, bell pepper, celery, gingerroot, beans, and zucchini. Bring mixture to a boil, reduce heat to medium low, and simmer for 15 minutes, stirring occasionally. Sprinkle Beef Not! into the soup. Combine the boiling water with the broth powder and add to the soup. Spoon tomato paste into the broth, stirring after each addition, and cook for 10 minutes. Combine miso and wine in a small bowl and blend with a fork. Add to the soup with the granulated garlic, ginger, basil, and thyme. Remove kombu and reserve for another use. Simmer soup gently for 5 minutes, stirring occasionally. Do not boil.

Beef Not!, which is TVP, or Textured Vegetable Protein, is made from soy. Easy to use and widely available, this credible ground beef alternative reconstitutes quickly and is fat-free!

---

NUTRITION ANALYSIS: PER 2-CUP SERVING

**Enlightened Chunky Vegetable "Beef" Soup**
Protein 5 g, carbohydrate 12 g, fiber 3 g, fat 1 g,
saturated fat 0 g, cholesterol 0 mg,
calcium 52 mg, sodium 295 mg
Calories 76: from protein 28%,
from carbohydrate 65%, from fat 7%

**Traditional Vegetable Beef Soup**
Protein 7 g, carbohydrate 7 g, fiber 2 g, fat 13 g,
saturated fat 4 g, cholesterol 24 mg,
calcium 32 mg, sodium 439 mg
Calories 171: from protein 16%,
from carbohydrate 16% , from fat 68%

# Easy and Delicious Miso Soup

*I love miso soup. This version is made with wakame, a very tender*
*and delicate seaweed that looks like curly black threads.*

*6*
*Servings*

⅓ cup wakame
7 cups cold water
4 cloves garlic, minced
⅓ cup sliced scallions (about 3
    scallions)
⅓ cup chopped red bell pepper
1 tablespoon grated fresh gingerroot
¾ cup sliced cremini mushrooms

3 rounded tablespoons DDC onion
    broth powder
1 cup light silken tofu, cut into small
    cubes
¼ cup mellow white miso
2 tablespoons red miso
¼ cup dry sherry or vegetable broth

Place wakame in a medium bowl, cover with cold water, and set aside for 10 minutes. Place 7 cups of cold water in a 3-quart saucepan. Add garlic, scallions, bell pepper, gingerroot, mushrooms, and broth powder. Cover and bring to a boil.

Drain wakame, rinse, and add to the soup with the tofu. Reduce heat to medium low and simmer for 40 minutes or more, stirring occasionally. Combine the mellow white and red miso with sherry in a small bowl and blend with a fork. Stir miso mixture into the soup and simmer for 3 minutes. Do not boil.

NUTRITION ANALYSIS: PER PER 2-CUP SERVING

| Enlightened Easy and Delicious Miso Soup | Traditional Miso Soup |
| --- | --- |
| Protein 4 g, carbohydrate 9 g, fiber 0 g, fat 1 g, | Protein 7 g, carbohydrate 5 g, fiber 1 g, fat 5 g, |
| saturated fat 0 g, cholesterol 0 mg, | saturated fat 1 g, cholesterol 0 mg, |
| calcium 29 mg, sodium 375 mg | calcium 49 mg, sodium 445 mg |
| Calories 68: from protein 22%, | Calories 87: from protein 30%, |
| from carbohydrate 62%, from fat 16% | from carbohydrate 20%, from fat 50% |

# Gingered Acorn Squash Soup

*This soup can be an elegant first course or, accompanied by a colorful salad, the foundation of a satisfying meal.*

2 large acorn squash (3 pounds each)
2 teaspoons olive oil
¼ teaspoons crushed red pepper
7 cloves garlic, minced
1 medium yellow onion, chopped
2 tablespoons grated fresh gingerroot
2 medium russet potatoes, peeled and diced (2 cups)

3½ cups chicken-flavor vegetarian broth, boiling
½ cup enriched 1% fat soymilk
⅔ cup mellow white miso
½ cup dry sherry
1 teaspoon granulated garlic
1 teaspoon ground ginger
½ teaspoon ground nutmeg, plus additional for garnish

Preheat oven to 350°.

Cut the acorn squash in half crosswise; remove and discard seeds. Place cut side down in baking pans (you will need two) and add about 1 inch of water to each pan. Bake for 1 hour. Remove from pans and set aside to cool.

Warm the oil and crushed pepper in a 5-quart saucepan over medium-high heat for 1 minute. Add the minced garlic, onion, and gingerroot and cook for 3 minutes. Add potatoes and cook mixture, stirring frequently, for 5 minutes, or until the potatoes are beginning to soften. Add boiling broth and reduce heat to medium low. Scoop out cooked squash (you should have about 8 cups) into a large bowl and mash lightly before adding to the pot. Simmer for 15 minutes, stirring occasionally. Place soup in food processor in batches and process, adding some soymilk to each batch. Return

THE ENLIGHTENED approach to this rich-textured soup replaces fatty butter and cream with wholesome alternatives. Soymilk adds a silky mouthfeel and potatoes lend a hearty richness without adding extra fat. The velvety texture of this savory soup is heightened by the final addition of an enriching mellow white miso and sherry blend.

**Gingered Acorn Squash Soup** *(continued)*

the purée to the soup pot. Place miso and sherry in a small bowl and blend with a fork or small whisk. Add to the soup with the granulated garlic, ground ginger, and nutmeg. Simmer gently for 10 minutes. Do not boil. (Soup may be thinned with additional broth if desired) Sprinkle with a light dusting of nutmeg before serving.

---

NUTRITION ANALYSIS: PER 2-CUP SERVING

Enlightened Gingered Acorn Squash Soup
Protein 4 g, carbohydrate 48 g, fiber 12 g, fat 2 g,
saturated fat 0 g, cholesterol 0 mg,
calcium 137 mg, sodium 105 mg
Calories 211: from protein 8%,
from carbohydrate 85%, from fat 7%

Traditional Gingered Acorn Squash Soup
Protein 5 g, carbohydrate 41 g, fiber 11 g, fat 14 g,
saturated fat 6 g, cholesterol 23 mg,
calcium 157 mg, sodium 765 mg
Calories 282: from protein 6%,
from carbohydrate 53%, from fat 41%

# Tomato Vegetable Soup
# with Garbanzos

*This hearty tomato soup is creamy without the use of artery-clogging
dairy products. Instead, a richly flavorful mix of red and white
miso is added to the soup when the broth is hot, but not boiling, as
excessive cooking can destroy the beneficial enzymes.*

*8
Servings*

1 piece kombu
1½ quarts cold water
7 cloves garlic, minced
1 medium red onion, chopped
⅔ cup chopped green bell pepper
1 tablespoon grated fresh gingerroot
2 cups green beans, cut into 2-inch
  pieces
2 cups sliced baby-cut carrots
2 cups thinly sliced zucchini
2 cups chicken-flavor vegetarian
  broth, boiling

1 6-ounce can tomato paste
1 15-ounce can garbanzo beans
⅓ cup mellow white miso
⅓ cup red miso
½ cup dry vermouth or vegetable
  broth
1 teaspoon granulated garlic
1 teaspoon ground ginger
1 teaspoon dried basil
1 teaspoons dried thyme

In a large soup pot, combine kombu and water and set aside for 15
minutes. To the kombu stock, add the the minced garlic, onion,
bell pepper, gingerroot, green beans, carrots, and zucchini. Over
medium-high heat, bring mixture to a boil. Reduce heat to
medium and cook for 15 minutes, stirring occasionally. Add the
boiling broth, and spoon the tomato paste into the soup, stirring
after each addition. Reduce heat to low and add the garbanzo
beans. Place the mellow white and red miso in a small bowl, add

*THE ENLIGHTENED
KITCHEN* style of soup
making features a broth
started by soaking sea vegetables, such as kombu.
This nutritious sea veg-
etable simmers to a buttery
texture and is cut into delicious, bite-sized pieces and
returned to the soup.

**Tomato Vegetable Soup with Garbanzos** *(continued)*

the vermouth, and blend with a fork until smooth. Add to the soup with the granulated garlic, ground ginger, basil, and thyme. Remove kombu; cut it into bite-size pieces and return to soup, or reserve to add to a vegetable medley or stir fry. Simmer gently for 8 minutes, stirring occasionally. Do not boil.

---

NUTRITION ANALYSIS: PER 2-CUP SERVING

Enlightened Tomato Vegetable Soup
with Garbanzos
Protein 6 g, carbohydrate 23 g, fiber 6 g, fat 1 g,
saturated fat 0 g, cholesterol 0 mg,
calcium 79 mg, sodium 245 mg
Calories 132: from protein 18%,
from carbohydrate 75%, from fat 7%

Traditional Tomato Vegetable Soup
with Garbanzos
Protein 9 g, carbohydrate 22 g, fiber 5 g, fat 10 g,
saturated fat 2 g, cholesterol 8 mg,
calcium 144 mg, sodium 763 mg
Calories 205: from protein 16%,
from carbohydrate 41%, from fat 43%

# Cold Sesame Noodles

*A personal favorite, this is a*
*spicy Szechuan-style starter or side dish.*

1 recipe Szechuan Sesame Sauce
(page 201)

12 ounces thin spaghetti (not angel
hair)
⅓ cup thinly sliced scallions

Make the Szechuan Sesame Sauce, and set aside. Cook the spaghetti according
to package directions. Drain, rinse with cold water, and set aside in colander.
Toss with sauce and scallions and mix thoroughly. Chill.

---

## NUTRITION ANALYSIS: PER 1-CUP SERVING

**Enlightened Cold Sesame Noodles**
Protein 6 g, carbohydrate 21 g, fiber 2 g, fat 13 g,
saturated fat 1 g, cholesterol 0 mg,
calcium 25 mg, sodium 228 mg
Calories 151: from protein 12%,
from carbohydrate 37%, from fat 51%

**Traditional Cold Sesame Noodles**
Protein 7 g, carbohydrate 22 g, fiber 2 g, fat 15 g,
saturated fat 1 g, cholesterol 0 mg,
calcium 50 mg, sodium 575 mg
Calories 250: from protein 12%,
from carbohydrate 35%, from fat 53%

\* The percentage of calories from fat seems high because the calories are so low.

# Enticing Entrées

Elevate healthy eating to gourmet status with cutting-edge techniques, varietals, spices, herbs, and flavorful broths. We make it easy, too, with ingredients that are time-saving and convenient. Choose from a wide variety of entrées: elegant dishes such as Caribbean Mobay or Grilled Polenta with Tomato-Basil Cream; homey dishes like Roasted "Chicken" and Vegetables or Sloppy Joes; and delightful pasta dishes such as Neopolitan Pasta and Lentils and Linguine al Pesto.

The Chinese- and Japanese-style tofu called for in this chapter have different characteristics, and each has specific applications. Silken Japanese-style tofu is perfect for fillings such as quiche, lasagna, or stuffed shells, while, the firm, spongy texture of the Chinese-style makes excellent dishes like grilled marinated tofu.

You'll come to realize that plant-based meal planning doesn't have to differ from the traditional in terms of style. Enlightened meals are just as delicious, and virtually indiscernible from the traditional, but without the unhealthy baggage. You can create satisfying meals that are very low in fat and cholesterol-free effortlessly because of the many innovative new products. Forward-thinking manufacturers have developed hundreds of exciting new products made with soy protein and wheat gluten that meet the needs of today's health-conscious consumer. Versatile textured vegetable protein, tempeh, and numerous credible substitutes such as ready-to-use ground beef alternatives, Lightlife Lean Links Italian, Gimme Lean sausage, poultry and beef strips, Yves Veggie Canadian Bacon, and veggie pepperoni, make offering healthy "traditional" meals a snap!

# Recipes

Grilled Polenta with Tomato-Basil Cream

Kung Pao "Chicken"

Moroccan "Chicken" Tagine

Cassoulet

Tofu and Snow Peas

Grilled Marinated Tofu and Vegetables

Harvest Medley

Ginger Tempeh Wrap

Mexican Polenta

Hearty Stuffed Squash

Neapolitan Pasta and Lentils

Roasted "Chicken" and Vegetables

Hearty "Chicken" with Asparagus

Southern Greens and "Sausage"

Thai Tofu and Peanut Sauce

Marinated Tofu and Baby Bok Choy

Basque Stew

Caribbean Mobay

South of the Border Tofu

Sautéed Polenta with Sweet Italian "Sausage"

Tempeh Kebabs

Linguine al Pesto

Sloppy Joes

"Sausage" and Asparagus Fajitas

Yam Patties with Curry Sauce

Creamed Penne and "Ham"

"Beefy" Polenta Bake

Pineapple "Chicken"

Penne with Tofu Tomato Sauce

Vegetable Curry with Tofu
Open-Faced Grilled "Cheese" Triangles
Balsamic "Chicken"
Burmese Curry
Five-Spice Tofu and Snow Peas in Ginger "Cream"
Hearty Tempeh and Potato Roast
North African Stew (Sikbadj)
Balsamic "Beef" and Broccoli
Onion Okara Burgers
A-Maize-ing Okara Burgers
Quick Soy Burgers
Broccoli and Potato Curry
Braised Tempeh with Mushrooms and Tomatoes
"Beef" and Asparagus Oriental
Tempeh and Sweet Beans
"Beef" Vindaloo

# Grilled Polenta with Tomato-Basil Cream

*Grilled, sliced polenta is great topped with a tomato-basil cream.*

*8 servings*

1½ teaspoons olive oil
3 cloves garlic, minced
½ cup chopped yellow onion
¼ cup dry vermouth
2 cups Mori Nu Tomato Soup
¼ cup nutritional yeast
¼ cup soy Parmesan cheese

1 tablespoon capers, rinsed
1 teaspoon dried basil
olive oil cooking spray
2 18-ounce packages San Gennaro polenta

In a medium saucepan, warm oil over medium-high heat for 1 minute. Add garlic and onion and cook for 4 minutes, stirring frequently. Add vermouth and cook for 3 minutes, or until liquid is reduced by half. Add tomato soup, yeast, soy Parmesan, capers, and basil, stirring after each addition. Bring to a boil, then reduce heat to low, stirring well to dissolve yeast and Parmesan. Set aside; sauce will thicken as it sits.

Spray grill with olive oil cooking spray and preheat. Cut polenta into ¼-inch slices and place on hot grill. Cook 5 to 7 minutes on the first side. Spray polenta top with oil, flip and cook second side for 5 minutes, or until cooked through. Serve the polenta topped with the Tomato-Basil Cream.

Cooking polenta from scratch can be a time-consuming chore. Precooked, shelf-stable and so very convenient, San Gennaro polenta is a staple in my pantry.

---

NUTRITION ANALYSIS: PER SERVING (4 SLICES GRILLED POLENTA WITH SAUCE)

| Enlightened Grilled Polenta with Tomato-Basil Cream | Traditional Grilled Polenta with Tomato-Basil Cream |
|---|---|
| Protein 8 g, carbohydrate 28 g, fiber 1 g, fat 2 g, saturated fat 0 g, cholesterol 0 mg, calcium 52 mg, sodium 630 mg Calories 170: from protein 19%, from carbohydrate 68%, from fat 13% | Protein 7 g, carbohydrate 26 g, fiber 2 g, fat 21 g, saturated fat 13 g, cholesterol 69 mg, calcium 122 mg, sodium 787 mg Calories 323: from protein 8%, from carbohydrate 33%, from fat 59% |

# Kung Pao "Chicken"

*This spicy Szechuan dish is a popular favorite.*

### Kung Pao Sauce

1 cup chicken-flavor vegetarian
   broth, boiling
¼ cup tamari
1 teaspoon granulated garlic

½ teaspoon ground ginger
1 teaspoon sesame oil
⅛ teaspoon hot chile oil

### Sauté

1½ teaspoons olive oil
¼ teaspoon crushed red pepper
1 rounded tablespoon grated
   gingerroot
3 cloves garlic, minced
⅔ cup sliced scallions
1 small red bell pepper, cut into
   2-inch strips
1¼ cups coarsely shredded
   carrots

2 6-ounce packages Smart Chick'n
   Strips
½ cup dry sherry or vegetarian broth
4 ounces fresh shitake mushrooms,
   stemmed and sliced
9 ounces fresh snow peas, strings
   removed
1½ teaspoons cornstarch
1½ teaspoons cold water
½ cup Tosteds soynuts

*For the sauce:* Combine broth, tamari, garlic, ginger, sesame oil, and chile oil in a medium liquid measuring cup and set aside.

*For the sauté:* In a 10-inch frying pan, heat oil and crushed pepper over medium-high heat for 1 minute. Add gingerroot, garlic, scallions, bell pepper, and carrots. Cook for 3 minutes. Add Chick'n strips and cook for 5 minutes, stirring frequently. Add sherry, stir, then add mushrooms and snow peas. Lower heat to simmer. Add Kung Pao Sauce to the pan and cook for 2 minutes. Blend cornstarch and water in a small bowl, then stir into the pan. Simmer for 5 minutes. Add soynuts and serve.

TOSTEDS SOYNUTS are my choice for this dish. They look and taste just like peanuts, but are lower in fat, and have the goodness of soy. In order to maintain a crunchy texture, be sure to add the soynuts just before serving.

---

## NUTRITION ANALYSIS: PER 1½-CUP SERVING

### Enlightened Kung Pao "Chicken"
Protein 19 g, carbohydrate 21 g, fiber 9 g, fat 5 g,
saturated fat 1 g, cholesterol 0 mg,
calcium 86 mg, sodium 778 mg
Calories 219: from protein 37%,
from carbohydrate 40%, from fat 23%

### Traditional Kung Pao Chicken
Protein 27 g, carbohydrate 15 g, fiber 4 g, fat 28 g,
saturated fat 5 g, cholesterol 54 mg,
calcium 52 mg, sodium 994 mg
Calories 423: from protein 26%,
from carbohydrate 15%, from fat 59%

# Moroccan "Chicken" Tagine

*Tagine, a slow-cooked meat, fruit, and vegetable dish,
is considered a hallmark of Moroccan cuisine.*

**8
Servings**

2 cups DDC Chicken Not! Strips
2 cups boiling water
2 tablespoons DDC original broth
  powder
½ cup dry sherry or hot vegetarian
  broth
1 teaspoon saffron threads
¼ cup pine nuts
1½ teaspoons olive oil
¼ teaspoon crushed red pepper
1 rounded tablespoon grated fresh
  gingerroot
4 cloves garlic, minced
1 cup sliced scallions
1 medium red bell pepper, cut into
  2-inch strips

1½ cups sliced baby-cut carrots
1 cup chicken-flavor vegetarian
  broth, boiling
3 tablespoons nutritional yeast
1 cinnamon stick
½ cup dried currants
1 15-ounce can garbanzo beans,
  drained
2 plum tomatoes, diced
¼ cup chopped fresh cilantro
1 teaspoon granulated garlic
1 tablespoon tamari
juice of 1 lime
dash hot pepper sauce (to taste)

THE SOY CHICKEN alternative in this dish (Chicken Not!) is TVP (Textured Vegetable Protein).

Preheat oven to 350°.

Combine Chicken Not! with boiling water and broth powder in a medium saucepan, bring to a boil, and simmer for 8 minutes. Set aside. Combine sherry and saffron in a small glass liquid measuring cup and set aside. Toast pine nuts in a small pan over medium heat, shaking pan until nuts are lightly brown and fragrant. Set aside.

In a 5-quart saucepan, heat oil with crushed pepper and gingerroot over medium-high heat for 1 minute. Add minced garlic, scallions, bell pepper, and carrots. Cook for 3 minutes. Add rehydrated "chicken" and cook mixture for 10 minutes, stirring frequently. Add broth, yeast, saffron/sherry mixture, cinnamon stick, currants, garbanzo beans, tomatoes, and cilantro. Stir in granulated garlic, tamari, and lime juice and pour mixture into a shallow 9-by-13-inch baking pan. Cover and bake for 25 minutes. Uncover, sprinkle with toasted pine nuts, and bake an for additional 10 minutes. Remove cinnamon stick before serving. Serve with couscous.

---

NUTRITION ANALYSIS: PER 2-CUP SERVING

**Enlightened Moroccan "Chicken" Tagine**
Protein 17 g, carbohydrate 32 g, fiber 9 g, fat 4 g,
saturated fat 1 g, cholesterol 0 mg,
calcium 110 mg, sodium 265 mg
Calories 221: from protein 29%,
from carbohydrate 55%, from fat 16%

**Traditional Moroccan Chicken Tagine**
Protein 17 g, carbohydrate 20 g, fiber 4 g, fat 20 g,
saturated fat 7 g, cholesterol 68 mg,
66 mg, sodium 366 mg
Calories 323: from protein 20%,
from carbohydrate 25%, from fat 55%

# Cassoulet

*Like many casseroles, this dish profits from advance preparation.*
*You can make Cassoulet a day or two in advance and reheat just*
*before serving. Serve with crusty French bread.*

*8*
*Servings*

2 teaspoons olive oil
5 cloves garlic, minced
1 large shallot, minced
1 medium red onion, chopped
1 6-ounce package veggie Canadian
    bacon, diced
1 14-ounce package Gimme Lean,
    sausage style

1½ cups sliced baby-cut carrots
1½ cups thinly sliced zucchini
2 15-ounce cans small white beans,
    drained
⅓ cup white wine
1 teaspoon Bragg Liquid Aminos
¾ teaspoon dried thyme
1 bay leaf

*Topping*

2 tablespoons whole wheat bread
    crumbs

1 teaspoon dried marjoram
⅛ teaspoon lemon pepper

Cassoulet
IS A French country-
style baked dish. The
cornerstone of this
main dish casserole is
small white beans, but
Great Northern or lima
beans may also be used.

Preheat oven to 350°.

    In a medium saucepan, heat oil for 1 minute over medium-high heat. Add garlic, shallot, and onion. Sauté for 2 minutes, then add veggie bacon. Cook 3 minutes, then add Gimme Lean, stirring often and breaking apart with a spoon. Continue cooking for 3 minutes. Stir in carrots, zucchini, and beans. Reduce heat to low and add the wine, liquid aminos, thyme, and bay leaf. Transfer the mixture to a 2-quart baking dish and set aside.

    *For the topping:* In a small bowl, mix together the bread crumbs, marjoram, and lemon pepper. Sprinkle topping over casserole and place, uncovered, in preheated oven. Bake for 30 to 35 minutes, or until brown.

## NUTRITION ANALYSIS: PER 2-CUP SERVING

| Enlightened Cassoulet | Traditional Cassoulet |
|---|---|
| Protein 23 g, carbohydrate 54 g, fiber 8 g, fat 2 g, | Protein 20 g, carbohydrate 34 g, fiber 7 g, fat 24 g, |
| saturated fat 0 g, cholesterol 0 mg, | saturated fat 7 g, cholesterol 45 mg, |
| calcium 141 mg, sodium 848 mg | calcium 189 mg, sodium 1130 mg |
| Calories 264: from protein 29%, | Calories 454: from protein 18%, |
| from carbohydrate 67%, from fat 4% | from carbohydrate 32%, from fat 50% |

# Tofu and Snow Peas

*Marinating contributes flavor and texture
to firm, Chinese-style tofu.*

1 recipe Fragrant Soy Marinade,
    (page 211)
1 16-ounce package firm nigari tofu
1 tablespoon olive oil
1/8 teaspoon crushed red pepper
1 tablespoon dried minced garlic
1 tablespoon grated fresh gingerroot
1 medium red onion, quartered, then
    thinly sliced

2 slices veggie Canadian bacon, cut
    into thin strips
1 8-ounce package button
    mushrooms, sliced
12 ounces fresh snow peas, rinsed
    and trimmed
3 cups cooked brown rice

Prepare the marinade. Cut tofu into 1-inch cubes and place in a nonreactive (preferably glass) bowl. Pour marinade over tofu, cover, and refrigerate at least 1 hour or overnight.

In a wok or electric frying pan, heat oil, crushed red pepper, garlic, and gingerroot over medium-high heat for 2 minutes. Add onion and veggie bacon and sauté for 2 minutes. Remove tofu, discarding marinade, and add tofu to the pan with the mushrooms. Cook for 5 minutes, stirring frequently. Add the snow peas and cook mixture just until peas are heated through, about 1 minute. Serve immediately with brown rice.

SNOW PEAS ARE similar to fresh green peas, but much more delicate. This legume is entirely edible, including the pod, which accounts for its French name, *mange-tout,* or "eat it all."

---

NUTRITION ANALYSIS: PER 2-CUP SERVING WITH 1/2 CUP RICE

**Enlightened Tofu and Snow Peas**
Protein 19 g, carbohydrate 39 g, fiber 7 g, fat 5 g,
saturated fat 1 g, cholesterol 0 mg,
calcium 63 mg, sodium 200 mg
Calories 272: from protein 28%,
from carbohydrate 56%, from fat 16%

**Traditional Beef and Snow Peas**
Protein 23 g, carbohydrate 41 g, fiber 3g, fat 25 g,
saturated fat 7 g, cholesterol 0 mg,
calcium 32 mg, sodium 725 mg
Calories 484: from protein 19%,
from carbohydrate 34%, from fat 47%

# Grilled Marinated Tofu and Vegetables

*Make this dish with firm nigari tofu, which is low in fat and has a sweet flavor. You will find this type of tofu in clear vacuum packages in the refrigerated case in health food stores.*

*8
Servings*

1 recipe Red Miso Marinade
(page 216)

*Recommended vegetables for the grill*
4 ears of corn, quartered
4 Japanese eggplants, cut to ½-inch
rounds
1 pound fresh asparagus spears,
tough ends trimmed
2 whole red onions, cut to ¾-inch-
thick wedges

2 12-ounce packages firm nigari tofu,
cut into 2-inch pieces

2 whole bell peppers, cut to ½-inch
strips
4 large carrots, cut diagonally to
½-inch slices

GRILLING TOFU gives
it a firmer, chewier texture.

Combine marinade ingredients. Place tofu in a nonreactive bowl (preferably glass) and cover with marinade. Cover and refrigerate for up to 36 hours, stirring occasionally. Grill the tofu and veggies until brown, brushing with marinade frequently.

NUTRITION ANALYSIS: PER 2-CUP SERVING

Enlightened Grilled Marinated
Tofu and Vegetables
Protein 16 g, carbohydrate 24 g, fiber 8 g, fat 2 g,
saturated fat 0 g, cholesterol 0 mg,
calcium 80 mg, sodium 179 mg
Calories 166: from protein 36%,
from carbohydrate 54%, from fat 11%

Traditional Grilled Marinated
Beef and Vegetables
Protein 18 g, carbohydrate 19 g, fiber 5 g, fat 29 g,
saturated fat 12 g, cholesterol 64 mg,
calcium 33 mg, sodium 572 mg
Calories 397: from protein 17%,
from carbohydrate 19%, from fat 64%

# Harvest Medley

*This dish combines tender, chewy tempeh with chunks of golden
butternut squash and russet potatoes in an enticing fusion
of textures, color, and flavor.*

olive oil cooking spray
2 teaspoons olive oil, divided
2 8-ounce packages tempeh, cubed
    and steamed
¼ teaspoon crushed red pepper
2 tablespoons dried minced garlic
1 large shallot, minced (about ⅓
    cup)
1 large leek, rinsed thoroughly and
    sliced

1 medium red bell pepper, chopped
1 medium butternut squash, peeled
    and cubed (about 6 cups)
5 small red bliss potatoes, halved
    crosswise and cut into ¼-inch
    slices (about 2 cups)
8 cherry tomatoes, quartered
⅓ cup chopped flat-leaf parsley
½ cup dry vermouth
2 tablespoons tamari

Spray an electric frying pan or Dutch oven with olive oil spray. Add
1 teaspoon of the oil and warm over medium-high heat. Add tempeh and brown on all sides. Remove from pan and set aside. Spray
pan again with oil and add the remaining teaspoon of oil with
crushed pepper and dried garlic. Heat for 1 minute and add the
shallot, leek, and bell pepper. Sauté for 3 minutes. Add squash and
potatoes and cook for 10 minutes, stirring frequently. Add tempeh,
tomatoes, and parsley. Cook for 3 minutes, then add vermouth and
tamari. Reduce heat to low and simmer, stirring occasionally, for 5
minutes or until veggies are tender.

Butternut squash
has a characteristic bell-
shaped, pale tan shell,
sweet orange flesh, and
usually weighs between two
and three pounds.

---

NUTRITION ANALYSIS: PER 2-CUP SERVING

**Enlightened Harvest Medley**
Protein 13 g, carbohydrate 50 g, fiber 10 g, fat 5 g,
saturated fat 1 g, cholesterol 0 mg,
calcium 90 mg, sodium 223 mg
Calories 291: from protein 18%,
from carbohydrate 68%, from fat 14%

**Traditional Harvest Medley**
Protein 14 g, carbohydrate 38 g, fiber 7 g, fat 15 g,
saturated fat 6 g, cholesterol 0 mg,
calcium 94 mg, sodium 330 mg
Calories 340: from protein 16%,
from carbohydrate 45%, from fat 39%

# Ginger Tempeh Wrap

*Enjoy this delicious wrap made with healthy alternatives that reduce the calories, sodium, and fat content dramatically.*

2 8-ounce packages tempeh, cubed
olive oil cooking spray
1/8 teaspoon crushed red pepper
1 tablespoon minced dried garlic
2 tablespoons grated fresh gingerroot
1 medium red onion, chopped
1/2 cup chopped red bell pepper

1/2 cup veggie pepperoni, diced
1 cup diced portobello mushroom
1/2 cup dry sherry
2 tablespoons tamari
1 cup halved cherry tomatoes.
6 whole wheat tortillas (without
  hydrogenated oils)

Place tempeh in a steamer basket over boiling water for 15 minutes. Set aside. Spray a 4-quart saucepan or electric frying pan with olive oil. Add crushed pepper and dried garlic and heat over medium-high heat for 1 minute. Add gingerroot, onion, bell pepper, and pepperoni. Sauté for 3 minutes, stirring frequently. Crumble tempeh into the pan and add mushrooms. Cook for 8 minutes, stirring to keep the mixture from sticking to the pan. Add sherry, tamari, and tomatoes. Reduce heat and simmer for 10 minutes, stirring occasionally. Warm tortillas in microwave for 1 minute, or conventional oven for 5 minutes, and keep warm. Add 1½ cups filling to each tortilla and fold.

SPREAD TORTILLAS with dairy-free Creamy Dill Dressing (page 93), and garnish with fresh salad greens.

NUTRITION ANALYSIS: PER SERVING (1 TORTILLA WITH 1 1/2 CUPS FILLING)

**Enlightened Ginger Tempeh Wrap**
Protein 25 g, carbohydrate 34 g, fiber 6 g, fat 5 g,
saturated fat 2 g, cholesterol 0 mg,
calcium 140 mg, sodium 295 mg
Calories 644: from protein 37%,
from carbohydrate 48%, from fat 15%

**Traditional Ginger Beef Wrap**
Protein 22 g, carbohydrate 27 g, fiber 3 g, fat 35 g,
saturated fat 16 g, cholesterol 68 mg,
calcium 67 mg, sodium 962 mg
Calories 482: from protein 19%,
from carbohydrate 23%, from fat 58%

# Mexican Polenta

*Precooked polenta can be used right from the package. I slice the polenta and blend it with a little soymilk. Voila! Soft polenta !*

olive oil cooking spray
1½ teaspoons olive oil
¼ teaspoon crushed red pepper
4 cloves garlic, minced
½ cup sliced scallions
½ cup chopped green bell pepper
2 12-ounce packages Smart Ground,
   Taco & Burrito style

1 15-ounce can black beans, drained
1 14½-ounce can diced tomatoes
   with mild green chilies
1 24-ounce package precooked
   polenta, chile and cilantro
¼ cup enriched 1% fat soymilk
paprika for garnish

Preheat oven to 350°. Lightly spray a 2-quart baking dish with olive oil.

Place oil and crushed red pepper in a 10-inch frying pan and warm over medium-high heat for 1 minute. Add the garlic, scallions, and bell pepper. Cook for 3 minutes, then add the Smart Ground. Cover, with lid set slightly ajar, lower heat, and simmer for 10 minutes, stirring frequently. Place the beans in a medium bowl and add the diced tomatoes. Stir to mix and set aside. Turn the taco mixture into the prepared baking dish. Top with the black bean and tomato mixture. Cut the polenta into 1-inch slices, and place in the food processor with soymilk. Process until smooth. Spread the polenta over the beans and sprinkle with paprika. Bake for 30 minutes, or until brown.

MEXICAN CUISINE IS bursting with flavor. In this dish, I used a flavored, wholesome alternative that is delicious, easy to use, and fat-free.

NUTRITION ANALYSIS: PER 1½-CUP SERVING

**Enlightened Mexican Polenta**
Protein 21 g, carbohydrate 33 g, fiber 9 g, fat 1 g,
saturated fat 0 g, cholesterol 0 mg,
calcium 101 mg, sodium 614 mg
Calories 221: from protein 37%,
from carbohydrate 59%, from fat 4%

**Traditional Mexican Polenta**
Protein 22 g, carbohydrate 22 g, fiber 5 g, fat 30 g,
saturated fat 11 g, cholesterol 77 mg,
calcium 41 mg, sodium 800 mg
Calories 221: from protein 19%,
from carbohydrate 22%, from fat 59%

# Hearty Stuffed Squash

*Serve with jellied cranberry sauce and a salad.*

2 medium acorn squash
1½ teaspoons olive oil
⅛ teaspoon crushed red pepper
4 cloves garlic, minced
½ cup sliced scallions
1 cup coarsely shredded carrots
1 12-ounce package ground beef
    alternative

1 medium Granny Smith apple,
    peeled and diced
3 tablespoons fresh lime juice
1 cup dried cranberries
¼ cup mirin cooking wine

ACORN SQUASH HAS a ribbed shell and moist, sweet, tender flesh. When cut in half crosswise, this delicious winter squash makes very attractive scalloped bowls.

Preheat oven to 375°.

Halve squash crosswise and remove seeds. Place squash halves cut side down in 1 inch of water in a 9-by-13-inch pan. Bake 1 hour while preparing stuffing.

Heat oil and crushed pepper in a 10-inch frying pan over medium-high heat. Add garlic, scallions, and shredded carrots. Sauté for 3 minutes. Add ground beef alternative and cook for 5 minutes, stirring frequently. Drizzle diced apple with lime juice. Add to pan with cranberries and mirin. Lower heat to simmer and cook for 5 minutes.

Remove squash from oven, leaving oven on. Discard water and replace squash in pan, cut side up. Spray the flesh of each squash half with olive oil and divide the filling between the four halves. Cover the baking dish with foil and bake for 10 minutes, or until heated through.

---

NUTRITION ANALYSIS: PER SERVING (1 STUFFED SQUASH HALF)

**Enlightened Hearty Stuffed Squash**
Protein 7 g, carbohydrate 63 g, fiber 11 g, fat 2,
saturated fat 0 g, cholesterol 0 mg,
calcium 114 mg, sodium 86 mg
Calories 155: from protein 9%,
from carbohydrate 85%, from fat 6%

**Traditional Hearty Stuffed Squash**
Protein 16 g, carbohydrate 57 g, fiber 10 g, fat 34 g,
saturated fat 16 g, cholesterol 104 mg,
calcium 95 mg, sodium 544 mg
Calories 603: from protein 11%,
from carbohydrate 38%, from fat 51%

# Neapolitan Pasta and Lentils

*Pasta and lentils are
often combined in Italian cooking.*

2 teaspoons olive oil
¼ teaspoon crushed red pepper
5 cloves garlic, minced
1 medium yellow onion, chopped
4 slices veggie Canadian bacon, diced
2 cups cooked lentils
¼ cup dry sherry
1 25-ounce jar roasted red pepper
   tomato sauce

1 14½-ounce can Mexican-style
   stewed tomatoes, diced
1 teaspoon dried marjoram
12 ounces penne, cooked according
   to package directions
⅓ cup soy Parmesan cheese

In a 5-quart saucepan, heat oil and crushed pepper over medium-high heat for
1 minute. Add garlic, onion, and veggie bacon and cook for 5 minutes. Add
lentils and cook, stirring for 3 minutes. Add sherry and reduce heat to low. Add
tomato sauce, stewed tomatoes, and marjoram. Simmer for 15 minutes. Combine with cooked pasta and soy Parmesan cheese.

NUTRITION ANALYSIS: PER 2-CUP SERVING

**Enlightened Neapolitan Pasta and Lentils**
Protein 16 g, carbohydrate 37 g, fiber 6 g, fat 3 g,
saturated fat 0 g, cholesterol 0 mg,
calcium 40 mg, sodium 653 mg
Calories 242: from protein 26%,
from carbohydrate 61%, from fat 13%

**Traditional Neapolitan Pasta and Lentils**
Protein 17 g, carbohydrate 33 g, fiber 5 g, fat 15 g,
saturated fat 5 g, cholesterol 29 mg,
calcium 124 mg, sodium 929 mg
Calories 334: from protein 21%,
from carbohydrate 39%, from fat 40%

# Roasted "Chicken" and Vegetables

*This dish has hearty Midwestern appeal.*

1 5.1-ounce package DDC Roasted
    Chicken Not!
3¼ cups water
2 large russet potatoes, cut in eighths
1½ cups baby-cut carrots, sliced in
    half vertically

1½ teaspoons olive oil
1 tablespoon dried minced garlic
½ cup chopped red onion
6 ounces sliced cremini mushrooms
½ cup vermouth
2 teaspoons dried thyme

Preheat oven to 400°.

Combine Chicken Not! mix with water in a medium saucepan and bring to a boil. Lower heat to medium low and simmer for 12 minutes. Set aside.

Parboil potatoes and carrots for 5 minutes, drain, and set aside.

Heat oil and garlic over medium-high heat in a 5-quart ovenproof pan for 1 minute. Add onion and mushrooms and cook for 3 minutes. Add vermouth and cook for 2 minutes. Lower heat, add potatoes, carrots, and reconstituted Chicken Not! Cook for 5 minutes. Sprinkle with thyme, and place, uncovered, in preheated oven. Bake for 25 minutes or until tender. Serve hot.

ROASTED CHICKEN Not! is a no-fuss soy product with great texture and flavor.

## NUTRITION ANALYSIS: PER 2-CUP SERVING

**Enlightened "Roasted Chicken" and Vegetables**
Protein 10 g, carbohydrate 35 g, fiber 6 g, fat 3 g,
saturated fat 0 g, cholesterol 0 mg,
calcium 65 mg, sodium 360 mg
Calories 214: from protein 15%,
from carbohydrate 65%, from fat 20%

**Traditional Roasted Chicken and Vegetables**
Protein 19 g, carbohydrate 27 g, fiber 3 g, fat 17 g,
saturated fat 9 g, cholesterol 76 mg,
calcium 47 mg, sodium 441 mg
Calories 356: from protein 22%,
from carbohydrate 31%, from fat 47%

# Hearty "Chicken" with Asparagus

*Marinated seitan gives this dish its
exceptional flavor and texture.*

1 recipe Lively Marinade (page 212)
2 16-ounce packages seitan, drained
1½ teaspoons olive oil
¼ teaspoon crushed red pepper
3 cloves garlic, minced
1 cup sliced scallions
1 yellow bell pepper, chopped
1 cup sliced baby-cut carrots
3 slices veggie Canadian bacon, diced

6 ounces cremini mushrooms, sliced
12 ounces fresh asparagus, trimmed
    and cut to 2-inch pieces
⅓ cup dry sherry
1¼ cups chicken-flavor vegetarian
    broth, boiling
1 cup frozen corn, thawed
½ cup nutritional yeast
1 teaspoon dried oregano

Prepare marinade and set aside. Drain seitan and place in a medium nonreactive (preferably glass) bowl, tearing into smaller pieces where necessary. Pour marinade over seitan, cover, and refrigerate for at least 1 hour.

In a Dutch oven or electric frying pan, heat oil with crushed red pepper over medium-high heat, for 1 minute. Add garlic, scallions, bell pepper, carrots, and veggie bacon. Cook for 5 minutes, stirring frequently. Remove seitan from marinade, reserving the liquid. Add seitan to pan and cook for 5 minutes, stirring occasionally. Add mushrooms and asparagus, reduce heat to low, and simmer for 4 more minutes. Add sherry, broth, ½ cup of the reserved marinade, and corn. Stir for 2 minutes, then add yeast and oregano. Simmer for 5 minutes, or until asparagus is crisp-tender.

WHEN DRAINED, a 16-ounce package of seitan packed in broth will yield 8 ounces of seitan. This dish calls for 16 ounces of seitan, so two packages are necessary.

NUTRITION ANALYSIS: PER 1½-CUP SERVING

**Enlightened Hearty "Chicken" with Asparagus**
Protein 15 g, carbohydrate 19 g, fiber 7 g, fat 2 g,
saturated fat 0 g, cholesterol 0 mg,
calcium 58 mg, sodium 461 mg
Calories 147: from protein 41%,
from carbohydrate 50%, from fat 9%

**Traditional Hearty Chicken with Asparagus**
Protein 16 g, carbohydrate 11 g, fiber 2 g, fat 24 g,
saturated fat 8 g, cholesterol 71 mg,
calcium 52 mg, sodium 976 mg
Calories 324: from protein 20%,
from carbohydrate 14%, from fat 66%

# Southern Greens and "Sausage"

*I make this dish New Orleans style, with vegetarian
sausage and a prepackaged mix of mustard, collard,
and turnip greens with spinach. Terrific!*

6
*Servings*

1½ teaspoons olive oil
¼ teaspoon crushed red pepper
3 cloves garlic, minced
1 medium red onion, chopped
1 14-ounce package Gimme Lean,
  sausage style

1 pound mixed greens
2 cups chicken-flavor vegetarian
  broth, hot
1 14½-ounce can Mexican-style
  stewed tomatoes

Heat oil and crushed red pepper in a Dutch oven or electric frying pan over
medium-high heat for 1 minute. Add garlic and onion. Cook for 3 minutes. Add
sausage, stirring and breaking apart with a large spoon, and cook
mixture for 10 minutes, stirring frequently until browned. Add
greens and broth, lower heat to medium low, and cook for 1 minute.
Stir to mix, and add tomatoes. Cover and simmer for 30 minutes or
until greens are tender, stirring occasionally.

LOOK FOR PACKAGED
Cut 'n Clean Greens. A
time saver, they are conveniently washed, precut, and
ready to use.

NUTRITION ANALYSIS: PER 1½-CUP SERVING

**Enlightened Greens and "Sausage"**
Protein 14 g, carbohydrate 20 g, fiber 4 g, fat 1 g,
saturated fat 0 g, cholesterol 0 mg,
calcium 26 mg, sodium 583 mg
Calories 149: from protein 38%,
from carbohydrate 55%, from fat 7%

**Traditional Greens and Sausage**
Protein 17 g, carbohydrate 10 g, fiber 2 g, fat 28 g,
saturated fat 8 g, cholesterol 55 mg,
calcium 48 mg, sodium 1256 mg
Calories 363: from protein 19%,
from carbohydrate 11%, from fat 70%

# Thai Tofu and Peanut Sauce

*This spirited dish could be called "Curry in-a-Hurry"*

1 recipe Spicy Peanut Sauce
  (page 200)
1 16- to 19-ounce package firm
  nigari tofu, cubed
olive oil cooking spray
1 teaspoon olive oil
2 cups julienned baby-cut carrots
1 medium red bell pepper, cut into
  3-inch strips

2 Japanese eggplants, sliced
¼ cup dry sherry
1 8-ounce can sliced water chestnuts,
  drained
1½ cups frozen peas, thawed
¼ cup chopped fresh cilantro

Make the Spicy Peanut Sauce, and set aside.

Rinse the tofu and pat dry. Spray a wok or electric frying pan with olive oil cooking spray. Add oil and heat for 30 seconds over medium-high heat. Add tofu and cook on all sides for 8 minutes, or until brown. Remove tofu from the pan and set aside.

Spray pan with oil and add carrots, bell pepper, and eggplant. Cook for 5 minutes, stirring occasionally. Return the tofu to the pan, stir to mix, then add sherry, water chestnuts, and peas. Reduce heat to medium low and add Spicy Peanut Sauce and cilantro. Simmer mixture for 10 minutes, or until tofu and vegetables are coated with sauce and heated through.

> JULIENNE BABY-CUT carrots by making about 4 vertical cuts in each carrot, to produce ¼-inch strips.

---

NUTRITION ANALYSIS: PER 1½-CUP SERVING

**Enlightened Thai Tofu and Peanut Sauce**
Protein 14 g, carbohydrate 22 g, fiber 7 g, fat 6 g,
saturated fat 0 g, cholesterol 0 mg,
calcium 71 mg, sodium 240 mg
Calories 193: from protein 27%,
from carbohydrate 45%, from fat 28%

**Traditional Thai Chicken and Peanut Sauce**
Protein 18 g, carbohydrate 18 g, fiber 5 g, fat 20 g,
saturated fat 11 g, cholesterol 0 mg,
calcium 46 mg, sodium 347 mg
Calories 431: from protein 23%,
from carbohydrate 22%, from fat 55%

# Marinated Tofu and Baby Bok Choy

*Tofu absorbs marinade like a sponge,*
*adding flavor and dimension to most any dish.*

*8*
*Servings*

1 recipe Asian Marinade (page 208)

1 16- to 19-ounce package very firm tofu

*Sauté*

2 teaspoons olive oil, divided
1 tablespoon grated gingerroot
¾ cup sliced scallions
½ cup minced shallot
1 cup sliced baby-cut carrots
1 pound baby bok choy, cut to
　　1-inch pieces (about 5 to 6 cups)

1 8-ounce package button mush-
　　rooms, sliced
1 15-ounce can baby corn
2 tablespoons cornstarch
2 tablespoons cold water
⅓ cup chopped fresh cilantro
1 cup bean sprouts

Baby bok choy is more tender and delicate than the mature version. However, regular bok choy is an option here as well.

Prepare marinade and set aside. Rinse tofu, pat dry, and cut into 1-inch cubes. Place in a nonreactive medium bowl. Pour marinade over tofu, cover, and set aside for at least an hour.

*For the sauté:* In a wok or electric frying pan, heat 1 teaspoon of oil over medium-high heat for 1 minute. Remove tofu from marinade (reserve marinade), and sauté for 5 minutes, browning on all sides. Remove tofu from pan and set aside. Add the remaining 1 teaspoon oil to the pan, and sauté gingerroot, scallions, shallots, and carrots for 5 minutes. Add tofu back to the pan, along with the bok choy, mushrooms, and baby corn. Cook mixture for 5 minutes, stirring occasionally. Add reserved marinade, lower heat to medium low, and cook mixture for 3 minutes. Combine cornstarch and water in a small bowl. Blend until smooth, and stir into the pan. Add cilantro and bean sprouts. Simmer for 5 minutes and serve with steamed brown rice.

NUTRITION ANALYSIS: PER 2-CUP SERVING

**Enlightened Tofu and Baby Bok Choy**
Protein 9 g, carbohydrate 16 g, fiber 4 g, fat 5 g,
saturated fat 1 g, cholesterol 0 mg,
calcium 151 mg, sodium 388 mg
Calories 138: from protein 25%,
from carbohydrate 43%, from fat 32%

**Traditional Beef and Baby Bok Choy**
Protein 16 g, carbohydrate 13 g, fiber 3 g, fat 19 g,
saturated fat 6 g, cholesterol 48 mg,
calcium 89 mg, sodium 583 mg
Calories 289: from protein 22%,
from carbohydrate 18%, from fat 60%

# Basque Stew

*Stews are very popular in Basque cooking, and the bold
tastes in this delightful dish profit from long simmering.
Soy-based ground sausage, and chicken-style seitan made
from wheat gluten add authentic flavor and texture.*

1 1-pound, 2-ounce package
chicken-flavor seitan, packed in
broth
1 16-ounce package baby-cut carrots,
halved vertically
1½ teaspoons olive oil
8 cloves garlic, minced
1 medium red onion, chopped
1 medium red bell pepper, chopped
1 14-ounce package Gimme Lean,
sausage style

1 14½-ounce can Mexican-style
stewed tomatoes
1 13¾-ounce can quartered
artichoke hearts
1 6-ounce can low-sodium tomato
paste
3 ounces red wine
1 teaspoon dried thyme
1 teaspoon dried marjoram
1 teaspoon granulated garlic
Tabasco sauce to taste

Remove the seitan from the broth and set aside. Place the carrots and seitan broth in a Crock-Pot and turn indicator to high.

Warm olive oil in a 10-inch frying pan over medium-high heat for 1 minute. Sauté the minced garlic, onion, and red pepper for 3 minutes. Add sausage and seitan and cook for 10 minutes, stirring occasionally. Add mixture to the Crock-Pot with the stewed tomatoes and artichoke hearts. Spoon tomato paste into the mixture. Fill tomato paste can halfway (3 ounces) with red wine, then add water to fill can. Stir into the pot, cover, and cook for 6 to 8 hours. Add thyme, marjoram, and granulated garlic 10 minutes before serving. You may season with a touch of Tabasco or serve the hot sauce on the side.

ANYONE WITH A busy lifestyle can appreciate the convenience of setting up the Crock-Pot when you leave for work, then coming home to find dinner ready and waiting. And the other bonus? The whole house smells like someone has been cooking all day in the kitchen!

---

NUTRITION ANALYSIS: PER 2-CUP SERVING

**Enlightened Basque Stew**
Protein 15 g, carbohydrate 27 g, fiber 7 g, fat 1 g,
saturated fat 0 g, cholesterol 0 mg,
calcium 67 mg, sodium 515 mg
Calories 181: from protein 33%,
from carbohydrate 61%, from fat 6%

**Traditional Basque Stew**
Protein 21 g, carbohydrate 16 g, fiber 4 g,
fat 26 g, saturated fat 9 g, cholesterol 70 mg,
calcium 62 mg, sodium 1219 mg
Calories 392: from protein 22%,
from carbohydrate 17%, from fat 61%

# Caribbean Mobay

*"Mobay" is Island shorthand for Montego Bay (Jamaica).*
*This version of the classic curry is rich in flavor and nutrients, and*
*much lower in calories and fat than the traditional dish.*

*8*
*Servings*

1½ teaspoons olive oil
¼ teaspoon crushed red pepper
1 tablespoon grated gingerroot
6 cloves garlic, minced
1 large onion, chopped
⅓ cup chopped red bell pepper
1 cup diced parsnips
1⅓ cups sliced baby-cut carrots
1 medium zucchini, cut in half
    vertically, then crosswise into
    ¼-inch slices
1 medium Japanese eggplant, cut in
    half vertically, then crosswise to
    ¼-inch slices
1 medium plum tomato, diced

1 cup chicken-flavor
    vegetarian broth, boiling
1 cinnamon stick
1 15-ounce can garbanzo beans,
    drained
1 14-ounce can lite coconut milk
juice of 1 lime
2 tablespoons tamari
1 teaspoon ground turmeric
2½ tablespoons nutritional yeast
⅛ teaspoon ground nutmeg
1 cup dried currants
½ cup chopped flat-leaf parsley
1 tablespoon cornstarch
1½ tablespoons cold water

Refresh WITH about a half cup of hot vegetarian broth when reheating leftovers.

Heat oil and crushed red pepper in a 5-quart saucepan over medium-high heat for 1 minute. Add gingerroot, garlic, onion, and bell pepper. Sauté for 2 minutes, then add parsnips, carrots, zucchini, and eggplant. Cook for 5 minutes, stirring frequently. Add tomato, broth, cinnamon stick, and beans. Reduce heat to medium low and add coconut milk, lime juice, tamari, turmeric, and nutritional yeast. Stir to mix, and add nutmeg, currants, and parsley. Cook mixture for 5 minutes. In a small bowl, combine cornstarch and water, and add to curry. Simmer for 10 minutes, stirring occasionally. Remove cinnamon stick before serving.

## NUTRITION ANALYSIS: PER 2-CUP SERVING

**Enlightened Caribbean Mobay**
Protein 8 g, carbohydrate 33 g, fiber 6 g, fat 5 g,
saturated fat 2 g, cholesterol 0 mg,
calcium 67 mg, sodium 244 mg
Calories 192: from protein 15%,
from carbohydrate 65%, from fat 20%

**Traditional Caribbean Mobay**
Protein 8 g, carbohydrate 28 g, fiber 6 g, fat 20 g,
saturated fat 17 g, cholesterol 0 mg,
calcium 67 mg, sodium 743 mg
Calories 294: from protein 9%,
from carbohydrate 33%, from fat 58%

# South of the Border Tofu

*Serve this zesty entrée with brown rice.*

1 tablespoon olive oil
1 tablespoon dried minced garlic
1 16- to 19-ounce package firm tofu, cut into 1-inch cubes
olive oil cooking spray
1 medium red onion, halved, then cut into ¼-inch-thick wedges
1¼ cups sliced celery hearts with leaves

1 cup coarsely shredded carrots
⅓ cup vermouth
1 14½-ounce can Mexican-style stewed tomatoes
1 cup frozen corn, thawed
2½ Melissa's Fire Roasted Chiles, diced
¼ cup chopped fresh cilantro

Heat oil and garlic in a Dutch oven or electric frying pan for 1 minute. Add tofu and sauté for 5 minutes, browning cubes on all sides. Push tofu to one side, and coat exposed surface of pan with olive oil cooking spray. Add onion, celery, and carrots to the pan and cook for 4 minutes, stirring frequently. Stir tofu and softened veggies together and add vermouth. Cook for 1 minute, then add tomatoes. Reduce heat and simmer for 2 minutes. Add corn, chiles, and cilantro. Simmer for 5 minutes. Serve with brown rice.

I USE CHINESE-STYLE tofu (available both water packed and vacuum packed) for this dish. This style of tofu is much lower in fat these days, often averaging about 3 grams of fat per serving.

---

## NUTRITION ANALYSIS: PER 2-CUP SERVING

**Enlightened South of the Border Tofu**
Protein 16 g, carbohydrate 24 g, fiber 6 g, fat 4 g, saturated fat 0 g, cholesterol 0 mg, calcium 38 mg, sodium 214 mg
Calories 203: from protein 32%, from carbohydrate 50%, from fat 18%

**Traditional South of the Border Chicken**
Protein 20 g, carbohydrate 20 g, fiber 3 g, fat 22 g, saturated fat 7 g, cholesterol 86 mg, calcium 89 mg, sodium 409 mg
Calories 353: from protein 22%, from carbohydrate 22%, from fat 56%

# Sautéed Polenta with Sweet Italian "Sausage"

*Italian Sausage and Peppers is traditionally served on a crisp Kaiser roll.
I serve it spooned over browned slices of polenta.*

*8
Servings*

olive oil cooking spray
2 teaspoons olive oil, divided
1 11.2-ounce package Smart Links, Italian
3 garlic cloves, minced
1 red bell pepper, cut into 3-inch strips
1 green bell pepper, cut into 3-inch strips

1 yellow onion, quartered, then cut into ¼-inch wedges
1 cup dry white wine
1 25-ounce jar fat-free tomato sauce
1 teaspoon dried basil
1 teaspoon dried thyme
1 18-ounce package San Genarro Basil and Garlic Polenta

CONVENIENT
AND widely available, precooked polenta is a versatile time-saver.

Spray an electric frying pan or Dutch oven with olive oil spray. Add 1 teaspoon of oil, and brown the links over medium-high heat, turning gently. Remove from pan and set aside. Refresh the pan with oil spray. Add the garlic, bell peppers, and onion and cook for 3 minutes. Return the browned links to the pan and cook for 3 minutes. Add the wine and reduce heat to medium low. Cook for 2 minutes, then add tomato sauce, basil, and thyme. Reduce heat to low and simmer for 15 minutes, stirring occasionally.

While mixture is simmering, slice polenta into ½-inch slices. Spray a 10-inch frying pan with olive oil and add remaining 1 teaspoon of oil. Over medium-high heat, sauté polenta, about 3 minutes on each side, or until brown. Remove sausage and slice into bite-size pieces. Arrange polenta and sausage on plate and top with sauce and peppers. Serve immediately.

NUTRITION ANALYSIS: PER SERVING (2 SLICES OF POLENTA WITH SAUSAGE)

| Enlightened Sautéed Polenta and Sweet Italian "Sausage" | Traditional Sautéed Polenta and Sweet Italian Sausage |
|---|---|
| Protein 8 g, carbohydrate 27 g, fiber 3 g, fat 4 g, saturated fat 1 g, cholesterol 0 mg, calcium 33 mg, sodium 500 mg Calories 189: from protein 24%, from carbohydrate 58%, from fat 18% | Protein 10 g, carbohydrate 23 g, fiber 3 g, fat 22 g, saturated fat 6 g, cholesterol 30 mg, calcium 37 mg, sodium 1092 mg Calories 338: from protein 11%, from carbohydrate 29%, from fat 60% |

# Tempeh Kebabs

*Made either on the barbecue grill or in the oven, these tasty
kebabs are delicious! You will want to have six bamboo
(or other type) of skewers on hand.*

1 recipe Roasted Chile Marinade
(page 217)
2 8-ounce packages tempeh, cubed
and steamed
3 medium Granny Smith apples,
peeled and cut into 1-inch wedges
2 medium yellow onions, cut into
¼-inch wedges

1 medium red bell pepper, cut into
2-inch pieces
1 medium yellow bell pepper, cut
into 2-inch pieces
12 cherry tomatoes

If using bamboo skewers, soak them in hot water for 20 minutes. Prepare the marinade and set aside.

Thread steamed tempeh onto skewers, with apples, onions, peppers, and tomatoes. Place in a 9-by-13-inch baking dish. Pour marinade over the kebabs and turn to coat. Set aside, covered, in the refrigerator, for at least 1 hour.

Preheat oven to 400°. Bake kebabs for 20 minutes, turning kebobs and basting several times during baking. When cooking on the barbecue, simply place Tempeh Kebabs on the preheated grill, turn and baste until brown and cooked through, about 20 minutes.

## NUTRITION ANALYSIS: PER SERVING (1 KEBAB)

| Enlightened Tempeh Kebobs | Traditional Beef Kebobs |
|---|---|
| Protein 19 g, carbohydrate 28 g, fiber 3 g, fat 5 g, cholesterol 0 mg, saturated fat 1 g, calcium 120 mg, sodium 193 mg Calories 216: from protein 34%, from carbohydrate 49%, from fat 17% | Protein 17 g, carbohydrate 20 g, fiber 3 g, fat 24 g, saturated fat 7 g, cholesterol 60 mg, calcium 32 mg, sodium 327 mg Calories 357: from protein 19%, from carbohydrate 22%, from fat 59% |

# Linguine al Pesto

*Traditionally pesto is very high in fat, because it is made with lots of oil. Not this delicious pesto!*

*8*
*Servings*

⅓ cup pine nuts
1 large bunch fresh basil leaves
4 cloves garlic, peeled
¾ cup Mori Nu Pea Soup
½ cup soy Parmesan cheese

2 tablespoons nutritional yeast
⅛ teaspoon coarse black pepper
¼ teaspoon sea salt
1 16-ounce package linguine, cooked
   according to package directions

WHOLESOME alternative ingredients combine to create a delightful pesto with all of the flavor and texture you expect—without a *drop* of oil!

Toast pine nuts in a small, dry frying pan. Place the basil and garlic in food processor and process to chop coarsely. Add pine nuts and pea soup and process. Add the soy Parmesan, nutritional yeast, black pepper, and salt. Process until well mixed, and set aside. Drain cooked pasta, and toss with pesto. Mix thoroughly and serve immediately.

NUTRITION ANALYSIS: PER 1½-CUP SERVING

**Enlightened Linguine al Pesto**
Protein 12 g, carbohydrate 50 g, fiber 4 g, fat 5 g,
saturated fat 0 g, cholesterol 0 mg,
calcium 122 mg, sodium 261mg
Calories 283: from protein 17%,
from carbohydrate 69%, from fat 14%

**Traditional Linguine al Pesto**
Protein 10 g, carbohydrate 46 g, fiber 4 g, fat 34 g,
saturated fat 5 g, cholesterol 5 mg,
calcium 148 mg, sodium 381 mg
Calories 518: from protein 8%,
from carbohydrate 35%, from fat 57%

# Sloppy Joes

*This simple dish makes a great quick lunch.*
*Use any leftovers as a tasty topping for noodles or a baked potato.*

2 cups boiling water
1 tablespoon DDC original broth
  powder
2 cups DDC Beef Not! ground
1½ teaspoons olive oil
¼ teaspoon crushed red pepper
4 cloves garlic, minced
1 cup chopped red bell pepper

1 14½-ounce can Mexican-style
  stewed tomatoes
1 6-ounce can tomato paste
2 tablespoons Dijon mustard
1 teaspoon granulated onion
1 tablespoon chile powder
1 teaspoon dried Mexican oregano
¼ cup nutritional yeast
8 whole wheat buns

Combine boiling water, broth powder, and Beef Not! in a 4-quart saucepan and set aside.

In a medium frying pan, heat oil and crushed red pepper over medium-high heat for 1 minute. Add garlic and bell pepper, and cook for 5 minutes. Add to "beef" in saucepan, stirring to mix, over medium heat. Place stewed tomatoes in food processor or blender and pulse to chop. Add chopped tomatoes to the pan with tomato paste, mustard, granulated onion, chile powder, oregano, and nutritional yeast and one tomato paste can of cold water. Stir after each addition. Reduce heat and simmer for 10 minutes. Serve over split whole wheat buns.

---

NUTRITION ANALYSIS: PER 1-CUP SERVING

| Enlightened Sloppy Joes | Traditional Sloppy Joes |
|---|---|
| Protein 16 g, carbohydrate 18 g, fiber 7 g, fat 2 g, saturated fat 0 g, cholesterol 0 mg, calcium 97 mg, sodium 296 mg Calories 134: from protein 42%, from carbohydrate 46%, from fat 12% | Protein 17 g, carbohydrate 18 g, fiber 2 g, fat 18 g, saturated fat 7 g, cholesterol 64 mg, calcium 42 mg, sodium 942 mg Calories 300: from protein 22%, from carbohydrate 24%, from fat 54% |

# "Sausage" and Asparagus Fajitas

*Boasting the culinary heritage of Mexico, fajitas have evolved to include a wide spectrum of ingredients, but with the fragrant and colorful filling still served sizzling hot!*

*8 Servings*

2 teaspoons olive oil
¼ teaspoon crushed red pepper
1 tablespoon dried minced garlic
1 large red onion, quartered, then cut into ¼-inch slices
1 large red bell pepper, cut into 2-inch strips
3 medium russet potatoes, peeled, quartered, and cut into ¼-inch slices

⅔ cup dry vermouth, divided
1 14-ounce package Gimme Lean, sausage style
12 ounces of fresh asparagus with thin stalks, cut into 3-inch pieces
3 tablespoons mango or pineapple salsa
8 whole wheat tortillas (nonhydrogenated)

Sold bulk style, sausage-flavored Gimme Lean is a wholesome alternative that adds a delicious flavor and texture to this dish, while eliminating excess fat and cholesterol.

Heat olive oil, crushed red pepper, and dried garlic over medium-high heat in a cast-iron skillet or electric frying pan for 1 minute. Add onion and bell pepper, and cook for 3 minutes. Add potatoes and cook for 8 minutes, stirring frequently. Add ⅓ cup of the vermouth and cook for 3 minutes. Add Gimme Lean, breaking it up with a large spoon. Continue to cook, stirring frequently for 5 minutes. Add asparagus pieces and reduce heat. Add the salsa and remaining ⅓ cup vermouth and simmer for 10 minutes, stirring occasionally. Warm tortillas in preheated 300° oven or microwave. Serve hot.

---

NUTRITION ANALYSIS: PER SERVING (1 TORTILLA WITH 1 CUP FILLING)

**Enlightened "Sausage" and Asparagus Fajitas**
Protein 13 g, carbohydrate 43 g, fiber 6 g, fat 2 g, saturated fat 0 g, cholesterol 0 mg, calcium 28 mg, sodium 444 mg
Calories 236: from protein 22%, from carbohydrate 71%, from fat: 7%

**Traditional Sausage and Asparagus Fajitas**
Protein 16 g, carbohydrate 36 g, fiber 3 g, fat 25 g, saturated fat 8 g, cholesterol 47 mg, calcium 77 mg, sodium 876 mg
Calories 435: from protein 14%, from carbohydrate 34%, from fat 52%

# Yam Patties with Curry Sauce

*The tasty curry sauce brings out the rich flavor*
*and texture of the yams in this dish.*

olive oil cooking spray
2 medium yams, peeled and grated
   (about 2 cups)
1 cup coarsely grated carrots
1½ cups okara, drained
1 tablespoon grated gingerroot
4 cloves garlic, minced
⅓ cup thinly sliced scallions
⅓ cup whole wheat flour

2 tablespoons egg replacer powder
⅓ cup cold water
1 26-gram package Tofu Hero Italian
   Herb Medley
¼ cup Dijon mustard
⅓ cup nutritional yeast
1 recipe Coconut Curry Sauce
   (page 198)

Preheat oven to 400°. Spray baking pan with olive oil.

In a large bowl, combine the grated yams and carrots with the okara, gingerroot, garlic, scallions, and flour. In a small bowl, whisk egg replacer with the water until foamy, then add to the vegetable mixture with the Italian Herb Medley, mustard, and nutritional yeast. Mix thoroughly. Form into 12 patties and place on prepared pan. Bake for 30 minutes, or until brown. Make Coconut Curry Sauce and serve with yam patties.

NUTRITION ANALYSIS: PER SERVING (2 PATTIES WITH ½ CUP CURRY SAUCE)

| Enlightened Yam Patties with Curry Sauce | Traditional Yam Patties with Curry Sauce |
|---|---|
| Protein 8 g, carbohydrate 38 g, fiber 5 g, fat 5 g, saturated fat 2 g, cholesterol 0 mg, calcium 50 mg, sodium 322 mg Calories 229: from protein 15%, from carbohydrate 65%, from fat 20% | Protein 8 g, carbohydrate 23 g, fiber 0 g, fat 27 g, saturated fat 7 g, cholesterol 53 mg, calcium 70 mg, sodium 827 mg Calories 362: from protein 8%, from carbohydrate 25%, from fat 67% |

# Creamed Penne and "Ham"

*Toss the cream sauce with the pasta just before serving.*

*8
Servings*

1½ teaspoons olive oil
¼ teaspoon crushed red pepper
4 cloves garlic, minced
½ cup chopped red bell pepper
1 6-ounce package veggie Canadian
    bacon, diced
⅓ cup vermouth
4 medium plum tomatoes, diced

1 16-ounce package penne
1 12.3-ounce package lite silken tofu
2 tablespoons mellow white miso
1½ cups enriched 1% fat soymilk
1 tablespoon lemon juice
½ cup nutritional yeast
1 teaspoon granulated garlic
1 teaspoon Bragg Liquid Aminos

WHEN REHEATING leftovers, mix in a little hot vegetable broth, as the starch in the pasta will thicken the sauce as it sits.

In a stovetop- and oven-safe casserole, heat oil and crushed red pepper for 1 minute. Add minced garlic, bell pepper, and veggie Canadian bacon. Cook for 3 minutes, stirring frequently. Add vermouth and tomatoes and lower heat to medium low. Simmer for 10 minutes, stirring frequently. Cook pasta according to package directions, drain, and add to bacon and tomato mixture. Set aside and keep warm.

Place tofu in food processor and process until smooth, about 1 minute. Add miso, soymilk, and lemon juice. Blend. Add yeast, granulated garlic, and aminos. Set aside and fold into the pasta mixture just before serving.

NUTRITION ANALYSIS: PER 1½-CUP SERVING

| Enlightened Creamed Penne and "Ham" | Traditional Creamed Penne and Ham |
|---|---|
| Protein 16 g, carbohydrate 38 g, fiber 3 g, fat 3 g, saturated fat 0 g, cholesterol 0 mg, calcium 84 mg, sodium 279 mg. Calories 194: from protein 26%, from carbohydrate 64%, from fat 10% | Protein 15 g, carbohydrate 24 g, fiber 2 g, fat 22 g, saturated fat 12 g, cholesterol 63 mg, calcium 223 mg, sodium 685 mg Calories 356: from protein 17%, from carbohydrate 27%, from fat 56% |

# "Beefy" Polenta Bake

*This dish features a hearty stew baked under a*
*basil and garlic polenta crust. Yummy!*

Enticing
Entrées

141

8
*Servings*

1½ teaspoons DDC original broth powder

1½ cups DDC Beef Not! strips

2½ cups boiling water, divided

¾ cup diced dry packed sun-dried tomatoes

1½ teaspoons olive oil

¼ teaspoon crushed red pepper

2 cloves garlic, minced

1 small red onion, chopped

2 stalks celery, halved vertically, then cut into ¼-inch slices

2 medium zucchini, cut into ¼-inch slices

1 15-ounce can cannellini beans or white kidney beans

2 tablespoons nutritional yeast

¼ cup chopped flat-leaf parsley

2½ teaspoons dried marjoram, divided

1 18-ounce package San Gennaro precooked Basil and Garlic polenta

1 14½-ounce can Mexican-style tomatoes

1 tablespoon soy Parmesan cheese

Preheat oven to 350°.

Over medium-high heat, combine broth powder, "beef" strips, and 1½ cups boiling water in a medium saucepan. Bring to a second boil, reduce heat to simmer, and cook for 15 minutes, stirring occasionally. Set aside. Combine sun-dried tomatoes and 1 cup boiling water in a small bowl and set aside.

In a 5-quart stovetop- and oven-safe casserole dish, heat oil and crushed red pepper over medium-high heat for 1 minute. Add garlic, onion, and celery. Cook for 3 minutes. Add zucchini and cook for 2 minutes. Add reconstituted "beef strips" and sun-dried tomatoes with their soaking liquid. Lower heat and simmer mixture for 5 minutes, stirring occasionally. Add beans, yeast, parsley,

**"Beefy" Polenta Bake** *(continued)*

and 1½ teaspoons marjoram. Slice polenta into ¼-inch slices and layer, over-lapping, on top of zucchini mixture. Place tomatoes in food processor and process to blend, but not purée. Pour over polenta. Sprinkle with Parmesan and remaining 1 teaspoon marjoram. Bake, uncovered 35 minutes.

---

NUTRITION ANALYSIS: PER 2-CUP SERVING

Enlightened "Beefy" Polenta Bake
Protein 16 g, carbohydrate 34 g, fiber 8 g, fat 2 g,
saturated fat 0 g, cholesterol 0 mg,
calcium 87 mg, sodium 447 mg
Calories 205: from protein 30%,
from carbohydrate 63%, from fat 7%

Traditional Beefy Polenta Bake
Protein 19 g, carbohydrate 28 g, fiber 5 g, fat 21 g,
saturated fat 6 g, cholesterol 79 mg,
calcium 105 mg, sodium 755 mg
Calories 373: from protein 20%,
from carbohydrate 30%, from fat 50%

# Pineapple "Chicken"

*Serve this tasty dish with whole wheat couscous.*

1 recipe Pacific Blend Marinade
    (page 214)
2 6-ounce packages Smart Chick'n
    Strips
1½ teaspoons olive oil
4 cloves garlic, minced
1 tablespoon freshly grated
    gingerroot
1 medium yellow onion, chopped

⅓ cup chopped green bell pepper
1 cup sliced baby-cut carrots
1 8-ounce can pineapple chunks,
    drained, reserving syrup
1 6-ounce package fresh baby spinach
⅓ cup dry sherry
½ cup chopped fresh cilantro
2 tablespoon cornstarch
2 tablespoon cold water

Combine the marinade ingredients in a glass liquid measuring cup. Place Chick'n Strips in a medium nonreactive bowl and add marinade. Cover and refrigerate for 30 minutes to an hour.

In a Dutch oven or electric frying pan, heat oil for 1 minute over medium-high heat. Add garlic, gingerroot, onion, bell pepper, and carrots. Cook for 5 minutes. Add Chick'n Strips and pineapple to the pan, reserving marinade and syrup. Cook mixture for 5 minutes, stirring frequently. Add spinach and reduce heat to medium low. Cook until spinach has softened, about 3 minutes. Add sherry and cilantro and cook for 5 minutes, stirring occasionally. In a small bowl, blend cornstarch and water and stir into the reserved pineapple syrup. Set aside. Pour marinade into pan and stir in cornstarch mixture. Simmer for 5 minutes, or until ready to serve.

MARINATING THE soy-based Chick'n Strips enhances the complementary balance of flavors in this dish.

---

NUTRITION ANALYSIS: PER 1½-CUP SERVING

**Enlightened Pineapple "Chicken"**
Protein 9 g, carbohydrate 19 g, fiber 4 g, fat 4 g,
saturated fat 0 g, cholesterol 0 mg,
calcium 69 mg, sodium 758 mg
Calories 128: from protein 27%,
from carbohydrate 64%, from fat 9%

**Traditional Pineapple Chicken**
Protein 12 g, carbohydrate 17 g, fiber 2 g, fat 22 g,
saturated fat 7 g, cholesterol 59 mg,
calcium 53 mg, sodium 836 mg
Calories 316: from protein 15%,
from carbohydrate 22%, from fat 63%

# Penne with Tofu Tomato Sauce

*Chunks of firm tofu smothered in tomato sauce
and tossed with pasta taste delicious!*

1½ teaspoons olive oil
¼ teaspoon crushed red pepper
1 tablespoon dried minced garlic
⅔ cup chopped yellow onion
olive oil cooking spray
16 to 19 ounces firm Chinese-style
   tofu, cubed
½ cup vermouth

1 25-ounce jar tomato sauce
1 tablespoon nutritional yeast
1 teaspoon dried thyme
½ teaspoon dried marjoram
1 cup frozen peas, thawed
1 16-ounce package penne
⅓ cup soy Parmesan cheese

In a 5-quart saucepan or electric frying pan, heat oil and crushed red pepper. Add garlic and onion and cook over medium-high heat for 2 minutes. Push veggies to one side, spray clear side with olive oil cooking spray, and add cubed tofu. Sauté, turning frequently, for 8 minutes, or until tofu is brown on all sides. Add vermouth and tomato sauce, and lower heat to medium low. Add nutritional yeast, thyme, marjoram, and peas. Simmer for 10 minutes, stirring frequently.

Cook pasta according to package directions, drain, and toss with soy Parmesan and just enough of the tomato/tofu mixture to moisten. Reserve the remainder of the sauce to top individual servings. Keep warm until ready to serve.

NUTRITION ANALYSIS: PER 1½-CUP SERVING

**Enlightened Pasta
with Tofu Tomato Sauce**
Protein 15 g, carbohydrate 32 g, fiber 4 g, fat 6 g,
saturated fat 0 g, cholesterol 0 mg,
calcium 101 mg, sodium 254 mg
Calories 206: from protein 22%,
from carbohydrate 53%, from fat 25%

**Traditional Pasta with Beef Cubes
and Tomato Sauce**
Protein 15 g, carbohydrate 24 g, fiber 3 g, fat 20 g,
saturated fat 7 g, cholesterol 46 mg,
calcium 50 mg, sodium 490 mg
Calories 349: from protein 18%,
from carbohydrate 28%, from fat 54%

# Vegetable Curry with Tofu

*Broccoli, carrots, and corn add color, texture, and balance to the tofu in this easy curry. However, you may use any mix of vegetables you have on hand.*

---

1 recipe Coconut Curry Sauce,
   (page 198)
olive oil cooking spray
1 tablespoon dried minced garlic
16 ounces firm nigari tofu, cubed
1 teaspoon olive oil

⅓ cup minced shallots
1½ cups chopped carrots
3 cups broccoli florets, cut to bite size
¼ cup vegetable broth
1 cup frozen white corn, thawed

Prepare curry sauce and set aside.

  Spray an electric frying pan or Dutch oven with olive oil cooking spray and add garlic. Warm pan over medium-high heat for 1 minute. Add tofu and brown on all sides, refreshing again with oil spray if necessary. Remove tofu and set aside. Add olive oil to the pan and add shallots, carrots, and broccoli. Cook for 5 minutes, stirring frequently. Add tofu, cook for 3 minutes, then add vegetable broth and corn. Lower heat to medium low, add curry sauce, and simmer for 10 minutes, stirring occasionally.

---

NUTRITION ANALYSIS: PER 1½-CUP SERVING

**Enlightened Vegetable Curry with Tofu**
Protein 12 g, carbohydrate 19 g, fiber 5 g, fat 6 g,
saturated fat 2 g, cholesterol 0 mg,
calcium 67 mg, sodium 130 mg
Calories 172: from protein 26%,
from carbohydrate 44%, from fat 30%

**Traditional Vegetable Curry with Beef**
Protein 14 g, carbohydrate 16 g, fiber 3 g, fat 23 g,
saturated fat 13 g, cholesterol 51 mg,
calcium 48 mg, sodium 469 mg
Calories 318: from protein 17%,
from carbohydrate 19%, from fat 64%

# Open-Faced Grilled "Cheese" Triangles

*Before I kicked dairy out of my life for good more than ten years
ago, my favorite breakfast was grilled cheese and tomato slices, with
strong coffee. I still drink the coffee, but now it is accompanied by
a far healthier, and just as delicious, grilled "cheese."*

*4
Servings*

8 slices whole grain bread
2½ tablespoons Dijon mustard
1 tomato, quartered and cut into
 slices, or 4 whole Melissa's Fire
 Roasted Chiles, diced

½ cup Homemade Dairy-Free
 "Cheese" (page 202)

Preheat broiler.

Cut each slice of bread in half diagonally, creating triangles. Spread bread
with about ½ teaspoon Dijon mustard, and top with tomato or chiles. Place on
broiler pan and spoon "cheese" over all. Place under preheated
broiler for a few minutes, or until brown.

LOOK FOR multi-grain
bread that is fat-free,
dairy-free, and sweetened
with molasses.

## NUTRITION ANALYSIS: PER SERVING (4 TRIANGLES)

| Enlightened Grilled "Cheese" | Traditional Grilled Cheese |
|---|---|
| Protein 8 g, carbohydrate 34 g, fiber 4 g, fat 0 g, | Protein 15 g, carbohydrate 31 g, fiber 2 g, fat 26 g, |
| saturated fat 0 g, cholesterol 0 mg, | saturated fat 16 g, cholesterol 72 mg, |
| calcium 32 mg, sodium 218 mg | calcium 300 mg, sodium 890 mg |
| Calories 173: from protein 19%, | Calories 426: from protein 15%, |
| from carbohydrate 79%, from fat 2% | from carbohydrate 30%, from fat 55% |

# Balsamic "Chicken"

*In this recipe we replace chicken with Textured Vegetable Protein, or TVP.
Using this delicious soyfood alternative instead of animal products
eliminates unhealthy saturated fat and cholesterol from the diet.*

2 tablespoons DDC original broth
    powder
2 cups DDC Chicken Not! Strips
2 cups boiling water
2 teaspoons olive oil
¼ teaspoon crushed red pepper
4 cloves garlic, minced
⅓ cup minced shallots

3 cups sliced fresh green beans
6 ounces cremini mushrooms, sliced
3 large plum tomatoes, diced
⅓ cup dry sherry
1 tablespoon balsamic vinegar
¼ cup chopped fresh basil
2 teaspoons Bragg Liquid Aminos
3 tablespoons pine nuts

In a medium saucepan, combine broth powder and Chicken Not!
Strips with boiling water. Bring to a second boil, cover, and reduce
heat. Simmer for 10 minutes and set aside.

In a 5-quart saucepan or Dutch oven, heat oil and crushed red
pepper over medium-high heat for 1 minute. Add garlic and shallots, sauté for 3 minutes, then add green beans and mushrooms.
Cook for 5 minutes, then add reconstituted "chicken" with any
liquid that remains. Reduce heat to medium low and cook mixture
for 10 minutes, stirring frequently. Add tomatoes, sherry, and balsamic vinegar. Reduce heat further and add chopped basil and liquid aminos.
Simmer for 5 minutes, stirring occasionally. In a small, dry frying pan, toast
pine nuts over medium heat, shaking pan, until nuts are fragrant and lightly
brown, about 3 minutes. Sprinkle over Balsamic "Chicken" just before serving.

BALSAMIC vinegar is a
study in balance and con-
trast. This classic dish
takes full advantage of the
dramatic flavor notes of
this fragrant seasoning.

---

### NUTRITION ANALYSIS: PER 2-CUP SERVING

**Enlightened Balsamic "Chicken"**
Protein 18 g, carbohydrate 58 g, fiber 9 g, fat 5 g,
saturated fat 1 g, cholesterol 0 mg,
calcium 107 mg, sodium 236 mg
Calories 191: from protein 21%,
from carbohydrate 66%, from fat 13%

**Traditional Balsamic Chicken**
Protein 24 g, carbohydrate 13 g, fiber 4 g, fat 21 g,
saturated fat 6 g, cholesterol 72 mg,
calcium 50 mg, sodium 592 mg
Calories 323: from protein 28%,
from carbohydrate 16%, from fat 56%

# Burmese Curry

*I chose a wholesome soy-based
poultry alternative for this delicious dish.*

*8
Servings*

1½ teaspoons olive oil
¼ teaspoon crushed red pepper
1 tablespoon dried minced garlic
1 rounded tablespoon grated
  fresh gingerroot
⅓ cup minced shallots
1 medium red onion, chopped
⅓ cup chopped red bell pepper
3 cups diced, peeled potatoes
2 6-ounce packages Smart Chick'n
  Strips

1 15-ounce can garbanzo beans
2 plum tomatoes, chopped
1 teaspoon turmeric
1 teaspoon ground ginger
1 teaspoon ground coriander
2 cinnamon sticks
1 cup hot chicken-flavor vegetarian
  broth
1 14-ounce can lite coconut milk

Myanmar, formerly
known as Burma, provides
the inspiration for this
dish. This cuisine tends to
fall somewhere between
Chinese and Thai. It is
richer than Chinese food,
and less spicy than Thai
food.

Heat oil, crushed red pepper, and garlic over medium-high heat in
an electric frying pan or Dutch oven for 1 minute. Add gingerroot,
shallots, onion, and bell pepper. Sauté for 3 minutes, then add
potatoes. Cook for 8 minutes, or until potatoes are softening, stirring frequently. Add Chick'n Strips to the pan along with garbanzo
beans, chopped tomatoes, turmeric, ground ginger, coriander, and
cinnamon sticks. Cook mixture for 5 minutes. Lower heat and add
broth and coconut milk. Simmer for 10 minutes, stirring occasionally. Discard cinnamon sticks before serving.

NUTRITION ANALYSIS: PER 1½-CUP SERVING

**Enlightened Burmese Curry**
Protein 10 g, carbohydrate 25 g, fiber 5 g, fat 4 g,
saturated fat 2 g, cholesterol 0 mg,
calcium 56 mg, sodium 247 mg
Calories 176: from protein 23%,
from carbohydrate 56%, from fat 21%

**Traditional Burmese Curry**
Protein 11 g, carbohydrate 16 g, fiber 3 g, fat 35 g,
saturated fat 16 g, cholesterol 45 mg,
calcium 33 mg, sodium 132 mg
Calories 302: from protein 14%,
from carbohydrate 20%, from fat 66%

# Five-Spice Tofu and Snow Peas in Ginger "Cream"

*A unique combination of flavors is used to make this luscious ginger "cream" sauce. Serve with basmati rice.*

1 ounce dried shitake mushrooms
2 cups boiling water
2 teaspoons olive oil
4 cloves garlic, minced
2 tablespoons grated fresh gingerroot
1 small leek, thinly sliced
1 medium red bell pepper, cut into 2-inch strips
1 8-ounce package Five-Spice Baked Tofu, sliced on an angle
1 9-ounce package fresh snow peas

1 8-ounce can sliced water chestnuts, drained
¼ cup dry sherry
1¾ cups Mori Nu Butternut Squash Soup
¼ cup Mori Nu Tomato Soup
2 tablespoons chopped fresh cilantro
1 teaspoon ground ginger
1 teaspoon granulated onion
1 teaspoon granulated garlic
1 tablespoon tamari lite

Rinse shitake mushrooms and combine with boiling water in a small saucepan. Bring to a second boil, reduce heat, and simmer for 5 minutes. Set aside to soak.

In a 5-quart stovetop-safe casserole, warm oil over medium-high heat for 1 minute. Add minced garlic, gingerroot, leek, and bell pepper, and cook for 3 minutes. Remove mushrooms from soaking water and cut into ¼-inch slices. Add mushrooms and tofu to casserole dish, cook for 2 minutes, then add snow peas, water chestnuts, and sherry. Reduce heat, add soups, and simmer for 3 minutes. Add cilantro, ginger, onion, granulated garlic, and tamari, and simmer for 5 minutes. Serve with basmati rice.

---

NUTRITION ANALYSIS: PER 2-CUP SERVING

| Enlightened Five-Spice Tofu and Snow Peas in Ginger "Cream" | Traditional Five-Spice Duck and Snow Peas in Ginger Cream |
|---|---|
| Protein 13 g, carbohydrate 27 g, fiber 6 g, fat 4 g, saturated fat 1 g, cholesterol 0 mg, calcium 39 mg, sodium 536 mg | Protein 8 g, carbohydrate 29 g, fiber 5 g, fat 27 g, saturated fat 15 g, cholesterol 0 mg, calcium 81 mg, sodium 535 mg |
| Calories 194: from protein 26%, from carbohydrate 56%, from fat 18% | Calories 386: from protein 8%, from carbohydrate 30%, from fat 62% |

# Hearty Tempeh and Potato Roast

*This tasty casserole is rich in flavor,
texture, and eye appeal.*

1 recipe Sweet 'n' Sassy Marinade
(page 210)
2 8-ounce packages tempeh, cubed
and steamed
olive oil cooking spray
4 medium russet potatoes, peeled
and cut into ¼-inch slices

1 medium yellow onion, cut into
¼-inch wedges
3 bell peppers, (1 each red, yellow,
and green) cut into 3-inch strips
12 ripe cherry tomatoes, cut in half

Tempeh can be steamed in
advance. Store, covered, in
the refrigerator for up to
5 days.

Prepare marinade. Place tempeh and marinade in a large, nonreactive bowl (preferably glass), cover, and set aside for at least 1 hour.

Preheat oven to 400°. Spray a 9-by-13-inch baking pan with olive oil cooking spray. Add potatoes, onions, peppers, and tomatoes to tempeh, and stir to mix. Turn mixture into prepared baking pan. Cover with foil and bake for 20 minutes. Remove foil and bake for 10 minutes longer, or until lightly browned.

## NUTRITION ANALYSIS: PER 2-CUP SERVING

**Enlightened Hearty Tempeh and Potato Roast**
Protein 11 g, carbohydrate 34 g, fiber 5 g, fat 3 g,
saturated fat 0 g, cholesterol 0 mg
calcium 130 mg, sodium 194 mg
Calories 205: from protein 23%,
from carbohydrate 63%, from fat 14%

**Traditional Beef and Potato Roast**
Protein 13 g, carbohydrate 22 g, fiber 2 g, fat 18 g,
saturated fat 5 g, cholesterol 40 mg,
calcium 24 mg, sodium 664 mg
Calories 297: from protein 18%,
from carbohydrate 29%, from fat 53%

# North African Stew (Sikbadj)

*This delicious Moroccan stew is rich in healthful soy,
replacing unhealthy traditional ingredients that are notoriously
high in saturated fat and unnecessary cholesterol.*

2 8-ounce packages tempeh, cubed
2 teaspoons olive oil
¼ teaspoon crushed red pepper
4 cloves garlic, minced
1 large yellow onion, chopped
3 cups sliced zucchini, cut into half
   circles
1 15-ounce can garbanzo beans,
   drained
1 14½-ounce can Italian-style,
   stewed tomatoes, diced

½ cup beef-flavored vegetarian broth,
   boiling
2 cinnamon sticks
1 cup chopped dried apricots
1 cup date pieces
½ teaspoon ground coriander
¼ teaspoon ground allspice
⅓ cup chopped fresh cilantro
2 tablespoons toasted sesame seeds
   (optional)

Steam cubed tempeh for 15 minutes and set aside.

In a 5-quart saucepan, heat oil and crushed red pepper over medium-high heat for 1 minute. Add garlic and onion and sauté for 3 minutes. Add tempeh and cook for 10 minutes, stirring frequently. Add zucchini, garbanzo beans, and tomatoes. Reduce heat to medium and cook mixture for 3 minutes, then add broth and cinnamon sticks. Add apricots, dates, coriander, allspice, and cilantro. Lower heat and simmer, stirring occasionally, for 15 minutes. Sprinkle with toasted sesame seeds, if desired. Remove cinnamon sticks before serving.

---

### NUTRITION ANALYSIS: PER 1½-CUP SERVING

| Enlightened North African Stew | Traditional North African Stew |
| --- | --- |
| Protein 17 g, carbohydrate 51 g, fiber 9 g, fat 5 g, saturated fat 1 g, cholesterol 0 mg, calcium 159 mg, sodium 147 mg Calories 308: from protein 22%, from carbohydrate 64%, from fat 14% | Protein 23 g, carbohydrate 35 g, fiber 6 g, fat 27 g, saturated fat 8 g, cholesterol 78 mg, calcium 88 mg, sodium 370 mg Calories 468: from protein 19%, from carbohydrate 30%, from fat 51% |

*8
Servings*

# Balsamic "Beef" and Broccoli

*Serve this hearty dish, with its fusion of flavors
and textures, over brown rice or pasta.*

1½ teaspoons olive oil
1 tablespoon dried minced garlic
1 14-ounce package Gimme Lean,
   ground beef style
6 cups fresh broccoli florets
   (1 medium head)
1 15-ounce can garbanzo beans,
   drained

1 6-ounce can tomato paste
¾ cup boiling water
1 tablespoon balsamic vinegar
¼ cup chopped fresh basil
¼ cup fruity red wine, such as Sirah,
   Shiraz, or Grenach
1 25-ounce jar tomato and basil
   sauce
½ cup pitted kalamata olives, sliced

Heat oil and garlic in a 5-quart saucepan for 1 minute. Add Gimme Lean and
cook for 5 minutes, breaking apart with a large spoon. Add broccoli and cook
for 3 minutes, stirring frequently. Add garbanzo beans and lower heat to
medium low. In a large glass measuring cup, combine tomato paste, boiling
water, vinegar, and basil. Stir into the broccoli mixture. Add the wine, tomato
sauce, and olives. Simmer for 5 minutes.

## NUTRITION ANALYSIS: PER 2-CUP SERVING

**Enlightened Balsamic "Beef" and Broccoli**
Protein 17 g, carbohydrate 29 g, fiber 10 g, fat 4 g,
saturated fat 0 g, cholesterol 0 mg,
calcium 61 mg, sodium 534 mg
Calories 206: from protein 30%,
from carbohydrate 53%, from fat 17%

**Traditional Balsamic Beef and Broccoli**
Protein 17 g, carbohydrate 25 g, fiber 7 g, fat 25 g,
saturated fat 7 g, cholesterol 49 mg,
calcium 48 mg, sodium 869 mg
Calories 389: from protein 17%,
from carbohydrate 26%, from fat 57%

# Onion Okara Burgers

*These delicious burgers use
onion broth powder for extra flavor.*

olive oil cooking spray
1½ cups beef-flavor vegetarian broth, boiling
¾ cup quick-cooking barley
2 cups okara
¼ cup whole wheat flour
¼ cup Barbara's mashed potato flakes
1 tablespoon DDC onion broth powder
½ cup nutritional yeast
½ tablespoon nonaluminum baking powder
½ cup thinly sliced scallions
½ cup shredded carrots
4 cloves garlic, minced
1 teaspoon dried thyme
paprika for garnish

Preheat oven to 400°. Spray a baking pan with olive oil spray.

Combine boiling broth and barley, bring to a second boil, and reduce heat to low. Simmer for 12 minutes, or until liquid is absorbed. Set aside. In a large bowl, combine okara, cooked barley, flour, potato flakes, broth powder, yeast, and baking powder, mixing well after each addition. Add scallions, carrots, garlic, and thyme and mix thoroughly. Form into patties and place on prepared pan. Sprinkle with paprika and bake for 30 minutes, or until brown. Serve with tomato sauce or salsa.

YOU CAN combine the ingredients and set aside in the refrigerator for up to 24 hours in advance. If you do this, do not add the baking powder until just before shaping and baking the patties.

---

NUTRITION ANALYSIS: PER SERVING (1 BURGER)

**Enlightened Onion Okara Burgers**
Protein 8 g, carbohydrate 28 g, fiber 6 g, fat 1 g,
saturated fat 0 g, cholesterol 0 mg,
calcium 95 mg, sodium 169 mg
Calories 147: from protein 20%,
from carbohydrate 72%, from fat 8%

**Traditional Onion Burgers**
Protein 14 g, carbohydrate 14 g, fiber 0 g, fat 24 g,
saturated fat 8 g, cholesterol 83 mg,
calcium 69 mg, sodium 489 mg
Calories 311: from protein 18%,
from carbohydrate 14%, from fat 68%

# A-Maize-ing Okara Burgers

*Okara, the by-product of soymilk making, is a hearty and nutritious ingredient that adds protein, fiber, and the goodness of soy to any dish.*

olive oil cooking spray
1½ cups okara
¼ cup whole wheat flour
2 tablespoons whole grain yellow cornmeal
2 tablespoons Barbara's mashed potato flakes
2 cups cooked brown rice

⅓ cup nutritional yeast
1 26-gram package Tofu Hero Italian Herb Medley
1 teaspoon nonaluminum baking powder
½ teaspoon granulated garlic
1 teaspoon dried marjoram
1 cup frozen corn, thawed

Preheat oven to 400°. Spray a baking pan with olive oil cooking spray.

Combine okara, flour, cornmeal, and potato flakes in a large bowl. Add rice, yeast, Italian Herb Medley, baking powder, garlic, and marjoram. Mix thoroughly and add corn. Form into 8 equal patties and place on prepared baking pan. Bake for 25 minutes, or until brown. Serve with ketchup or applesauce.

## NUTRITION ANALYSIS: PER SERVING (1 BURGER)

| Enlightened A-Maize-ing Okara Burgers | Traditional Hamburgers |
| --- | --- |
| Protein 6 g, carbohydrate 28 g, fiber 4 g, fat 1 g, saturated fat 0 g, cholesterol 0 mg, calcium 63 mg, sodium 178 mg Calories 133: from protein 16%, from carbohydrate 76%, from fat 8% | Protein 13 g, carbohydrate 3 g, fiber 0 g, fat 23 g, saturated fat 8 g, cholesterol 107 mg, calcium 46 mg, sodium 266 mg Calories 271: from protein 19%, from carbohydrate 4%, from fat 77% |

# Quick Soy Burgers

*These tasty burgers are high in protein and fiber, and low in
fat and calories. With a little leftover rice and wholesome
TVP, you can mix and bake these in no time.*

olive oil cooking spray
1½ cups boiling water
1 tablespoon DDC original broth
    powder
1½ cups DDC Beef Not! ground
1 cup cooked brown rice
¼ cup tomato paste

¼ cup nutritional yeast
1 teaspoons granulated garlic
1 26-gram package Tofu Hero Italian
    Herb Medley
1 tablespoon egg replacer powder
¼ cup cold water
⅓ cup barbecue sauce

Preheat oven to 400°. Spray baking pan with olive oil.

Combine the boiling water, broth powder, and Beef Not! in a medium
saucepan. Bring to a second boil, reduce heat to low, and simmer for 15 minutes. Set aside.

Combine brown rice, tomato paste, yeast, garlic, and Italian Herb Medley,
mixing well after each addition. Add reconstituted "beef." In a small bowl,
whisk egg replacer with water until foamy, and add to "beef" mixture. Mix
thoroughly. Form into 8 patties and place on prepared pan. Top with barbecue
sauce and bake for 20 minutes, or until brown.

NUTRITION ANALYSIS: PER SERVING (1 BURGER)

| Enlightened Soy Burgers | Traditional Burgers |
|---|---|
| Protein 18 g, carbohydrate 26 g, fiber 7 g, fat 2 g, | Protein 20 g, carbohydrate 11 g, fiber 0 g, fat 28 g, |
| saturated fat 0 g, cholesterol 0 mg, | saturated fat 11 g, cholesterol 119 mg, |
| calcium 83 mg, sodium 255 mg | calcium 67 mg, sodium 585 mg |
| Calories 165: from protein 38%, | Calories 381: from protein 22%, |
| from carbohydrate 55%, from fat 7% | from carbohydrate 12%, from fat 66% |

*6
Servings*

# Broccoli and Potato Curry

*Broccoli is often paired with potatoes in curry dishes,
as it provides a good balance of texture, color, and flavor.*

olive oil cooking spray
1 teaspoon olive oil
¼ teaspoon crushed red pepper
2 tablespoons grated fresh gingerroot
4 cloves garlic, minced
1 medium red onion, cut into
  ¼-inch wedges
½ cup chopped red bell pepper
2 medium russet potatoes, peeled
  and cubed

2 medium plum tomatoes, diced
½ cup dry vermouth
½ teaspoon turmeric
4 cups fresh broccoli florets
1 14-ounce can lite coconut milk
1 tablespoon Thai green curry paste
⅓ cup chopped fresh cilantro

Spray a Dutch oven or electric frying pan with olive oil cooking spray, and heat over medium-high heat. Add oil and crushed red pepper, heat for 1 minute, then add gingerroot, garlic, onion, and bell pepper. Cook for 3 minutes. Add potatoes and cook for 8 minutes, stirring frequently and spraying lightly with oil spray as needed. Add tomatoes, vermouth, and turmeric, and cook mixture for 5 minutes. Add broccoli and cook for 3 minutes. Heat coconut milk in microwave-safe bowl for 2 minutes, or on stovetop for 3 minutes. Add curry paste, stirring to blend. Add coconut milk mixture and chopped cilantro to the vegetable mixture and reduce heat to low. Simmer 4 minutes, or until broccoli is tender but not overcooked. Serve with basmati rice.

## NUTRITION ANALYSIS: PER 1½-CUP SERVING

**Enlightened Broccoli and Potato Curry**
Protein 5 g, carbohydrate 21 g, fiber 4 g, fat 5 g,
saturated fat 3 g, cholesterol 0 mg,
calcium 44 mg, sodium 78 mg
Calories 155: from protein 19%,
from carbohydrate 53%, from fat 28%

**Traditional Burgers**
Protein 7 g, carbohydrate 21 g, fiber 4 g, fat 23 g,
saturated fat 18 g, cholesterol 27 mg,
calcium 72 mg, sodium 159 mg
Calories 321: from protein 9%,
from carbohydrate 26%, from fat 65%

# Braised Tempeh
# with Mushrooms and Tomatoes

*Braising combines two cooking techniques: sautéing to develop flavor and
color, and slow cooking in a small amount of liquid.*

2 8-ounce packages tempeh, cubed
1½ teaspoons olive oil
¼ teaspoon crushed red pepper
4 cloves garlic, minced
½ cup sliced scallions
1 cup coarsely shredded carrots

6 ounces cremini mushrooms, sliced
½ cup dry sherry
1 14½-ounce can Mexican-style
   stewed tomatoes
1 cup frozen corn, thawed

Steam cubed tempeh for 15 minutes and set aside.

Place oil and crushed red pepper in a 5-quart saucepan or electric frying pan, and warm over medium-high heat, for 1 minute.
Add garlic, scallions, and carrots, and sauté for 3 minutes. Add
tempeh and cook mixture for 8 minutes, stirring frequently. Add
mushrooms, stir 1 minute, then add sherry and tomatoes. Reduce
heat to medium low. Add corn and simmer for 10 minutes, stirring
occasionally.

YOU MAY USE any
variety of tempeh in this
dish, but it is best made
with tempeh that contains
"sea vegetables." Rich in
minerals like calcium and
iodine, such seaweed is very
low in calories and fat.

---

NUTRITION ANALYSIS: PER 1½-CUP SERVING

Enlightened Braised Tempeh
with Mushrooms and Tomatoes.
Protein 15 g, carbohydrate 30 g, fiber 7 g, fat 5 g,
saturated fat 0 g, cholesterol 0 mg,
calcium 199 mg, sodium 184 mg
Calories 230: from protein 26%,
from carbohydrate 53%, from fat 21%

Traditional Braised Beef
with Mushrooms and Tomatoes
Protein 16 g, carbohydrate 14 g, fiber 3 g, fat 24 g,
saturated fat 7 g, cholesterol 53 mg,
calcium 40 mg, sodium 385 mg
Calories 348: from protein 19%,
from carbohydrate 17%, from fat 64%

# "Beef" and Asparagus Oriental

*The flavorful marinade is reserved and added at the finish in this healthy Asian-style entrée.*

*6
Servings*

1 recipe Orient Express Marinade
  (page 213)
2 8-ounce packages seitan (not
  packed in broth)
1½ teaspoons olive oil
4 cloves garlic, minced
½ cup thinly sliced scallions
½ cup chopped red bell pepper
1 tablespoon grated fresh gingerroot

1½ cups julienned baby-cut carrots
1 pound asparagus spears, trimmed
  and sliced into 3-inch pieces
1 fresh tomato, diced
¼ cup dry sherry
1 8-ounce can sliced water chestnuts,
  drained
2 tablespoons cornstarch
2 tablespoons cold water

Combine the marinade ingredients in a glass liquid measuring cup and set aside. Tear the seitan into bite-size pieces and place in a medium, nonreactive bowl. Add marinade, cover, and refrigerate for at least 1 hour.

Heat oil in a Dutch oven or electric frying pan over medium-high heat for 1 minute. Add garlic, scallions, bell pepper, gingerroot, and carrots. Cook for 3 minutes, stirring frequently. Add seitan to the pan, reserving marinade. Cook for 3 minutes, then add asparagus, tomato, and sherry. Lower heat and simmer for 5 minutes, stirring ocassionally. Add the reserved marinade and water chestnuts. Combine cornstarch and water in a small bowl and stir into the pan. Simmer for 5 minutes and serve with rice.

---

NUTRITION ANALYSIS: PER 2-CUP SERVING

**Enlightened "Beef" and Asparagus Oriental**
Protein 15 g, carbohydrate 26 g, fiber 10 g, fat 2 g,
saturated fat 0 g, cholesterol 0 mg,
calcium 69 mg, sodium 674 mg
Calories 188: from protein 34%,
from carbohydrate 57%, from fat 9%

**Traditional Beef and Asparagus Oriental**
Protein 18 g, carbohydrate 19 g, fiber 4 g, fat 29 g,
saturated fat 8 g, cholesterol 53 mg,
calcium 56 mg, sodium 1641 mg
Calories 408: from protein 18%,
from carbohydrate 18%, from fat 64%

# Tempeh and Sweet Beans

*This easy to assemble dish combines hearty tempeh with edamame.*
*Serve over brown rice or pasta.*

olive oil cooking spray
¼ teaspoon crushed red pepper
1 tablespoon dried minced garlic
1 8-ounce package tempeh, cubed
    and steamed for 15 minutes
1 10-ounce package edamame (ready
    to eat, or cooked and drained)

⅓ cup dry sherry
1 25-ounce jar roasted red pepper
    tomato sauce (or your personal
    favorite)

*6*
*Servings*

Spray a 2-quart stovetop- and oven-safe casserole with olive oil cooking spray. Add crushed red pepper and garlic and heat for 1 minute over medium-high heat. Add tempeh and cook, turning often, for 5 minutes or until lightly browned. Add edamame, cook for 2 minutes, then add sherry. Lower heat to medium and add tomato sauce. Cook mixture for 10 minutes or until heated through.

EDAMAME, sometimes called sweet beans, are actually immature soybeans.

## NUTRITION ANALYSIS: PER 1½-CUP SERVING

**Enlightened Tempeh and Sweet Beans**
Protein 13 g, carbohydrate 22 g, fiber 7 g, fat 5 g,
saturated fat 1 g, cholesterol 0 mg,
calcium 111 mg, sodium 406 mg
Calories 197: from protein 28%,
from carbohydrate 47%, from fat 25%

**Traditional Beef and Beans**
Protein 16 g, carbohydrate 21 g, fiber 4 g, fat 16 g,
saturated fat 6 g, cholesterol 60 mg,
calcium 58 mg, sodium 952 mg
Calories 295: from protein 22%,
from carbohydrate 29%, from fat 49%

# "Beef" Vindaloo

*Originally created by Portuguese settlers in the tiny Indian
state of Goa, vindaloo is a fragrant, spicy stew.
Serve with Pineapple Basmati Pilaf (page 176).*

*6*
*Servings*

1½ teaspoons olive oil
½ teaspoon crushed red pepper
   (or to taste)
1 tablespoon dried minced garlic
2 tablespoons grated fresh gingerroot
1 large onion, halved, then sliced
   into ¼-inch wedges
1 6-ounce package baked, marinated
   tofu, sliced on an angle
1 12-ounce package vegetarian
   ground beef alternative
1 cinnamon stick
¼ cup dry sherry

½ teaspoon ground ginger
½ teaspoon ground cumin
1 teaspoon turmeric
⅛ teaspoon ground cloves
1 14½-ounce can Mexican-style
   stewed tomatoes
1 6-ounce package fresh baby spinach
½ cup beef-flavor vegetarian broth,
   boiling
1 cup dried currants
2 tablespoons nutritional yeast
¼ cup chopped fresh cilantro

In a 5-quart saucepan, heat oil, crushed red pepper, dried garlic, and gingerroot over medium-high heat for 1 minute. Add onion and tofu, and cook for 3 minutes, stirring frequently. Add "beef" and cinnamon stick. Cook mixture for 2 minutes and add sherry, ground ginger, cumin, turmeric, and cloves. Stir to blend. Place stewed tomatoes in food process or blender, and pulse to chop. Lower heat to medium low, and add tomatoes, spinach, and broth. Stir to mix thoroughly. Cover and cook mixture for 3 minutes, or until spinach begins to wilt. Add currants, yeast, and cilantro. Simmer for 10 minutes, stirring occasionally. Remove cinnamon stick before serving.

NUTRITION ANALYSIS: PER 2-CUP SERVING

| Enlightened "Beef" Vindaloo | Traditional Beef Vindaloo |
| --- | --- |
| Protein 13 g, carbohydrate 35 g, fiber 6 g, fat 2 g, saturated fat 0 g, cholesterol 0 mg, calcium 112 mg, sodium 405 mg Calories 207: from protein 25%, from carbohydrate 65%, from fat 10% | Protein 19 g, carbohydrate 18 g, fiber 4 g, fat 24 g, saturated fat 12 g, cholesterol 124 mg, calcium 80 mg, sodium 571 mg Calories 757: from protein 18%, from carbohydrate 28%, from fat 54% |

# Savory Side Dishes

These dishes will most often be chosen as accompaniments to the main course. However, you may also assemble a delicious meal from several complementary side dishes. For instance, Hearty Yams and Lentils is a dish that is perfect on the sideboard at a multicourse holiday meal, but it also makes a terrific entrée when accompanied by a crisp salad.

You will find innovative side dishes here, like Edamame Succotash and Crumbled Tofu with Peas, Tomatoes, and Bell Pepper, as well as traditional-style dishes like "Pepperoni" Potatoes, Red Beans and Rice with "Sausage, " and Cauliflower in "Cheese" Sauce. All these fabulous dishes are healthy because of the many wholesome alternatives used. We've also offered a few dishes with kale, a wonderful vegetable that is all too often overlooked by cooks who just haven't tried it. Delicious leafy greens like kale are incredibly satisfying and really good for you. Kale is high in vitamins A and C, folic acid, calcium, and cancer-fighting phytochemicals. So try Mexicali Kale with spicy soy chorizo; Kale with Toasted Pine Nuts and Raisins, and rich-tasting Kale, White Beans, and "Ham."

Many of these dishes also are driven by new and exciting health-supporting products. A versatile new ingredient is the line of tofu purée–based soups from Mori Nu. These creamy soups make creating richly flavorful accompaniments a snap. Curried Brussels Sprouts and Baby Carrots, drenched in a richly flavored sauce is made with one of these creamy soups. Dilled Asparagus and Wild Mushrooms is another, to be served over rice or couscous or as a fabulous filling for an elegant crepe.

# Recipes

Cauliflower in "Cheese" Sauce
Curried Brussels Sprouts and Baby Carrots
Dilled Asparagus and Wild Mushrooms
Edamame Succotash
Kale with Toasted Pine Nuts and Raisins
Mexicali Kale
Kale, White Beans, and "Ham"
Oven Roasted Balsamic Veggies
Savory Corn Medallions
Broken Pasta Casserole
Brown Rice and Tomato Pilaf
Kasha Pilaf
Whole Wheat Couscous Pilaf
Pineapple Basmati Pilaf
Brown Rice with Broccoli and Pine Nuts
Hearty Yams and Lentils
Yams, "Bacon," Pears, and Raisins
"Pepperoni" Potatoes
Hawaiian Unbaked Beans
Creamy Mushroom Cauliflower Bake
Couscous, Golden Raisin, and Soynut Pilaf
Roasted Garlic Couscous with Blueberries and Walnuts
Crumbled Tofu with Peas, Tomatoes, and Bell Pepper
Red Beans and Rice with "Sausage"
Roasted Corn and Potato Gratin
Vegetable Medley with Edamame
Braised Veggies with Baked Tofu and Okara

# Cauliflower in "Cheese" Sauce

*This favorite is "cheesy," delicious, and dairy-free!*

1½ teaspoons olive oil
1 tablespoon dried minced garlic
¼ teaspoon crushed red pepper
1 large shallot, minced
1 medium yellow bell pepper, cut
   into 2-inch strips
1 medium head cauliflower, cut into
   florets (about 6 cups)
1 medium plum tomato, diced

1 cup frozen peas, thawed
1 12.3-ounce package lite silken tofu
¼ cup dry sherry
½ cup chicken-flavor vegetarian
   broth
2 teaspoons Bragg Liquid Aminos
⅔ cup nutritional yeast
½ teaspoon granulated garlic
1½ teaspoon dried thyme

Over medium-high heat, warm oil, dried minced garlic, and crushed red pepper for 1 minute in a 5-quart saucepan. Add shallot and bell pepper strips, and cook for 3 minutes. Add cauliflower and tomato, and cook for 8 minutes, stirring occasionally. Reduce heat to medium low, add peas, and simmer while making sauce, about 3 minutes.

Place tofu in food processor and blend, scraping down once. Add sherry, broth, liquid aminos, yeast, and granulated garlic. Blend until smooth. Pour over cauliflower mixture and stir to mix. Sprinkle with thyme and simmer for 10 minutes.

---

NUTRITION ANALYSIS: PER 1½-CUP SERVING

| Enlightened Cauliflower in "Cheese" Sauce | Traditional Cauliflower in Cheese Sauce |
|---|---|
| Protein 12 g, carbohydrate 51 g, fiber 5 g, fat 2 g, saturated fat 0 g, cholesterol 0 mg, calcium 74 mg, sodium 205 mg Calories 131: from protein 18%, from carbohydrate 74%, from fat 8% | Protein 10 g, carbohydrate 17 g, fiber 4 g, fat 16 g, saturated fat 10 g, cholesterol 46 mg, calcium 227 mg, sodium 550 mg Calories 243: from protein 17%, from carbohydrate 27%, from fat 56% |

# Curried Brussels Sprouts and Baby Carrots

*Brussels sprouts, baby carrots, and currants are bathed in
an intensely flavored curry sauce.*

*6
Servings*

1 tablespoon olive oil
¼ teaspoon crushed red pepper
3 cloves garlic, minced
⅓ cup minced shallots
½ cup thinly sliced scallions
1½ cups sliced baby-cut carrots
1 pound fresh brussels sprouts,
   trimmed and quartered

½ cup boiling vegetable broth
2 cups Mori Nu Creamy Corn Soup
½ cup dried currants
1 teaspoon mild curry powder
½ teaspoon turmeric
¼ cup nutritional yeast
1 teaspoon Bragg Liquid Aminos
2 tablespoons chopped fresh cilantro

Heat oil and crushed red pepper in a medium saucepan over medium-high heat
for 1 minute. Add garlic, shallots, and scallions. Cook for 3 minutes, then add
carrots and cook for 5 minutes, stirring frequently. Add brussels sprouts and
cook for 8 minutes, stirring often. Add broth and cook for 3 minutes, allowing
liquid to reduce. Lower heat to medium low and add corn soup, currants, curry
powder, turmeric, yeast, aminos, and cilantro, stirring after each addition. Simmer for 10 minutes. For a complete meal, serve with Pineapple Basmati Pilaf
(page 176).

NUTRITION ANALYSIS: PER 1½-CUP SERVING

**Enlightened Curried Brussels Sprouts
and Baby Carrots**
Protein 8 g, carbohydrate 47 g, fiber 7 g, fat 5 g,
saturated fat 1 g, cholesterol 0 mg,
calcium 85 mg, sodium 297 mg
Calories 179: from protein 12%,
from carbohydrate 72%, from fat 16%

**Traditional Curried Brussels Sprouts
and Baby Carrots**
Protein 6 g, carbohydrate 25 g, fiber 7 g, fat 25 g,
saturated fat 20 g, cholesterol 22 mg,
calcium 82 mg, sodium 445 mg
Calories 322: from protein 7%,
from carbohydrate 28%, from fat 65%

# Dilled Asparagus and Wild Mushrooms

*This dish makes an elegant filling for a crepe.*
*Top it off with your favorite salsa.*

1 1-ounce package dried mushroom medley, or any dried mushrooms

3 cups boiling water

1½ teaspoons olive oil

2 cloves garlic, minced

⅔ cup chopped red onion

⅓ cup chopped red bell pepper

12 ounces fresh asparagus, trimmed and cut into bite-size pieces

1⅔ cups Mori Nu Butternut Squash Soup

2 teaspoons dried dillweed

1 tablespoon tamari

½ teaspoon lemon pepper

Rinse mushrooms and combine with boiling water in a medium bowl. Set aside for 15 minutes.

In a 4-quart saucepan, heat oil over medium-high heat. Add garlic, onion, and bell pepper, and cook for 3 minutes. Drain mushrooms, discarding soaking liquid, and snip larger mushrooms with clean kitchen shears. Add softened mushrooms to the pan with the asparagus. Cook for 5 minutes, stirring frequently. Add squash soup, dillweed, tamari, and lemon pepper, stirring after each addition. Lower heat and simmer for 10 minutes.

## NUTRITION ANALYSIS: PER 1-CUP SERVING

### Enlightened Dilled Asparagus and Wild Mushrooms

Protein 3 g, carbohydrate 12, fiber 3 g, fat 2 g, saturated fat 0 g, cholesterol 0 mg, calcium 39 mg, sodium 292 mg
Calories 83: from protein 17%, from carbohydrate 58%, from fat 25%

### Traditional Dilled Asparagus and Wild Mushrooms

Protein 3 g, carbohydrate 10 g, fiber 2 g, fat 21 g, saturated fat 13 g, cholesterol 74 mg, calcium 85 mg, sodium 389 mg
Calories 243: from protein 6%, from carbohydrate 16%, from fat 78%

# Edamame Succotash

*Shelled edamame look somewhat like plump green lima beans.*
*Their hearty texture and delicious flavor add an interesting*
*dimension to this dish.*

*8*
*Servings*

1 16-ounce package frozen shelled
    edamame
1½ teaspoons olive oil
4 cloves garlic, minced
1 medium yellow onion, chopped
1 small green bell pepper, chopped
1 6-ounce package veggie Canadian
    bacon, diced
2 small sunburst squash or yellow
    summer squash, thinly sliced into
    bite-size pieces

1 16-ounce package frozen corn,
    thawed
3 medium tomatoes, diced
¼ cup nutritional yeast
½ cup dry sherry
3 tablespoons fresh lemon juice
1 tablespoon Bragg Liquid Aminos
1 teaspoon dried thyme

Cook frozen edamame according to package directions. Drain and set aside.

In an electric frying pan or Dutch oven, heat oil over medium-high heat and add garlic, onion, bell pepper, and diced veggie bacon. Cook for 3 minutes, then add squash. Cook mixture, stirring frequently, until crisp-tender, about 5 minutes. Add edamame, corn, and tomatoes. Reduce heat to medium low and cook for 5 minutes. Add nutritional yeast, sherry, lemon juice, aminos, and thyme. Simmer for 5 minutes.

NUTRITION ANALYSIS: PER 1½-CUP SERVING

| Enlightened Edamame Succotash | Traditional Succotash |
|---|---|
| Protein 18 g, carbohydrate 65 g, fiber 7 g, fat 4 g, saturated fat 1 g, cholesterol 0 mg, calcium 62 mg, sodium 297 mg Calories 213: from protein 20%, from carbohydrate 70%, from fat 10% | Protein 17 g, carbohydrate 30 g, fiber 7 g, fat 15 g, saturated fat 8 g, cholesterol 0 mg, calcium 42 mg, sodium 852 mg Calories 310: from protein 21%, from carbohydrate 37%, from fat 42% |

# Kale with Toasted Pine Nuts and Raisins

*This is a colorful dish with a lovely balance of flavor and texture.
Pine nuts, sweet raisins, and hickory baked tofu provide a counterpoint
to the flavorful, deep green lacy leaves of kale.*

*6*
*Servings*

3 tablespoons pine nuts
2 teaspoons olive oil
1 tablespoon dried minced garlic
¾ cup chopped red onion
¼ cup chopped green bell
  pepper
1½ cups sliced baby-cut carrots
1 large bunch kale, torn into
  bite-size pieces

1 6-ounce package hickory baked
  tofu, sliced on an angle
3 ounces portobello mushrooms,
  diced
1 cup frozen white corn, defrosted
½ cup golden raisins
¼ cup dry sherry
1 tablespoon tamari
1 tablespoon nutritional yeast

Toast pine nuts in a small, dry frying pan over medium-high heat, shaking the pan frequently until the nuts just begin to change color and are fragrant, about 3 minutes. Set aside.

Heat oil and garlic in a 14-inch stir-fry pan or wok for 1 minute. Add onion, bell pepper, and carrots. Sauté for 3 minutes, then add the kale. Cook for 3 minutes, then add tofu and mushrooms. Cook for 5 minutes, stirring frequently. Add the corn, raisins, pine nuts, sherry, tamari, and nutritional yeast. Reduce heat and simmer for 5 minutes, stirring occasionally.

To PREPARE kale, first rinse the leaves thoroughly. While many cooks like to use a sharp knife to strip the leaf from the rib, I prefer to tear the leaves away from the tough stalk.

---

NUTRITION ANALYSIS: PER 2-CUP SERVING

| Enlightened Kale with Toasted Pine Nuts and Raisins | Traditional Kale with Toasted Pine Nuts and Raisins |
|---|---|
| Protein 15 g, carbohydrate 43 g, fiber 8 g, fat 5 g, saturated fat 1 g, cholesterol 0 mg, calcium 185 mg, sodium 383 mg | Protein 22 g, carbohydrate 35 g, fiber 6 g, fat 25 g, saturated fat 7 g, cholesterol 66 mg, calcium 150 mg, sodium 456 mg |
| Calories 255: from protein 21 %, from carbohydrate 62%, from fat 17% | Calories 437: from protein 20%, from carbohydrate 31%, from fat 49% |

# Mexicali Kale

*In this tasty dish, kale is paired with potatoes and braised in
dry vermouth (if you prefer you may use vegetable broth).
Braising greens after wilting gives them a softer texture.*

*8
Servings*

olive oil cooking spray
8 ounces Soyrizo vegetarian chorizo
4 cloves garlic, minced
1 red onion, chopped
3 cups peeled and cubed potatoes

1 large bunch kale, torn into bite-size
   pieces
1 medium tomato, diced
¼ cup dry vermouth or vegetable
   broth

Spray a Dutch oven or electric frying pan with
olive oil and warm over medium-high heat.
Squeeze the veggie chorizo from its casing into pan
and cook for 8 minutes, or until crisp and brown,
stirring frequently. Remove chorizo from pan and
set aside.

Spray pan with oil, add garlic and onion, and
cook for 2 minutes. Add potatoes and cook for 10
minutes, stirring frequently. Add kale and cook
mixture, stirring often, for 5 minutes. Add tomato
and vermouth and reduce heat to low. Cook for 5
minutes, then return the chorizo to the pan. Simmer mixture for 3 minutes or until ready to serve.

MANY TRADITIONAL
recipes cook greens with
bacon or fatty meats. A
healthier approach livens
up greens with an authentic
vegetarian chorizo alternative. This recipe uses half a
16-ounce package of
Soyrizo. Save the rest for
another use.

---

NUTRITION ANALYSIS: PER 1-CUP SERVING

**Enlightened Mexicali Kale**
Protein 8 g, carbohydrate 27 g, fiber 5 g, fat 5 g,
saturate fat 3 g, cholesterol 0 mg,
calcium 152 mg, sodium 270 mg
Calories 182: from protein 17%,
from carbohydrate 58%, from fat 25%

**Traditional Mexicali Kale**
Protein 11 g, carbohydrate 25 g, fiber 4 g, fat 17 g,
saturated fat 5 g, cholesterol 25 mg,
calcium 129 mg, sodium 393 mg
Calories 294: from protein 15%,
from carbohydrate 34%, from fat 51%

# Kale, White Beans, and "Ham"

*Diced vegetarian bacon, Great Northern beans, and tofu-based tomato soup taste wonderful in this delicious kale dish.*

2 teaspoons olive oil
1 tablespoon dried minced garlic
½ cup chopped scallions
½ cup chopped red bell pepper
4 slices veggie Canadian bacon, diced
1 large bunch kale, torn into bite-size pieces

1 15-ounce can Great Northern beans
¼ cup dry sherry
⅔ cup Mori Nu Tomato Soup
1 tablespoon nutritional yeast
1 teaspoon dried basil
⅛ teaspoon lemon pepper

Heat oil and garlic over medium-high heat for 1 minute in a 14-inch stir-fry pan or wok. Add scallions, bell pepper, and veggie bacon. Cook for 5 minutes, then add the kale. Cook for 3 minutes, stirring frequently, then add the beans, sherry, and soup. Reduce heat to medium low and cook for 3 minutes, stirring occasionally. Add the nutritional yeast, basil, and lemon pepper. Reduce heat to low and simmer for 5 minutes, stirring occasionally.

NUTRITION ANALYSIS: PER 1½-CUP SERVING

Enlightened Kale, White Beans, and "Ham"
Protein 15 g, carbohydrate 28 g, fiber 7 g, fat 3 g,
saturated fat 1 g, cholesterol 0 mg,
calcium 171 mg, sodium 253 mg
Calories 195: from protein 30 %,
from carbohydrate 56%, from fat14%

Traditional Kale, White Beans, and Ham
Protein 14 g, carbohydrate 24 g, fiber 6 g, fat 17 g,
saturated fat 8 g, cholesterol 35 mg,
calcium 164 mg, sodium 344 mg
Calories 296: from protein 19%
from carbohydrate 31%, from fat 50%

# Oven Roasted Balsamic Veggies

*Classic roasting involves oven-cooking in an uncovered pan without the addition of liquid. However, this mix of hearty vegetables is enhanced with a tasty balsamic finish.*

*6*
*Servings*

olive oil cooking spray
4 cups peeled, cubed banana squash,
    or any variety of winter squash
2 cups peeled and cubed russet
    potatoes
2 medium yellow onions, halved,
    then cut into ¼-inch wedges
2 cups whole baby-cut carrots
½ cup minced shallots

3 medium plum tomatoes, diced
2 tablespoons olive oil
2 tablespoon balsamic vinegar
1 tablespoon tamari
1 teaspoon dried basil
1 teaspoon dried minced garlic
⅓ cup hot chicken-flavor vegetarian
    broth
paprika for garnish

Rasting produces intensely flavored vegetables that are moist and tender on the inside and brown and crispy on the outside.

Preheat oven to 450°. Spray a nonreactive 9-by-13-inch baking dish with olive oil cooking spray.

Combine squash, potatoes, onions, carrots, and shallots in prepared pan. Bake for 20 minutes. Remove from oven and add tomatoes, stirring to mix. Combine oil, vinegar, tamari, basil, garlic, and broth. Pour over vegetables, toss to mix, and sprinkle with paprika. Return to oven. Bake for an additional 25 minutes, stirring occasionally.

---

NUTRITION ANALYSIS: PER 2-CUP SERVING

**Enlightened Oven Roasted Balsamic Veggies**
Protein 5 g, carbohydrate 48 g, fiber 9 g, fat 5 g,
saturated fat 1 g, cholesterol 0 mg,
calcium 104 mg, sodium 221 mg
Calories 241: from protein 8%,
from carbohydrate 74%, from fat 18%

**Traditional Oven Roasted Balsamic Veggies**
Protein 5 g, carbohydrate 45 g, fiber 8 g, fat 14 g,
saturated fat 4 g, cholesterol 11 mg,
calcium 104 mg, sodium 465 mg
Calories 298: from protein 6%,
from carbohydrate 54%, from fat 40%

# Savory Corn Medallions

*Really delicious, these savory mini-muffins bake up to look like large gold
coins! Serve with soup or any entrée that features a savory sauce.*

---

olive oil cooking spray
1 12.3-ounce package lite silken tofu,
    extra firm
2 cloves garlic, peeled
⅓ cup sliced scallions
2 tablespoons Dijon mustard
1 tablespoon tamari lite
½ cup coarsely shredded carrots
⅔ cup frozen white corn, thawed

⅓ cup nutritional yeast
1 cup yellow cornmeal
½ tablespoon baking powder
1 teaspoon baking soda
1 tablespoon egg replacer powder
¼ cup cold water
3 tablespoons liquid Fruitsource
1 teaspoon lemon juice
paprika for garnish

Preheat oven to 400°. Spray mini-muffin pan cups with olive oil.

Place tofu in food processor and process for 2 minutes, scraping down
halfway through. Add garlic, scallions, mustard, and tamari. Blend. Add carrots
and corn, and pulse to mix. Add yeast, cornmeal, baking powder, and baking
soda. Blend. In a small bowl or measuring cup, combine egg replacer with
water, whisking until foamy. Add to tofu mixture with Fruitsource and lemon
juice. Blend. Spoon a scant ⅓ cup batter into each prepared muffin cup. Sprinkle with paprika. Bake 10 minutes. Reduce oven temperature to 350°, and bake
for 5 minutes or until golden brown.

---

NUTRITION ANALYSIS: PER SERVING (2 MINI-MUFFINS)

**Enlightened Corn Medallions**
Protein 5 g, carbohydrate 17 g, fiber 2 g, fat 1 g,
saturated fat 0 g, cholesterol 0 mg,
calcium 51 mg, sodium 252 mg
Calories 90: from protein 23%,
from carbohydrate 71%, from fat 6%

**Traditional Corn Mini-Muffins**
Protein 4 g, carbohydrate 17 g, fiber 1 g, fat 12 g,
saturated fat 7 g, cholesterol 65 mg,
calcium 89 mg, sodium 387 mg
Calories 191: from protein 8%,
from carbohydrate 35%, from fat 57%

# Broken Pasta Casserole

*Here's what to do with those dribs and drabs of leftover uncooked pasta (you know, when a recipe calls for 12 ounces and you have a 16-ounce package). Just place the various shapes in a zip-top plastic bag and rap with the edge of a rolling pin until you have broken the shapes into smaller pieces. They don't all have to be the exactly same size. Then—use this recipe!*

*6*
*Servings*

3 quarts water with 1 teaspoon salt and 1 tablespoon of olive oil, boiling
8 ounces broken pasta (about 2½ cups)
1 6-ounce package fresh baby spinach
1½ teaspoons olive oil
⅛ teaspoon crushed red pepper
⅓ cup minced shallots
⅓ cup chopped red bell pepper

½ cup sliced scallions
4 slices veggie Canadian bacon, diced
2 ounces baby portobello mushrooms, diced
1½ cups shelled edamame, cooked
2 cups enriched 1% fat soymilk
2 tablespoons lemon juice
½ cup nutritional yeast
½ teaspoon granulated garlic
1 tablespoon tamari

Preheat oven to 350°.

Add pasta to boiling water, bring to a second boil, and cook over medium-high heat for 6 minutes. Add spinach to the pot and cook for an additional 2 minutes. Drain and rinse with cold water occasionally.

In a 5-quart stovetop- and oven-safe casserole dish, heat oil and crushed red pepper over medium-high heat for 1 minute. Add shallots, bell pepper, scallions, and veggie bacon. Cook for 5 minutes, stirring frequently. Add mushrooms and edamame, reduce heat to medium low, and cook mixture for 4 minutes. Add pasta mixture. Place soymilk and lemon juice in a large bowl. Using a small wire whisk or fork, mix in the yeast, garlic, and tamari. Add sauce to the pasta and mix thoroughly. Cover and bake for 15 minutes.

NUTRITION ANALYSIS: PER 1½-CUP SERVING

**Enlightened Broken Pasta Casserole**
Protein 14 g, carbohydrate 20 g, fiber 4 g, fat 4 g, saturated fat 0 g, cholesterol 0 mg, calcium 148 mg, sodium 216 mg
Calories 164: from protein 31%, from carbohydrate 47%, from fat 22%

**Traditional Broken Pasta Casserole**
Protein 12 g, carbohydrate 20 g, fiber 3 g, fat 17 g, saturated fat 10 g, cholesterol 51 mg, calcium 163 mg, sodium 563 mg
Calories 277: from protein 17%, from carbohydrate 28%, from fat 55%

# Brown Rice and Tomato Pilaf

*This dish is easy to assemble,
especially when using a rice cooker!*

1½ cups raw brown rice
5 cups chicken-flavor vegetarian
broth, boiling
1 14½-ounce can Mexican-style
stewed tomatoes, chopped

1 15-ounce can Great Northern
beans
2 teaspoons Bragg Liquid Aminos
¼ cup chopped fresh cilantro

*Using rice cooker:* Place rice and broth in pan and press "start" (or "cook"). When liquid is absorbed (about 40 minutes) and cooker sets itself to warm, add the tomatoes, beans, aminos, and cilantro. Set to cook again for 10 minutes. Keep warm until ready to serve.

*Conventional method:* Add rice to boiling broth, stir, and bring to a second boil. Lower heat, cover, and simmer for 45 minutes, or until the liquid is absorbed. Add tomatoes, beans, aminos, and cilantro. Simmer for 10 minutes, stirring occasionally.

---

### NUTRITION ANALYSIS: 2-CUP SERVING

**Enlightened Brown Rice and Tomato Pilaf**
Protein 8 g, carbohydrate 55 g, fiber 5 g, fat 1 g,
saturated fat 0 g, cholesterol 0 mg,
calcium 62 mg, sodium 204 mg
Calories 214: from protein 12%,
from carbohydrate 84%, from fat 4%

**Traditional Rice and Tomato Pilaf**
Protein 11 g, carbohydrate 51 g, fiber 4 g, fat 11 g,
saturated fat 7 g, cholesterol 28 mg,
calcium 115 mg, sodium 938 mg
Calories 350: from protein 13%,
from carbohydrate 59%, from fat 28%

6
*Servings*

# Kasha Pilaf

*Kasha Pilaf, made with barley and portobello
mushrooms, is a substantial side dish.*

1 cup boiling vegetable broth
½ cup quick-cooking pearled barley
1½ teaspoons olive oil
⅛ teaspoon crushed red pepper
2 cloves garlic, minced
1 small yellow onion, chopped
1 cup coarsely shredded carrots
2 ounces baby portobello
    mushrooms, diced

1 tablespoon egg replacer powder
¼ cup cold water
1 cup kasha, medium granulation
2 cups boiling water
2 tablespoons DDC onion broth
    powder
¼ cup nutritional yeast
1 teaspoon Bragg Liquid Aminos
1 teaspoon granulated garlic

KASHA, HULLED grains of buckwheat that have been oven-toasted, has a hearty, nutlike flavor and is available in fine, medium, and coarse granulation.

Combine boiling broth and barley in a small saucepan, and bring to a second boil. Reduce heat to low, cover, and simmer for 12 minutes. Set aside.

In a medium saucepan, heat oil and crushed red pepper over medium-high heat for 1 minute. Add minced garlic, onion, and carrots, and cook for 3 minutes. Add mushrooms, and continue to cook vegetables for 5 minutes, stirring frequently. In a medium bowl, combine egg replacer powder and cold water. Blend with a wire whisk until foamy. Combine kasha and egg replacer mixture, and quickly add to the pan, stirring to mix. Quickly combine boiling water with broth powder, and stir into the mixture. Reduce heat to low and simmer for 10 minutes. Add cooked barley, yeast, aminos, and granulated garlic. Stir to mix, and simmer a few minutes, or until liquid is absorbed.

---

NUTRITION ANALYSIS: PER 2-CUP SERVING

**Enlightened Kasha Pilaf**
Protein 8 g, carbohydrate 63 g, fiber 5 g, fat 3 g,
saturated fat 0 g, cholesterol 0 mg,
calcium 19 mg, sodium 233 mg
Calories 239: from protein 11%,
from carbohydrate 81%, from fat 8%

**Traditional Kasha Pilaf**
Protein 11 g, carbohydrate 42 g, fiber 5 g, fat 21 g,
saturated fat 12 g, cholesterol 87 mg,
calcium 93 mg, sodium 347 mg
Calories 394: from protein 12%,
from carbohydrate 42%, from fat 46%

# Whole Wheat Couscous Pilaf

*Couscous is a type of pasta used throughout North Africa, especially in Morocco and Tunisia. Made from semolina, the variety commonly available in North America is precooked, making it quick and easy to prepare.*

2½ cups beef-flavor vegetarian broth, divided

1½ cups whole wheat couscous

1 teaspoon olive oil

1 tablespoon dried minced garlic

½ cup chopped yellow onion

⅓ cup chopped red bell pepper

2 ounces baby portobello mushrooms, diced

1 tablespoons balsamic vinegar

1 medium plum tomato, diced

1 cup frozen peas, thawed

⅓ cup golden raisins

2 tablespoons nutritional yeast

⅓ cup chopped flat-leaf Italian parsley

In a small saucepan, bring 1½ cups of the broth to a boil, stir in couscous, cover, and remove from heat. Set aside.

In a 5-quart saucepan, heat oil and garlic over medium-high heat for 1 minute. Add onion, bell pepper, and mushrooms, and sauté for 3 minutes. Add vinegar and tomato, and cook for 3 minutes. Add couscous, peas, raisins, yeast, parsley, and remaining 1 cup of broth. Lower heat and simmer for 5 minutes, stirring occasionally.

NUTRITION ANALYSIS: PER 1½-CUP SERVING

Enlightened Couscous Pilaf
Protein 11 g, carbohydrate: 56 g, fiber 9 g, fat 2 g, saturated fat 0 g, cholesterol 0 mg, calcium 41 mg, sodium 246 mg
Calories 270: from protein 15%, from carbohydrate 79%, from fat 6%

Traditional Couscous Pilaf
Protein 9 g, carbohydrate 53 g, fiber 3 g, fat 16 g, saturated fat 10 g, cholesterol 48 mg, calcium 40 mg, sodium 560 mg
Calories 387: from protein 10%, from carbohydrate 54%, from fat 36%

# Pineapple Basmati Pilaf

*The subtle fragrance of basmati is distinctive. When cooked, this delicate, aromatic rice elongates to twice its length.*

*6*
*Servings*

1½ cups raw white basmati rice
olive oil cooking spray
⅛ teaspoon crushed red pepper
1 clove garlic, minced
½ cup thinly sliced scallions
3 cups chicken-flavor vegetarian broth, boiling
½ cup coarsely shredded carrots
1 cinnamon stick

½ teaspoon ground ginger
½ teaspoon ground coriander
½ teaspoon turmeric
⅓ cup pineapple chunks packed in juice, sliced vertically
⅓ cup reserved pineapple juice
⅓ cup golden raisins
2 teaspoons Bragg Liquid Aminos
¼ cup chopped fresh cilantro

BASMATI RICE is a slender, long-grain rice, grown in the Himalayas. *Bas* means "fragrant" and *mati* means "of the earth."

Rinse basmati rice thoroughly in a small wire colander and set aside to drain.

Spray a 4-quart saucepan with olive oil, add crushed red pepper, garlic, and scallions, and cook over medium-high heat for 2 minutes. Add rice and cook for 3 minutes, stirring frequently. Add broth, carrots, and cinnamon stick. Add ginger, coriander, and turmeric, stirring after each addition. Lower heat and add pineapple chunks, reserved juice, raisins, aminos, and cilantro. Cover and simmer, undisturbed for 20 minutes, or until liquid is absorbed. Remove cinnamon stick before serving.

## NUTRITION ANALYSIS: PER 1-CUP SERVING

**Enlightened Pineapple Basmati Pilaf**
Protein 5 g, carbohydrate 82 g, fiber 6 g, fat 0 g,
saturated fat 0 g, cholesterol 0 mg,
calcium 24 mg, sodium 115 mg
Calories 222: from protein 5%,
from carbohydrate 94%, from fat 1%

**Traditional Pineapple Basmati Rice**
Protein 6 g, carbohydrate 43 g, fiber 2 g, fat 12 g,
saturated fat 6 g, cholesterol 22 mg,
calcium 31 mg, sodium 557 mg
Calories 309: from protein 8%,
from carbohydrate 57%, from fat 35%

# Brown Rice with Broccoli and Pine Nuts

*Here is a dish that is quick and delicious!*

¼ cup pine nuts
olive oil cooking spray
4 cups broccoli florets
3 cups cooked brown rice
3 tablespoons chopped fresh chives
⅔ cup hot chicken-flavor vegetarian
   broth

1 teaspoon Bragg Liquid Aminos
1 teaspoon granulated garlic
½ cup nutritional yeast
¼ cup chopped parsley

Place pine nuts in a small, dry saucepan and toast over medium-high heat, shaking pan constantly for 2 to 3 minutes, or until nuts are lightly browned. Set aside.

Spray a 2-quart microwave-safe casserole dish with olive oil cooking spray. Place broccoli in prepared dish, cover, and microwave on 100% power for 2 minutes. Add brown rice and chives, stir to mix, and set aside. Combine broth, aminos, garlic, and yeast. Add to rice mixture, stir, and sprinkle with parsley. Heat at 50% power for 2 minutes. Top with toasted pine nuts just before serving.

VEGETABLES cooked in the microwave retain their color better than steamed or boiled vegetables.

---

NUTRITION ANALYSIS: PER 1-CUP SERVING

| Enlightened Brown Rice with Broccoli and Pine Nuts | Traditional Rice with Broccoli and Pine Nuts |
|---|---|
| Protein 10 g, carbohydrate 46 g, fiber 5 g, fat 3 g, saturated fat 1 g, cholesterol 0 mg, calcium 47 mg, sodium 74 mg Calories 167: from protein 16%, from carbohydrate 74%, from fat 10% | Protein 9 g, carbohydrate 31 g, fiber 3 g, fat 16 g, saturated fat 8 g, cholesterol 32 mg, calcium 124 mg, sodium 346 mg Calories 297: from protein 11%, from carbohydrate 42%, from fat 47% |

# Hearty Yams and Lentils

*Leftover lentils? This tasty side
dish can be a hearty meal in itself.*

*8
Servings*

1½ teaspoons olive oil
¼ teaspoon crushed red pepper
4 cloves garlic, minced
¾ cup chopped red onion
3 slices veggie Canadian bacon, diced
2 medium yams, peeled and cut into
    1-inch cubes (4 cups)

¼ cup mirin cooking wine
⅔ cup boiling water
1 tablespoon DDC onion broth
    powder
2 cups cooked brown lentils
⅓ cup nutritional yeast
1 tablespoon tamari

Heat oil and crushed red pepper in a 4-quart saucepan over medium-high heat for 1 minute. Add garlic, onion, and bacon, and cook for 3 minutes. Add yams and cook for 5 minutes, stirring frequently. Reduce heat to medium, add mirin, and continue to cook for 8 minutes, stirring frequently. Combine boiling water and onion broth powder and add to the pan. Cook 5 minutes, stirring ocassionally. Lower heat to medium low and add lentils, nutritional yeast, and tamari. Simmer 5 minutes, or until yams are tender.

I ALWAYS PREFER yams over sweet potatoes, because of the rich color and much sweeter flesh, which has a very moist texture when cooked.

NUTRITION ANALYSIS: PER 1½-CUP SERVING

### Enlightened Yams and Lentils
Protein 10 g, carbohydrate 34 g, fiber 3 g, fat 1 g,
saturated fat 0 g, cholesterol 0 mg,
calcium 19 mg, sodium 323 mg
Calories 187: from protein 20%,
from carbohydrate 73%, from fat 7%

### Traditional Yams and Lentils
Protein 9 g, carbohydrate 34 g, fiber 3 g, fat 17 g,
saturated fat 7 g, cholesterol 28 mg,
calcium 51 mg, sodium 505 mg
Calories 326: from protein 11%,
from carbohydrate 42%, from fat 47%

# Yams, "Bacon," Pears, and Raisins

*Veggie Canadian bacon and yams make this dish
a natural for a holiday meal.*

1½ teaspoons olive oil
¼ teaspoon crushed red pepper
3 cloves garlic, minced
1 medium yellow onion, chopped
½ cup chopped red bell pepper
4 slices veggie Canadian bacon, diced
1 large yam, peeled and cubed
   (4 cups)

2 medium Bosc pears, peeled and
   diced (2 cups)
1 medium plum tomato, diced
¼ cup dry sherry
1 cup chicken-flavor vegetarian broth
½ cup golden raisins
¼ cup flat-leaf parsley
⅓ cup nutritional yeast

Place oil and crushed red pepper in a 5-quart saucepan or electric frying pan and warm over medium-high heat for 1 minute. Add garlic, onion, bell pepper, and diced bacon. Cook for 3 minutes. Add yams and cook mixture for 8 minutes, stirring frequently. Add pears, tomato, and sherry, and reduce heat to medium low. Add broth, raisins, parsley, and yeast. Continue to cook for 10 minutes, stirring occasionally.

## NUTRITION ANALYSIS: PER 1½-CUP SERVING

**Enlightened Yams "Bacon," Pears, and Raisins**
Protein 7 g, carbohydrate 43 g, fiber 5 g, fat 2 g,
saturated fat 0 g, cholesterol 0 mg,
calcium 43 mg, sodium 111 mg
Calories 205: from protein 12%,
from carbohydrate 81%, from fat 7%

**Traditional Yams, Bacon, Pears, and Raisins.**
Protein 7 g, carbohydrate 42 g, fiber 4 g, fat 12 g,
saturated fat 6 g, cholesterol 26 mg,
calcium 60 mg, sodium 243 mg
Calories 298: from protein 9%,
from carbohydrate 55%, from fat 36%

6
*Servings*

# "Pepperoni" Potatoes

*This zesty dish has character!*

1 tablespoon olive oil
1 tablespoon dried minced garlic
4 medium russet potatoes, quartered,
　then sliced into half circles

¼ cup chopped flat-leaf parsley
1 cup veggie pepperoni slices, cut
　into half circles
olive oil spray as needed

Heat oil and garlic in a Dutch oven or electric frying pan for 1 minute. Add potatoes and parsley and cook for 6 minutes, stirring frequently. Add pepperoni and cook mixture for 15 minutes, or until potatoes are tender, stirring often. Spray with olive oil cooking spray, as needed.

### NUTRITION ANALYSIS: PER 1-CUP SERVING

**Enlightened "Pepperoni" Potatoes**
Protein 12 g, carbohydrate 35 g, fiber 5 g, fat 2 g,
saturated fat 0 g, cholesterol 0 mg,
calcium 41 mg, sodium 295 mg
Calories 203: from protein 23%,
from carbohydrate 67%, from fat 10%

**Traditional Pepperoni Potatoes**
Protein 9 g, carbohydrate 33 g, fiber 3 g, fat 25 g,
saturated fat 9 g, cholesterol 38 mg,
calcium 22 mg, sodium 591 mg
Calories 393: from protein 9%,
from carbohydrate 34%, from fat 57%

# Hawaiian Unbaked Beans

*Baked beans are a barbecue standard, and an easy dish to take to
a potluck. Hawaiian Unbaked Beans give this popular dish a new spin.*

2 teaspoons olive oil
⅛ teaspoon crushed red pepper
4 cloves garlic, minced
1 stalk celery, sliced
½ cup sliced scallions
1 6-ounce package veggie Canadian
   bacon, diced
1⅔ cups shredded carrots
¼ cup mirin cooking wine
2 15-ounce cans low-sodium pinto
   beans

1 14½-ounce can Mexican-style
   stewed tomatoes
1 8-ounce can crushed pineapple,
   packed in juice
1 tablespoon Dijon mustard
1 teaspoon vegetarian Worcestershire
   sauce
2 tablespoons chopped fresh chives
2 tablespoons chopped fresh cilantro
2 tablespoons nutritional yeast

Heat oil and crushed red pepper in an electric frying pan or Dutch oven over
medium-high heat for 1 minute. Add garlic, celery, scallions, and veggie bacon.
Cook for 3 minutes, stirring frequently. Add carrots, cook for 2 minutes, then
add mirin. Cook mixture for 5 minutes. Add beans, tomatoes, and pineapple.
Lower heat to medium low, and add mustard, Worcestershire sauce, chives,
cilantro, and yeast. Cook for 10 to 15 minutes, or until heated through, stirring
occasionally.

---

NUTRITION ANALYSIS: PER 1½-CUP SERVING

**Enlightened Hawaiian Unbaked Beans**
Protein 14 g, carbohydrate 25 g, fiber 8 g, fat 1 g,
saturated fat 0 g, cholesterol 0 mg,
calcium 73 mg, sodium 359 mg
Calories 182: from protein 39%,
from carbohydrate 54%, from fat 7%

**Traditional Hawaiian Baked Beans**
Protein 16 g, carbohydrate 29 g, fiber 6 g, fat 13 g,
saturated fat 3 g, cholesterol 74 mg,
calcium 129 mg, sodium 378 mg
Calories 292: from protein 22%,
from carbohydrate 39%, from fat 39%

# Creamy Mushroom Cauliflower Bake

*Think you don't like cauliflower?*
*Try this richly flavorful casserole—dairy-free and delicious!*

*6*
*Servings*

1½ teaspoons olive oil
¼ teaspoon crushed red pepper
1 tablespoon dried minced garlic
1 medium red onion, coarsely
    chopped
8 ounces mushrooms, caps only,
    sliced in half
1 cup coarsely shredded carrots
1 medium head cauliflower, cut into
    florets (about 6 cups)

⅓ cup dry sherry
3 tablespoons DDC Crème of
    Mushroom Soup Mix
1 cup boiling water
½ cup nutritional yeast
3 tablespoons chopped flat-leaf
    parsley
2 tablespoons unsalted soynuts

Y OU MAY WANT to use Melissa's soynuts in this recipe. They are "sliced" before toasting, and retain their crunch when added to a sauced casserole such as this one.

Preheat oven to 400°.

Over medium-high heat, warm oil, crushed red pepper, and dried garlic for 1 minute in a 5-quart stovetop- and oven-safe casserole dish. Add onion and cook for 3 minutes, stirring frequently. Add mushrooms and cook for 3 minutes. Add cauliflower and cook for 5 minutes, stirring occasionally. Add sherry and reduce heat to medium low. Combine mushroom soup mix with boiling water, pour over cauliflower mixture, and stir to mix. Sprinkle with parsley and soynuts. Bake, uncovered, for 20 minutes, or until sauce has thickened and cauliflower is lightly browned.

NUTRITION ANALYSIS: PER 2-CUP SERVING

Enlightened Creamy Mushroom
Cauliflower Bake
Protein 9 g, carbohydrate 20 g, fiber 5 g, fat 4 g
saturated fat 1 g, cholesterol 0 mg,
calcium 45 mg, sodium 266 mg
Calories 146: from protein 23%,
from carbohydrate 54%, from fat 23%

Traditional Creamed Mushroom
Cauliflower Bake
Protein 13 g, carbohydrate 22 g, fiber 4 g, fat 23 g,
saturated fat 11 g, cholesterol 46 mg,
calcium 228 mg, sodium 757 mg
Calories 328: from protein 15%,
from carbohydrate 25%, from fat 60%

# Couscous, Golden Raisin, and Soynut Pilaf

*This simple dish has delightful flavor and texture.*

1¾ cups chicken-flavor vegetarian broth

1½ cups whole wheat couscous

⅓ cup golden raisins

⅓ cup soynuts

2 tablespoons chopped parsley

In a small saucepan, bring broth to a boil. Stir in couscous and raisins. Cover, remove from heat, and set aside for 5 minutes. Fluff with fork and stir in soynuts and parsley. Serve immediately.

NUTRITION ANALYSIS: PER 2-CUP SERVING

**Enlightened Couscous Pilaf**
Protein 11 g, carbohydrate 56 g, fiber 9 g, fat 2 g,
saturated fat 0 g, cholesterol 0 mg,
calcium 41 mg, sodium 246 mg
Calories 270: from protein 15%,
from carbohydrate 79%, from fat 6%

**Traditional Couscous Pilaf**
Protein 9 g, carbohydrate 53 g, fiber 3 g, fat 16 g,
saturated fat 10 g, cholesterol 48 mg,
calcium 40 mg, sodium 560 mg
Calories 387: from protein 10%,
from carbohydrate 54%, from fat 36%

# Roasted Garlic Couscous with Blueberries and Walnuts

*This light, appealing dish has an intriguing blend of flavors.*

1½ cups water
1 tablespoon DDC onion broth mix
1 6-ounce package roasted garlic
    couscous (1 cup)
1 tablespoon lemon juice

½ cup dried blueberries
⅓ cup chopped walnuts
1½ cups frozen peas, thawed
1 teaspoon dried tarragon

Boil water in a medium saucepan. Add broth powder and bring to a second boil. Stir in couscous, lemon juice, blueberries, and walnuts. Cover, remove from heat, and set aside for 5 minutes. Stir in peas and tarragon. Fluff with a fork, and serve.

## NUTRITION ANALYSIS: PER 1-CUP SERVING

**Enlightened Couscous Blueberries and Walnuts**
Protein 8 g, carbohydrate 42 g, fiber 4 g, fat 5 g,
saturated fat 0 g, cholesterol 0 mg,
calcium 18 mg, sodium 350 mg
Calories 239: from protein 13%,
from carbohydrate 69%, from fat 18%

**Traditional Couscous Blueberries and Walnuts**
Protein 11 g, carbohydrate 48 g, fiber 4 g, fat 14 g,
saturated fat 5 g, cholesterol 19 mg,
calcium 24 mg, sodium 568 mg
Calories 357: from protein 12%,
from carbohydrate 53%, from fat 35%

# Crumbled Tofu with Peas, Tomatoes, and Bell Pepper

*This dish is tasty, nutritious, and easy to make.*

2 teaspoons olive oil

1 tablespoon dried minced garlic

19 ounces extra-firm tofu

½ cup chopped red bell pepper

1 medium plum tomato, diced

1 cup frozen peas, thawed

2 tablespoons tamari

1 teaspoon granulated garlic

2 tablespoons nutritional yeast

Heat oil and minced garlic over medium-high heat in a 4-quart saucepan for 1 minute. Crumble tofu into pan and cook, stirring frequently, for 3 minutes. Add bell pepper. Cook for 5 minutes, stirring often. Add tomato, peas, tamari, granulated garlic, and yeast. Lower heat and simmer for 5 minutes, stirring occasionally.

NUTRITION ANALYSIS: PER ³/₄-CUP SERVING

| Enlightened Crumbled Tofu with Peas, Tomatoes, and Bell Pepper | Traditional Crumbled Beef with Peas, Tomatoes, and Bell Pepper |
|---|---|
| Protein 14 g, carbohydrate 12 g, fiber 4g, fat 5 g, saturated fat 0 g, cholesterol 0 mg, calcium 13 mg, sodium 301 mg | Protein 19 g, carbohydrate 6 g, fiber 1 g, fat 33 g, saturated fat 13 g, cholesterol 86 mg, calcium 76 mg, sodium 588 mg |
| Calories 145: from protein 36%, from carbohydrate 32%, from fat 32% | Calories 408: from protein 19%, from carbohydrate 6%, from fat 75% |

# Red Beans and Rice with "Sausage"

*Hearty and delicious, Red Beans and Rice is popular
in the South and in the Caribbean.*

2 teaspoons olive oil
¼ teaspoon crushed red pepper
1 tablespoon dried minced garlic
1 medium yellow onion, chopped
¼ cup chopped green bell pepper
1 stalk celery, chopped
1 14-ounce package Gimme Lean,
    sausage style

½ cup dry sherry
1 15-ounce can kidney beans,
    drained
2 cups cooked brown rice
¼ cup tomato paste mixed with ¼
    cup cold water
1 teaspoon dried thyme
½ cup chopped flat-leaf parsley

In a large saucepan, heat oil, crushed red pepper, and garlic over medium-high heat for 1 minute. Add onion, pepper, and celery, and sauté for 3 minutes. Add Gimme Lean and cook mixture, stirring frequently. Add sherry, reduce heat, and add beans. Stir in rice, tomato paste mixture, thyme, and parsley. Simmer, stirring occasionally, for 10 minutes.

NUTRITION ANALYSIS: PER 1½-CUP SERVING

| Enlightened Red Beans and Rice with "Sausage" | Traditional Red Beans, Rice and Sausage |
|---|---|
| Protein 13 g, carbohydrate 33 g, fiber 6 g, fat 2 g, saturated fat 0 g, cholesterol 0 mg, calcium 40 mg, sodium 330 mg Calories 208: from protein 26%, from carbohydrate 65%, from fat 9% | Protein 12 g, carbohydrate 30 g, fiber 5 g, fat 28 g, saturated fat 9 g, cholesterol 39 mg, calcium 50 mg, sodium 633 mg Calories 426: from protein 11%, from carbohydrate 28%, from fat 61 % |

# Roasted Corn and Potato Gratin

*Roasted sweet corn can add color and unique flavor and texture to many dishes.*

1 tablespoon olive oil
¼ teaspoon crushed red pepper
4 cloves garlic, minced
1 medium red onion, cut in half crosswise, then into ¼-inch wedges
½ cup chopped red bell pepper
4 cups peeled and thinly sliced potatoes
1 3-ounce package Melissa's roasted sweet corn
⅔ cup dry sherry
2½ cups Mori Nu Corn Soup
1 tablespoon tamari
3½ tablespoons Gratin Topping (page 196)
paprika for garnish

Preheat oven to 350°.

Heat oil and crushed red pepper in a 10-inch frying pan over medium-high heat for 1 minute. Add garlic, onion, and bell pepper and cook for 3 minutes. Add potatoes and cook for 10 minutes, stirring frequently. Add roasted corn and mix thoroughly. Add sherry and lower heat to medium low. Add corn soup and tamari and simmer for 5 minutes. Turn into a shallow 2-quart baking dish. Top with gratin topping and sprinkle with paprika. Bake, covered, 30 minutes. Uncover and bake an additional 15 minutes, or until potatoes are cooked through. Serve hot.

## NUTRITION ANALYSIS: PER 1½-CUP SERVING

**Enlightened Roasted Corn and Potato Gratin**
Protein 7 g, carbohydrate 33 g, fiber 4 g, fat 4 g, saturated fat 1 g, cholesterol 0 mg, calcium 36 mg, sodium 315 mg
Calories 190: from protein 14%, from carbohydrate 70%, from fat 16%

**Traditional Roasted Corn and Potato Gratin**
Protein 7 g, carbohydrate 28 g, fiber 3 g, fat 22 g, saturated fat 14 g, cholesterol 74 mg, calcium 129 mg, sodium 378 mg
Calories 339: from protein 8%, from carbohydrate 33%, from fat 59%

# Vegetable Medley with Edamame

*Rich in health-supporting soy protein and fiber, this delicious medley is an
interesting fusion of complementary texture, color, and flavor.*

*8
Servings*

1 16-ounce package shelled edamame
2 teaspoons olive oil
⅛ teaspoon crushed red pepper
1 tablespoon dried minced garlic
1 medium red onion, chopped
¼ cup red bell pepper, cut into
1½-inch strips
3 medium unpeeled Yellow Finn or
Yukon Gold potatoes, cubed

2 cups baby-cut carrots, sliced
lengthwise
2 baby portobello mushrooms, diced
(about 2 ounces)
2 medium tomatoes, diced
½ cup dry vermouth
2 tablespoons tamari
3 tablespoons chopped fresh chives
1 teaspoon dried thyme

If edamame is frozen, cook according to package directions, then drain and set
aside.

In an electric frying pan or Dutch oven, heat oil, crushed red pepper, and
garlic over medium-high heat for 1 minute. Add onion and bell pepper, and
cook for 2 minutes. Add potatoes and carrots and cook, stirring frequently, for
10 minutes. Add edamame, mushrooms, and tomatoes. Reduce heat to
medium low and cook for 8 minutes. Add vermouth, tamari, chives, and
thyme, and simmer for 5 minutes, or until potatoes and carrots are tender.

## NUTRITION ANALYSIS: PER 1-CUP SERVING

**Enlightened Vegetable Medley with Edamame**
Protein 11 g, carbohydrate 26 g, fiber 7 g, fat 5 g
saturated fat 1 g, cholesterol 0 mg,
calcium 73 mg, sodium 245 mg
Calories 202: from protein 22%,
from carbohydrate 53%, from fat 25%

**Traditional Vegetable Medley with Chicken**
Protein 18 g, carbohydrate 12 g, fiber 2 g, fat 16 g,
saturated fat 6g, cholesterol 62 mg,
calcium 42 mg, sodium 534 mg
Calories 264: from protein 27%,
from carbohydrate 18%, from fat 55%

# Braised Veggies with
# Baked Tofu and Okara

*This is a great way to use okara, but if you don't have any on hand, simply
add a cup of cooked couscous or increase the amount of vegetables.*

1 tablespoon olive oil, divided
1 tablespoon dried minced garlic
⅓ cup minced shallots
1 large red onion, chopped
⅓ cup chopped red bell pepper
1 cup coarsely shredded carrots
1 8-ounce package baked tofu, sliced
    on an angle
olive oil cooking spray
1 cup dry roasted okara (see page 39)

2½ cups broccoli florets, cut into
    bite-size pieces
⅔ cup boiling water
2 teaspoons DDC onion broth
    powder
2 tablespoons tomato paste
2 tablespoons nutritional yeast
½ cup dry sherry
1 tablespoon tamari

Heat ½ tablespoon of the oil over medium-high heat in a 4-quart
saucepan for 1 minute. Add garlic, shallots, onion, and bell pepper,
and sauté for 2 minutes. Add carrots and sliced tofu, and cook for
5 minutes, stirring frequently. Push veggies and tofu to edge of pan,
spray cleared surface with olive oil cooking spray, and add remaining ½ tablespoon of oil. Add okara and broccoli to the cleared side
and cook mixture for 3 minutes. Reduce heat to low and stir the
okara/broccoli and tofu mixtures together. Combine boiling water
and broth powder and set aside. Spoon tomato paste into the pan
and add hot broth, stirring to blend. Add nutritional yeast, sherry, and tamari.
Simmer for 10 minutes, or until heated through.

WHILE BAKED tofu is available in a variety of flavors, I like the Hickory Baked for this dish. However, your personal favorite will work just as well.

NUTRITION ANALYSIS: PER 1¼-CUP SERVING

**Braised Veggies with Baked Tofu and Okara**
Protein 12 g, carbohydrate 18 g, fiber 5 g, fat 4 g,
saturated fat 0 g, cholesterol 0 mg,
calcium 48 mg, sodium 427 mg
Calories 164: from protein 31%,
from carbohydrate 46%, from fat 23%

**Traditional Braised Beef and Veggies**
Protein 13 g, carbohydrate 8 g, fiber 2 g, fat 21 g,
saturated fat 7 g, cholesterol 48 mg,
calcium 50 mg, sodium 511 mg
Calories 279: from protein 29%,
from carbohydrate 12%, from fat 59%

# Self-Sufficient Gourmet

This chapter includes recipes for basic items that are homemade and wholesome. You will be able to use these basics in dish upon dish as you expand your healthy cooking repertôire. For example, here you will find healthy baking mixes that are very convenient to have on hand. The Multi-Grain Baking Mix is wholesome in every sense of the word: Knowing that all of the ingredients, down to the Celtic sea salt and nonaluminum baking powder, are health-supporting is very reassuring. The best part is that if you only add water and one or two other items, pancakes, quickbread, muffins, or coffeecake are a snap to make!

You'll discover how easy it is to make homemade soymilk and tofu. All you need is one of the new soymilk makers that are as easy to use as an automatic coffee maker. It takes about 20 minutes to make rich, delicious homemade soymilk. Homemade tofu is also made easily with this innovative machine. View video clips on *www.vegtv.com* if you want a visual demonstration of just how easy it is. Once you try fresh homemade tofu, you won't want to buy commercially made Chinese-style tofu again!

The many tasty marinades and sauces in this section all have interesting and distinct flavor notes and characteristics. You will find specific recipes for how to make each, but be bold and try different variations using other ingredients. You'll find my favorite pie crust in here, as well as gratin and cookie toppings that can be used in a number of dishes. There are also some delectable fruit butters that are really easy to make, and fat-free! These wholesome spreads are fabulous on toasted homemade muffins and breads. After reviewing this chapter and learning some of these useful fundamentals, you'll be well on your way to becoming a self-sufficient enlightened gourmet!

# Recipes

Deep-Dish Whole Wheat Pie Crust

Multi-Grain Baking Mix

Gratin Topping

Cookie Crumb Topping

Coconut Curry Sauce

Creamy Dijon Sauce

Spicy Peanut Sauce

Szechuan Sesame Sauce

Homemade Dairy-Free "Cheese"

Homemade Soymilk

Homemade Tofu

Homemade Ginger Baked Tofu

Homemade Barbecue Baked Tofu

Asian Marinade

Balsamic Marinade

Sweet 'n' Sassy Marinade

Fragrant Soy Marinade

Lively Marinade

Orient Express Marinade

Pacific Blend Marinade

Pungent Ginger Marinade

Red Miso Marinade

Roasted Chile Marinade

Savory Sesame Marinade

Spring Onion Marinade

Zesty Barbecue Marinade

Pineapple Apricot Butter

Spiced Peach Butter

# Deep-Dish Whole Wheat Pie Crust

*This wholesome pastry handles well and is made with just two tablespoons of health-supporting olive oil. It is great with any kind of pie filling.*

*1 Single
Deep-Dish
Pie Shell*

olive oil cooking spray
2 cups whole wheat pastry flour
¼ teaspoon sea salt

⅓ cup lite silken tofu
2 tablespoons mild olive oil
⅓ cup ice water

Lightly spray a deep-dish pie pan with oil.

Place the pastry flour and salt in food processor and pulse to mix. Add tofu and oil and process. While motor is running, pour in ice water and process until mixture comes together in a ball. Turn out on a lightly floured sheet of wax paper. Sprinkle lightly with flour and top with a second sheet of wax paper. Roll out to between ⅛ and ¼ inch. Peel off top sheet of wax paper and use bottom sheet to move dough to prepared pan, then discard. Press dough into pan, trimming around edges. Using thumb and forefinger, press a decorative design along the dough edge.

*To bake blind:* Prick pastry several times with a fork, and bake for 15 minutes in the center of preheated 400° oven. Set aside to cool.

*To baking with filling:* Bake according to recipe instructions.

---

NUTRITION ANALYSIS: PER SERVING (⅛ PIE, CRUST ONLY)

**Enlightened Whole Wheat Pie Crust**
Protein 5 g, carbohydrate 23 g, fiber 3 g, fat 4 g,
saturated fat 0 g, cholesterol 0 mg,
calcium 20 mg, sodium 75 mg
Calories 143: from protein 13%,
from carbohydrate 63%, from fat 24%

**Traditional Pie Crust**
Protein 4 g, carbohydrate 23 g, fiber 1 g, fat 24 g,
saturated fat 14 g, cholesterol 62 mg,
calcium 12 mg, sodium 271 mg
Calories 317: from protein 4%,
from carbohydrate 30%, from fat 66%

# Multi-Grain Baking Mix

*Homemade baking mixes are convenient, economical, and a welcome timesaver. This recipe makes enough for about six or seven dishes, such as muffins, coffee cakes, and pancakes.*

4 cups whole wheat flour
2 cups rolled oats, processed to flour
   in blender or food processor
1 cup whole grain yellow cornmeal
1 cup unbleached white flour
2 tablespoons nonaluminum baking
   powder

2 tablespoons baking soda
¼ cup egg replacer powder
2 teaspoons sea salt
1½ cups dry soymilk

Combine all ingredients in a large covered container and store in a cool, dry place.

Traditional baking mixes contain shortening, a source of unhealthy transfats, and totally unnecessary in the Enlightened Kitchen.

---

NUTRITION ANALYSIS: ½ CUP OF MIX

**Enlightened Multi-Grain Baking Mix**
Protein 6 g, carbohydrate 30 g, fiber 3 g, fat 2 g,
saturated fat 0 g, cholesterol 0 mg,
calcium 74 mg, sodium 283 mg
Calories 152: from protein 15%,
from carbohydrate 73%, from fat 12%

**Traditional Multi-Grain Baking Mix**
Protein 6 g, carbohydrate 32 g, fiber 3 g, fat 10 g,
saturated fat 3 g, cholesterol 1 mg,
calcium 177 mg, sodium 492 mg
Calories 239: from protein 10%,
from carbohydrate 52%, from fat 38%

# Gratin Topping

*Use this convenient make-ahead mix to transform most any
side dish into an elegant au gratin—style casserole, such as
Roasted Corn and Potato Gratin (page 187).*

*Makes
1¼ Cups*

½ cup whole wheat bread crumbs
   (nonhydrogenated)
½ cup soy Parmesan cheese

1 tablespoon granulated garlic
1 tablespoon dried parsley

In a small plastic container with a tight fitting lid, combine bread crumbs, soy
Parmesan, garlic, and parsley. Store, covered, in the freezer for up to 2 months.

---

NUTRITION ANALYSIS: ¼ CUP OF MIX

**Enlightened Gratin Topping**
Protein 10 g, carbohydrate 25 g, fiber 1 g, fat 1 g,
saturated fat 0 g, cholesterol 0 mg
calcium 87 mg, sodium 206 mg
Calories 65: from protein 27%,
from carbohydrate 66%, from fat 7%

**Traditional Gratin Topping**
Protein 7 g, carbohydrate 11 g, fiber 1 g, fat 5 g,
saturated fat 3 g, cholesterol 10 mg,
calcium 207 mg, sodium 342 mg
Calories 114: from protein 25%,
from carbohydrate 40%, from fat 35%

# Cookie Crumb Topping

*Add a sweet crunch to fillings, puddings, and baked goods with this quick mix.*

*Makes
1¼ Cups*

1 7-ounce package amaranth
   graham crackers
⅓ cup Sucanat, unrefined cane sugar

1 teaspoon ground cinnamon
½ teaspoon ground nutmeg

Place crackers in food processor and process to crumbs. Add Sucanat, cinnamon, and nutmeg, and pulse to mix. Topping may be stored in a covered container in the freezer for several months.

H EALTH VALLEY makes three styles of wholesome graham crackers: amaranth, oat bran, and rice bran. Any of these can be used for this topping mix.

NUTRITION ANALYSIS: PER 2 TABLESPOONS

**Enlightened Cookie Crumb Topping**
Protein 4 g, carbohydrate 31 g, fiber 0 g, fat 0 g,
saturated fat 0 g, cholesterol 0 mg,
calcium 33 mg, sodium 101 mg
Calories 164: from protein 15%,
from carbohydrate 75%, from fat 10%

**Traditional Cookie Crumb Topping**
Protein 2 g, carbohydrate 18 g, fiber 0 g, fat 11 g,
saturated fat 7 g, cholesterol 29 mg,
calcium 12 mg, sodium 108 mg
Calories 173: from protein 3%,
from carbohydrate 40 %, from fat 57%

# Coconut Curry Sauce

*This aromatic, rich-tasting sauce can add pizzazz
to a tofu stir fry or vegetable medley.*

*Makes
3 Cups*

2 tablespoons olive oil
1 tablespoon grated gingerroot
¼ cup minced scallions
¼ cup whole wheat flour
1 14-ounce can lite coconut milk
¼ cup tomato paste

½ cup dry sherry
1 teaspoon liquid Fruitsource
1 teaspoon curry powder
½ teaspoon turmeric
½ teaspoon granulated garlic
½ teaspoon sea salt

In a medium saucepan, heat oil over medium heat for 1 minute. Add ginger-root and scallions, sauté for 2 minutes, then stir in flour. Add coconut milk gradually. Reduce heat to low.

In a small bowl, blend tomato paste and sherry and add to the saucepan with Fruitsource, curry powder, turmeric, garlic, and salt. Simmer 5 minutes or until sauce has thickened.

NUTRITION ANALYSIS: PER ⅓-CUP SERVING

**Enlightened Coconut Curry Sauce**
Protein 1 g, carbohydrate 5 g, fiber 1 g, fat 5 g,
saturated fat 2 g, cholesterol 0 mg,
calcium 7 mg, sodium 115 mg
Calories 77: from protein 15%,
from carbohydrate 27%, from fat 58%*

**Traditional Coconut Curry Sauce**
Protein 1 g, carbohydrate 5 g, fiber 1 g, fat 14 g,
saturated fat 11 g, cholesterol 13 mg,
calcium 14 mg, sodium 165 mg
Calories 148: from protein 4%,
from carbohydrate 13%, from fat 83%

\* The percentage of calories from fat seems high because the calories are so low.

# Creamy Dijon Sauce

*Richly favorful without heart-heavy dairy ingredients, this creamy
sauce is made with Mori Nu Corn Soup, which contains nutritious tofu
purée. Serve with lightly steamed vegetables and brown
rice or Black Bean Cakes (page 91).*

2 cups Mori Nu Corn Soup
3 tablespoons Dijon mustard
3 rounded tablespoons soy Parmesan
  cheese
1 teaspoon granulated garlic

1 teaspoon granulated onion
¼ cup Barbara's mashed potato flakes
2 teaspoons tamari
1 tablespoon chopped fresh cilantro

Place soup in a medium pan over medium heat. Add mustard, soy Parmesan,
garlic, onion, potato flakes, tamari, and cilantro. Cook mixture for 5 minutes,
stirring frequently. Reduce heat to low, and simmer until ready to serve.

NUTRITION ANALYSIS: PER ½-CUP SERVING

**Enlightened Creamy Dijon Sauce**
Protein 5 g, carbohydrate 12 g, fiber 1 g, fat 2 g,
saturated fat 1 g, cholesterol 0 mg,
calcium 43 mg, sodium 262 mg
Calories 84: from protein 25%,
from carbohydrate 54%, from fat 21%

**Traditional Creamy Dijon Sauce**
Protein 5 g, carbohydrate 7 g, fiber 0 g, fat 30 g,
saturated fat 19 g, cholesterol 111 mg,
calcium 96 mg, sodium 444 mg
Calories 308: from protein 5%,
from carbohydrate 8%, from fat 87%

# Spicy Peanut Sauce

*This peanut sauce is far lower in fat, especially saturated fat, than its traditional counterpart. It's delicious with tofu; tempeh; cold noodles; or a mix of vegetables such as Japanese eggplant, broccoli, carrots, and zucchini.*

*Makes 3 Cups*

4 cloves garlic, peeled
1 large shallot, quartered
¼ cup sliced scallions
3 tablespoons chopped red bell pepper
1 tablespoon grated fresh gingerroot
1 cup Mori Nu Butternut Squash Soup

1 teaspoon Thai green curry paste
¼ cup vegetable broth, boiling
¼ cup peanut butter
2 tablespoons lime juice
½ tablespoon tamari

FOR THAI-STYLE dishes, use green curry paste and lime juice; for Szechuan-style dishes, substitute chile oil and lemon juice.

Place garlic, shallot, scallions, bell pepper, and ginger in the food processor. Add soup and process. Combine the curry paste with the broth and add to the soup mixture with peanut butter, lime juice, and tamari. Sauce may be made a day in advance.

### NUTRITION ANALYSIS: PER ⅓-CUP SERVING

**Enlightened Peanut Sauce**
Protein 4 g, carbohydrate 8 g, fiber 1 g, fat 5 g,
saturated fat 0 g, cholesterol 0 mg,
calcium 24 mg, sodium 224 mg
Calories 94: from protein 16%,
from carbohydrate 33%, from fat 51%*

**Traditional Peanut Sauce**
Protein 6 g, carbohydrate 7 g, fiber 2 g, fat 28 g,
saturated fat 17 g, cholesterol 14 mg,
calcium 23 mg, sodium 263 mg
Calories 289: from protein 8%,
from carbohydrate 9%, from fat 83%

* The percentage of calories from fat seems high because the calories are so low.

# Szechuan Sesame Sauce

*This spicy signature sauce for the classic Cold Sesame Noodles (page 109).
This spicy sauce is lower in calories and fat than the traditional, because
Mori Nu Corn Soup imparts a full, rich mouthfeel without excessive fat.*

*Makes
2²/₃ Cups*

3 cloves garlic, peeled
1 medium yellow onion, chopped
1 tablespoon grated fresh gingerroot
2 tablespoons chopped fresh cilantro
1¼ cups Mori Nu Corn Soup,
  divided

1½ teaspoons sesame oil
2 teaspoons rice vinegar
¼ cup chunky peanut butter, divided
1 tablespoon tamari
¼ teaspoon hot pepper sauce

Place garlic, onion, gingerroot, cilantro, and 1 cup of the soup in a
food processor, and pulse. Add sesame oil, vinegar, and 2 tablespoons of the peanut butter. Process. Place remaining 2 tablespoons
of peanut butter in a small bowl, and add the reserved ¼ cup of
soup, tamari, and hot pepper sauce. Blend with a fork and add to
the sauce. Do not process. Mix thoroughly when combining the
sauce with other ingredients, such as pasta, veggies, or tofu.

FOR A delicious side
dish or entrée, top sautéed
tofu or lightly steamed
vegetables, such as broc-
coli, snow peas, and baby
corn with this sauce.

---

### NUTRITION ANALYSIS: PER ¹/₃-CUP SERVING

| Enlightened Szechuan Sesame Sauce | Traditional Szechuan Sesame Sauce |
|---|---|
| Protein 4 g, carbohydrate 8 g, fiber 2 g, fat 5 g, | Protein 6 g, carbohydrate 11 g, fiber 2 g, fat 16 g, |
| saturated fat 0 g, cholesterol 0 mg, | saturated fat 2 g, cholesterol 0 mg, |
| calcium 71 mg, sodium 240 mg | calcium 50 mg, sodium 631 mg |
| Calories 91: from protein 15%, | Calories 210: from protein 11%, |
| from carbohydrate 34%, from fat 51% | from carbohydrate 20%, from fat 69% |

# Homemade Dairy-Free "Cheese"

*It's a spread, it's a filling . . . by gosh, you'd
swear it was soft cheddar cheese!*

*Makes
about
4¹/₂ Cups*

olive oil cooking spray
²/₃ cup enriched 1% fat soymilk
2 tablespoons lemon juice
1 12.3-ounce package lite silken tofu
¹/₄ cup white wine

¹/₄ cup mellow white miso
1 cup nutritional yeast
2 tablespoons DDC Créme-It
¹/₂ cup cold water
¹/₄ cup agar flakes

Spray a square lidded container (glass is optimal) with olive oil cooking spray. Combine soymilk and lemon juice in a glass measuring cup and set aside.

Dishes using this delicious Dairy-Free "Cheese" include Open-Faced Grilled "Cheese" Triangles (page 146) and Creamy "Cheese" Bites (page 63). Try spreading it on your favorite crackers, too.

Place tofu in food processor and process until smooth. In a small glass bowl, combine the wine and miso, blending with a fork. Add to tofu and blend. Add yeast, soymilk mixture, and Crème-It, and blend. Combine water and agar flakes in a glass measuring cup or microwave-safe bowl. Microwave on 100% power for about a minute or so, watching that it does not boil over, until mixture has thickened. Add to tofu mixture. Blend for a few minutes until mixture is smooth and has a satiny texture. Pour into prepared container, cover, and refrigerate overnight. "Cheese" can be stored for up to 5 days.

---

NUTRITION ANALYSIS: PER 2¹/₂-TABLESPOONS SERVING

**Enlightened Dairy-Free "Cheese"**
Protein 6 g, carbohydrate 4 g, fiber 1 g, fat 1 g,
saturated fat 0 g, cholesterol 0 mg,
calcium 35 mg, sodium 36 mg
Calories 45: from protein 51%,
from carbohydrate 35%, from fat 14%

**Traditional Cheese**
Protein 16 g, carbohydrate 1 g, fiber 0 g, fat 23 g,
saturated fat 15 g, cholesterol 72 mg,
calcium 495 mg, sodium 426 mg
Calories 276: from protein 25%,
from carbohydrate 1%, from fat 74 %

# Homemade Soymilk

*This recipe produces thick, rich soymilk without the use of additives such as thickeners. The reader is invited to go to www.vegtv.com to view a video clip demonstrating this technique.*

2 measures (70 grams each) Laura Beans (see page 38)
50 ounces cold water (6¼ cups)
½ teaspoon sea salt

3 rounded tablespoons liquid Fruitsource
1 teaspoon pure vanilla
Soyajoy automatic soymilk maker (see Sanlinx, page 272)

*Makes 1½ Quarts Soymilk*

Measure out soybeans using the plastic cup packaged with the soymilk maker. Rinse the soybeans thoroughly several times and place in a medium bowl. Cover with about 6 cups cold water and set aside to soak for 6 to 16 hours.

Rinse presoaked beans several times, then place half of the beans (about ¾ cup) in the filter cup and attach to the machine by turning to the left. Fill the canister with water to between the two water marks, and place the top machine assembly, with the filter cup attached, on the canister. Insert the plug, and press Start. The machine will go through its preprogrammed cycle, and beep in 15 minutes.

Remove the top assembly and run cold water over the coils, then remove the filter cup by turning to the right. The filter now holds the *okara,* a byproduct of soymilk-making process. Okara is a wonderful ingredient that adds fiber and soy protein to many dishes. If you are planning to use the okara, scoop it into a container and set aside. Okara can also be dry roasted (see page 39).

HOMEMADE soymilk is fresh, delicious, and quite cost-effective; about forty-two cents per gallon! Making soymilk in your own kitchen is as easy as using an automatic coffee maker. It takes just 22 minutes from start to finish with the new automatic soymilk makers.

The soymilk maker used in *The Enlightened Kitchen* makes terrific soymilk using presoaked soybeans. Soaking the beans produces a higher quality soymilk with a far greater yield. Soymilk made using this method will also be more successful in making homemade tofu. There are automatic soymilk makers available that use dry beans (not presoaked) but I do not recommend such machines. Besides, it is easy to set the beans to soak before bedtime, or in the morning, and making the soymilk as much as 16 hours later.

## Homemade Soymilk *(continued)*

Set top assembly aside, and remove and empty filter cup. Clean cup and coils *thoroughly,* using brush supplied with the machine and a scouring pad.

Leaving the first batch of soymilk in the canister, add the remaining soaked beans to the filter cup. Replace the assembly on the canister, plug in, and press Start. The second cycle will take only 7 minutes, as the milk in the canister is already hot. When machine beeps, remove the assembly, and pour the soymilk into a pitcher. Add salt, Fruitsource, and vanilla. Stir and set aside to cool, uncovered, for about an hour or so. When cool, store, covered, in refrigerator for up to 5 days.

### Chocolate-Flavored Homemade Soymilk

½ cup warm liquid Fruitsource or
   brown rice syrup
3 tablespoons cocoa powder
2 tablespoons pure vanilla extract

1 teaspoon almond extract
50 ounces Homemade Soymilk
   (6¼ cups)
½ teaspoon sea salt

Place the Fruitsource in a glass liquid measure and warm in the microwave for 20 seconds. Add the cocoa and blend. Stir in the vanilla and almond extracts and mix thoroughly. Scrape the mixture into the soymilk, using a rubber spatula, and add the sea salt.

---

### NUTRITION ANALYSIS: PER 1-CUP SERVING

**Enlightened Soymilk**
Protein 6 g, carbohydrate 11 g, fiber 2 g, fat 3 g,
saturated fat .5 g, cholesterol 0 mg,
calcium 53 mg, sodium 163 mg
Calories 97: from protein 25%,
from carbohydrate 44%, from fat 31%*

**Traditional Cow's Milk**
Protein 8 g, carbohydrate 11 g, fiber 0 g, fat 8 g,
saturated fat 5 g, cholesterol 13 mg,
calcium 290 mg, sodium 120 mg
Calories 150: from protein 21%,
from carbohydrate 30%, from fat 49%

* The percentage of calories from fat seems high because the calories are so low.

# Homemade Tofu

*It's really easy to take homemade soymilk a step further and make tofu in your own kitchen. You will need a tofu press, cheesecloth, and nigari. Everything you need is available in a nifty tofu-making kit that you can get online at www.fairviewfarms.com.*

3 quarts of Homemade Soymilk (page 203)

1 cup very warm water (about 100°)
2 teaspoons nigari

Pour soymilk into a covered 6-quart saucepan and keep it warm. Stir the nigari into the warm water. It will dissolve in less than a minute. Stir the hot soymilk in one direction, stop the spoon, and pour in half of the nigari mixture. Cover and set aside for 5 minutes. Pour in the rest of the nigari, stir, and cover. Set aside for 10 minutes. The soymilk will have separated into curds and whey. For a firm-style tofu, set the pot over low heat for 4 minutes, stirring frequently. Set up the tofu press in a flat-bottomed colander, and dampen the pressing cloth. Using a small, handled, wire mesh colander, scoop the curds into the pressing cloth. Fold the cloth in over the curds. Cover with the pressing lid and top with a small, narrow weight. Let the tofu press for at lease 1 hour. For very firm tofu, press for several hours. Remove the block of tofu from the press and place it in a covered container, submerged in water. Change the water daily, and use within 5 days.

THE NEW automatic soymilk makers really simplify the process of making both soymilk and tofu. And once you have made tofu in your own kitchen, you will be amazed at just how easy and delicious it can be!

## NUTRITION ANALYSIS: PER ⅓-CUP SERVING

### Enlightened Firm Nigari Tofu
Protein 11 g, carbohydrate 3 g, fiber 0 g, fat 6 g, saturated fat 1 g, cholesterol 0 mg, calcium 38 mg, sodium 9 mg
Calories 97: from protein 40%, from carbohydrate 11%, from fat 49%

### Traditional Pork Cutlet
Protein 18 g, carbohydrate 0 g, fiber 0 g, fat 16 g, saturated fat 6 g, cholesterol 73 mg, calcium 12 mg, sodium 59 mg
Calories 222: from protein 35%, from carbohydrate 0%, from fat 65%

# Homemade Ginger Baked Tofu

*When marinated and baked, tofu takes on a meaty texture
and flavor. Marinate and baste: that's all there is to it!*

*6
Servings*

1 recipe Pungent Ginger Marinade
  (page 215)
1 19-ounce package Chinese-style
  extra-firm tofu, cut into 3-by-
  ½-inch slices

olive oil cooking spray
2 tablespoons cornstarch
2 tablespoons cold water
2 tablespoons nutritional yeast

Sliced marinated baked tofu is terrific in sandwiches and salads. It is also a fabulous addition to stir-fry, vegetable, rice, and pasta dishes.

Combine tofu and marinade in a nonreactive (preferably glass) bowl. Cover and refrigerate for 1 hour.

Preheat oven to 350°. Spray 9-by-13-inch baking pan with olive oil cooking spray. Remove tofu from bowl, reserving marinade, and place in prepared baking pan. Lightly spray tofu with olive oil cooking spray. Bake for 10 minutes. In a small bowl, combine cornstarch and water. Stir into reserved marinade and yeast. Turn tofu slices over. Pour ½ cup of the marinade over tofu and return to oven. Repeat this process several times during baking. Bake for approximately 70 minutes in all, or until marinade is absorbed. (It may take as long as 90 minutes, depending on the texture of the tofu—but it's well worth it!). Cool, then refrigerate, covered, for up to 3 days.

NUTRITION ANALYSIS: PER 3-OUNCE SERVING

**Enlightened Baked Tofu**
Protein 15 g, carbohydrate 12 g, fiber 4 g,
fat 2 g, cholesterol 0 mg,
calcium 55 mg, sodium 362 mg
Calories 116: from protein 49%,
from carbohydrate 39%, from fat 12%

**Traditional Baked Chicken**
Protein 23 g, carbohydrate 4 g, fiber 0 g, fat 15 g,
saturated fat 3 g, cholesterol 68 mg,
calcium 23 mg, sodium 610 mg
Calories 247: from protein 38%,
from carbohydrate 7%, from fat 55%

# Homemade Barbecue Baked Tofu

*This kind of tofu is great sliced in
sandwiches or on salads.*

1 recipe Zesty Barbecue Marinade
   (page 220)
1 19-ounce package Chinese-style,
   extra-firm tofu, cut into 3-by-
   ½-inch slices

olive oil cooking spray

Combine tofu and marinade in a nonreactive (preferably glass) bowl. Cover, and refrigerate for 1 hour.

Preheat oven to 350°. Spray 9-by-13-inch baking pan with olive oil cooking spray. Remove tofu from bowl, reserving marinade, and place in prepared baking pan. Lightly spray tofu with olive oil cooking spray. Bake 10 minutes. Turn tofu slices over and pour ½ cup of the marinade over tofu. Repeat this process several times during baking. Bake approximately 70 to 90 minutes, or until marinade is absorbed. Cool, then refrigerate, covered, for up to 3 days.

NUTRITION ANALYSIS: PER 3-OUNCE SERVING

| Enlightened Barbecue Baked Tofu | Traditional Barbecue Baked Chicken |
|---|---|
| Protein 13 g, carbohydrate 18 g, fiber 3 g, fat 2 g, saturated fat 0 g, cholesterol 0 mg, calcium 49 mg, sodium 67 mg | Protein 19 g, carbohydrate 3 g, fiber 1 g, fat 12 g, saturated fat 3 g, cholesterol 55 mg, calcium 14 mg, sodium 523 mg |
| Calories 138: from protein 37%, from carbohydrate 51%, from fat 12% | Calories 197: from protein 40%, from carbohydrate 5%, from fat 55% |

# Asian Marinade

*Add an eastern tone to any dish,
from teriyaki to bok choy, with this tasty marinade.*

*Makes
about
2 Cups*

2 rounded teaspoons chicken-flavor
   vegetarian broth powder
1 cup boiling water
2 tablespoons tamari lite
2 tablespoons liquid Fruitsource or
   rice syrup

1 teaspoon sesame oil
1 teaspoon vegetarian Worstershire
   sauce
¼ cup mirin cooking wine
3 cloves garlic, minced
1 tablespoon rice vinegar

Use this marinade for very firm tofu or steamed tempeh.

Combine broth powder and boiling water. Add tamari, Fruitsource, sesame oil, Worcestershire sauce, mirin, garlic, and vinegar. Mix thoroughly, using a small wire whisk or fork. Marinate ingredients of choice for at least 1 hour, covered, in the refrigerator. Turn ingredients at least once during the marinating process.

NUTRITION ANALYSIS: PER 2-TABLESPOONS SERVING

**Enlightened Asian Marinade**
Protein 1 g, carbohydrate 4 g, fiber 0 g, fat 1 g,
saturated fat 0 g, cholesterol 0 mg,
calcium 3 mg, sodium 214 mg
Calories 24: from protein 12%,
from carbohydrate 66%, from fat 22%

**Traditional Asian Marinade**
Protein 1 g, carbohydrate 4 g, fiber 0 g, fat 9 g,
saturated fat 1 g, cholesterol 0 mg, saturated fat 2 g,
calcium 7 mg, sodium 680 mg
Calories 93: from protein 3%,
from carbohydrate 18%, from fat 79%

# Balsamic Marinade

*Use this marinade to enhance cooked edamame or vegetables, such as broccoli, cauliflower, fresh mushrooms, and bell peppers.*

½ rounded tablespoon DDC onion
    broth powder
1 cup boiling water
¼ cup balsamic vinegar
2 cloves garlic, minced

1 tablespoon Dijon mustard
2 tablespoons tamari
¼ teaspoon coarse black pepper
1 rounded teaspoon dried basil
½ cup sliced scallions

Combine broth powder and boiling water. Add vinegar, garlic, mustard, tamari, pepper, basil, and scallions, stirring after each addition. Marinate ingredients of choice for at least 1 hour, covered, in the refrigerator. Turn ingredients at least once during the marinating process.

BALSAMIC vinegar adds a sweet and sour balance of flavor not found in other vinegars.

### NUTRITION ANALYSIS: PER 2-TABLESPOONS SERVING

**Enlightened Balsamic Marinade**
Protein 1 g, carbohydrate 4 g, fiber 0 g, fat 0 g,
saturated fat 0 g, cholesterol 0 mg,
calcium 17 mg, sodium 130 mg
Calories 19: from protein 17%,
from carbohydrate 77%, from fat 6%

**Traditional Balsamic Marinade**
Protein 1 g, carbohydrate 7 g, fiber 0 g, fat 7 g,
saturated fat 1 g, cholesterol 0 mg,
calcium 3 mg, sodium 634 mg
Calories 87: from protein 4%,
from carbohydrate 25%, from fat 66%

# Sweet 'n' Sassy Marinade

*Use this marinade to enhance very firm tofu, steamed tempeh,
or a mix of vegetables such as potatoes (sweet and white),
carrots, onions, and bell peppers.*

*Makes
2¹/₃ Cups*

2 rounded teaspoons chicken-flavor
  vegetarian broth powder
1 cup boiling water
¹/₃ cup fruit-sweetened apricot
  preserves

2 tablespoons tamari
1 tablespoon balsamic vinegar
2 teaspoons granulated garlic
¹/₃ cup pineapple salsa
juice of 1 lime

Combine broth powder and boiling water. Add preserves, tamari, vinegar, garlic, salsa, and lime juice. Mix thoroughly, using a fork. Marinate ingredients of your choice for at least 1 hour, covered, in the refrigerator. Turn ingredients at least once during the marinating process.

NUTRITION ANALYSIS: PER 2-TABLESPOONS SERVING

**Enlightened Sweet 'n' Sassy Marinade**
Protein 1 g, carbohydrate 8 g, fiber 0 g, fat 0 g,
saturated fat 0 g, cholesterol 0 mg,
calcium 2 mg, sodium 185 mg
Calories 33: from protein 10%,
from carbohydrate 90%, from fat 0%

**Traditional Sweet 'n' Sassy Marinade**
Protein 1 g, carbohydrate 7 g, fiber 0 g, fat 7 g,
saturated fat 1 g, cholesterol 0 mg,
calcium 3 mg, sodium 634 mg
Calories 87: from protein 4%,
from carbohydrate 25%, from fat 66%

# Fragrant Soy Marinade

*This marinade is particularly well-suited for enhancing the flavor of very firm tofu.*

*Makes
2 Cups*

1 rounded teaspoon chicken-flavor
   vegetarian broth powder
1½ cups boiling water
⅓ cup tamari

1 tablespoon balsamic vinegar
1 teaspoon granulated garlic
½ teaspoon dried thyme
½ teaspoon dried oregano

Combine broth powder and boiling water. Add tamari, vinegar, garlic, thyme, and oregano. Mix thoroughly, using a small wire whisk or fork. Marinate ingredients of your choice for up to 24 hours, covered, in the refrigerator. Turn ingredients at least once during the marinating process.

---

NUTRITION ANALYSIS: PER 2-TABLESPOON SERVING

**Enlightened Fragrant Soy Marinade**
Protein 1 g, carbohydrate 2 g, fiber 0 g, fat 0 g,
saturated fat 0 g, cholesterol 0 mg,
calcium 6 mg, sodium 560 mg
Calories 10: from protein 41%,
from carbohydrate 56%, from fat 3%

**Traditional Soy Marinade**
Protein 1 g, carbohydrate 3 g, fiber 0 g, fat 4 g,
saturated fat 1 g, cholesterol 0 mg,
calcium 10 mg, sodium 1387 mg
Calories 52: from protein 10%,
from carbohydrate 21%, from fat 69%

# Lively Marinade

*The delicate balance of flavors in this marinade are readily absorbed,
as in dishes like Hearty "Chicken" with Asparagus (page 127).
Marinate overnight for deepened flavor.*

*Makes
1¹/₂ Cups*

1 rounded tablespoon chicken-flavor
   vegetarian broth powder
1 cup boiling water
1 tablespoon liquid Fruitsource

¼ cup tamari
1 teaspoon granulated garlic
1 tablespoon red wine vinegar
½ teaspoon dried basil

USE THIS lively marinade to enhance seitan (chicken-flavor or traditional), very firm tofu, or steamed tempeh.

Combine broth powder and boiling water. Add Fruitsource, tamari, garlic, vinegar, and basil, stirring after each addition. Marinate ingredients of choice for at least 1 hour, covered, in the refrigerator. Turn ingredients at least once during the marinating process.

NUTRITION ANALYSIS: PER 2-TABLESPOON SERVING

**Enlightened Lively Marinade**
Protein 1 g, carbohydrate 2 g, fiber 0 g, fat 0 g,
saturated fat 0 g, cholesterol 0 mg,
calcium 4 mg, sodium 382 mg
Calories 11: from protein 26%,
from carbohydrate 73%, from fat 1%

**Traditional Lively Marinade**
Protein 1 g, carbohydrate 3 g, fiber 0 g, fat 10 g,
saturated fat 2 g, cholesterol 0 mg,
calcium 4 mg, sodium 431 mg
Calories 109: from protein 2%,
from carbohydrate 11%, from fat 87%

# Orient Express Marinade

*This marinade has a*
*robust flavor with an Asian accent.*

*Makes*
*1¹/₂ Cups*

1 rounded tablespoon beef-flavor
    vegetarian broth powder
1¼ cups boiling water
¼ cup tamari
1 teaspoon vegetarian Worcestershire
    sauce

1 teaspoon granulated garlic
1 teaspoon ground ginger
½ teaspoon sesame oil

Combine broth powder and boiling water. Add tamari, Worcestershire sauce, garlic, ginger, and sesame oil, stirring after each addition. Marinate ingredients of choice for at least 1 hour, covered, in the refrigerator. Turn ingredients at least once during the marinating process.

USE THIS tasty marinade to enhance seitan (chicken-flavor or traditional), very firm tofu, or steamed tempeh.

---

NUTRITION ANALYSIS: PER 2-TABLESPOON SERVING

**Enlightened Orient Express Marinade**
Protein 1 g, carbohydrate 2 g, fiber 0 g, fat 0 g,
saturated fat 0 g, cholesterol 0 mg,
calcium 2 mg, sodium 433 mg
Calories 18: from protein 25%,
from carbohydrate 33%, from fat 17%

**Traditional Oriental Marinade**
Protein 2 g, carbohydrate 2 g, fiber 0 g, fat 5 g,
saturated fat 1 g, cholesterol 0 mg,
calcium 6 mg, sodium 1037 mg
Calories 61: from protein 10%,
from carbohydrate 14%, from fat 76%

# Pacific Blend Marinade

*Marinate overnight to create an extremely rich flavor in dishes such as Caribbean Pasta Salad (page 96).*

*Makes
1²/₃ Cups*

1 rounded tablespoon DDC onion
    broth powder
1 cup boiling water
3 scallions

¼ cup tamari
½ teaspoon granulated garlic
½ teaspoon granulated onion
½ teaspoon ground ginger

Use this flavorful marinade to enhance seitan (chicken-flavor or traditional), very firm tofu, or steamed tempeh.

Combine broth powder and boiling water. Chop scallions, including 2 inches of green. Add to broth with tamari, garlic, onion, and ginger. Mix thoroughly. Marinate ingredients of choice for at least 1 hour, covered, in the refrigerator. Turn ingredients at least once during the marinating process.

NUTRITION ANALYSIS: PER 2-TABLESPOON SERVING

**Enlightened Pacific Blend Marinade**
Protein 1 g, carbohydrate 2 g, fiber 0 g, fat 0 g,
saturated fat 0 g, cholesterol 0 mg,
calcium 2 mg, sodium 367 mg
Calories 11: from protein 30%,
from carbohydrate 56%, from fat 14%

**Traditional Pacific Marinade**
Protein 1 g, carbohydrate 4 g, fiber 0 g, fat 8 g,
saturated fat 1 g, cholesterol 0 mg,
calcium 4 mg, sodium 726 mg
Calories 93: from protein 5%,
from carbohydrate 18%, from fat 77%

# Pungent Ginger Marinade

*In addition to being great for making homemade baked tofu,
this marinade can also be used to enhance seitan (chicken-flavor
or traditional), very firm tofu, or steamed tempeh.*

1 rounded tablespoon beef-flavor
   vegetarian broth powder
1 cup boiling water
1 tablespoon liquid Fruitsource

2½ tablespoons tamari
1 tablespoon red wine vinegar
1 tablespoon grated gingerroot
1 teaspoon granulated garlic

Combine broth powder and boiling water. Add Fruitsource, tamari, vinegar, gingerroot, and garlic. Mix thoroughly, using a small wire whisk or fork. Marinate ingredients of choice for 1 hour, covered, in the refrigerator. Turn ingredients at least once during the marinating process.

NUTRITION ANALYSIS: PER 2-TABLESPOON SERVING

Enlightened Pungent Ginger Marinade
Protein 1 g, carbohydrate 3 g, fiber 0 g, fat 0 g,
saturated fat 0 g, cholesterol 0 mg,
calcium 3 mg, sodium 357 mg
Calories 15: from protein 19%,
from carbohydrate 80%, from fat 1%

Traditional Ginger Marinade
Protein 2 g, carbohydrate 2 g, fiber 0 g, fat 9 g,
saturated fat 1 g, cholesterol 0 mg,
calcium 5 mg, sodium 863 mg
Calories 91: from protein 7%,
from carbohydrate 10%, from fat 83%

# Red Miso Marinade

*Richly flavorful, red miso adds a particular depth to this delicious
marinade. For best results, marinate overnight.*

*Makes
2¹/₂ cups*

2 rounded teaspoons beef-flavored
    vegetarian broth powder
1½ cups boiling water
¼ cup tamari
1 teaspoon vegetarian Worcestershire
    sauce

1 teaspoons granulated garlic
1 teaspoon dried thyme
3 tablespoons red miso
⅓ cup dry vermouth

THIS MARINADE is very
nice with seitan (chicken-
flavor or traditional), very
firm tofu, or steamed tempeh.

Combine broth powder and boiling water. Add tamari, Worcestershire sauce, garlic, and thyme, stirring after each addition.
Spoon miso into a small cup, add vermouth, and blend well with
a fork. Add to the broth mixture and mix thoroughly, using a
fork or small wire whisk. Marinate ingredients of choice for at
least 1 hour, covered, in the refrigerator. Turn ingredients at least
once during the marinating process.

NUTRITION ANALYSIS: PER 2-TABLESPOON SERVING

Enlightened Red Miso Marinade
Protein 0 g, carbohydrate 1 g, fiber 0 g, fat 0 g,
saturated fat 0 g, cholesterol 0 mg,
calcium 3 mg, sodium 205 mg
Calories 10: from protein 38%,
from carbohydrate 58%, from fat 4%

Traditional Marinade
Protein 0 g, carbohydrate 1 g, fiber 0 g, fat 27 g,
saturated fat 5 g, cholesterol 0 mg,
calcium 3 mg, sodium 205 mg
Calories 249: from protein 1%,
from carbohydrate 3%, from fat 98%

# Roasted Chile Marinade

*A terrific marinade for Tempeh Kebabs (page 135), corn on the cob,
or anything you might grill, bake, or broil.*

1 rounded teaspoon beef-flavor
    vegetarian broth powder
½ cup boiling water
1 cup roasted chile salsa
1 whole red or green fire-roasted
    chile, chopped
2 tablespoons Dijon mustard

3 tablespoons fruit-sweetened
    ketchup
2 tablespoons tamari
1 tablespoon balsamic vinegar
2 teaspoons granulated garlic
juice of 1 lime

Combine broth powder and boiling water. Add salsa, chopped chile, mustard, ketchup, tamari, vinegar, garlic, and lime juice, stirring after each addition. Marinate ingredients of choice for at least 2 hours, covered, in the refrigerator. Turn ingredients at least once during the marinating process.

---

NUTRITION ANALYSIS: PER 2-TABLESPOON SERVING

**Enlightened Roasted Chile Marinade**
Protein 1 g, carbohydrate 5 g, fiber 0 g, fat 0 g,
saturated fat 0 g, cholesterol 0 mg,
calcium 2 mg, sodium 127 mg
Calories 21: from protein 23%,
from carbohydrate 77%, from fat 0%

**Traditional Roasted Chile Marinade**
Protein 1 g, carbohydrate 3 g, fiber 0 g, fat 12 g,
saturated fat 2 g, cholesterol 0 mg,
calcium 3 mg, sodium 346 mg
Calories 118: from protein 4%,
from carbohydrate 10%, from fat 86%

# Savory Sesame Marinade

*A full-bodied and really delicious marinade, based on a
popular salad dressing available at most health food stores.
Marinate overnight for the best flavor.*

*Makes
about
²/₃ Cup*

⅓ cup sesame shitake salad dressing
3 scallions, chopped
½ teaspoon granulated garlic

½ teaspoon granulated onion
2 tablespoons tamari
¼ cup chopped fresh cilantro

THIS MARINADE is a
knock-out when used to
enhance cooked edamame
and sliced mushrooms.

Combine all ingredients in a medium-size glass bowl or measuring
cup. Mix thoroughly, using a fork. Marinate ingredients of choice
for at least 1 hour, covered, in the refrigerator. Turn ingredients at
least once during the marinating process.

---

NUTRITION ANALYSIS: PER 1-TABLESPOON SERVING

**Enlightened Savory Sesame Marinade**
Protein 1 g, carbohydrate 2 g, fiber 0 g, fat 5 g,
saturated fat 0 g, cholesterol 0 mg,
calcium 6 mg, sodium 821 mg
Calories 52: from protein 5%,
from carbohydrate 12%, from fat 83%

**Traditional Sesame Marinade**
Protein 1 g, carbohydrate 3 g, fiber 0 g, fat 11 g,
saturated fat 2 g, cholesterol 0 mg,
calcium 6 mg, sodium 766 mg.
Calories 109: from protein 5%,
from carbohydrate 10%, from fat 85%

# Spring Onion Marinade

*A very interesting marinade for raw vegetables.*

*Makes
2¹/₄ Cups*

1 rounded tablespoon DDC onion
   broth powder
1 cup boiling water
3 cloves garlic, minced
3 scallions, chopped

3 tablespoons tamari
3 tablespoons lemon juice
1 tablespoon olive oil
1 teaspoon marjoram
1 teaspoon dried thyme

Combine broth powder and boiling water. Add garlic, scallions, tamari, lemon juice, oil, marjoram, and thyme. Mix thoroughly. Marinate ingredients of choice overnight, covered, in the refrigerator. Turn ingredients at least once during the marinating process.

THIS MARINADE adds light flavor accents to cooked edamame or vegetables such as cauliflower, carrots, and broccoli or sliced mushrooms.

---

NUTRITION ANALYSIS: PER 2-TABLESPOON SERVING

**Enlightened Spring Onion Marinade**
Protein 1 g, carbohydrate 2 g, fiber 0 g, fat 2 g,
saturated fat 0 g, cholesterol 0 mg,
calcium 10 mg, sodium 295 mg
Calories 24: from protein 12%,
from carbohydrate 29%, from fat 59%

**Traditional Marinade**
Protein 1 g, carbohydrate 7 g, fiber 0 g, fat 7 g,
saturated fat 1 g, cholesterol 0 mg,
calcium 3 mg, sodium 634 mg
Calories 87: from protein 4%,
from carbohydrate 25%, from fat 66%

# Zesty Barbecue Marinade

*This marinade is great for grilled, baked,
or broiled dishes.*

*Makes
about
2 Cups*

1 teaspoon beef-flavor vegetarian
  broth powder
½ cup boiling water
2 tablespoon liquid Fruitsource or
  brown rice syrup
1¼ cups barbecue sauce, hot &
  smoky or hickory flavor

1 tablespoon Dijon mustard
2 garlic cloves, minced
1 teaspoon granulated onion
3 tablespoons nutritional yeast

THIS MARINADE is is
used to make Homemade
Barbecue Baked Tofu
(page 207). Use it also
with steamed tempeh, firm
tofu, or seitan.

Combine broth powder and boiling water. Add Fruitsource, barbecue sauce, mustard, garlic, granulated onion, and yeast. Mix thoroughly, using a small wire whisk or fork. Marinate ingredient of choice and refrigerate, covered, for 1 hour. Turn ingredients at least once during the marinating process.

---

NUTRITION ANALYSIS: PER 2-TABLESPOON SERVING

**Enlightened Barbecue Marinade**
Protein 2 g, carbohydrate 10 g, fiber 0 g, fat 0 g,
saturated fat 0 g, cholesterol 0 mg,
calcium 5 mg, sodium 45 mg
Calories 48: from protein 15%,
from carbohydrate 78%, from fat 7%

**Traditional Barbecue Marinade**
Protein 1 g, carbohydrate 9 g, fiber 0 g, fat 8 g,
saturated fat 1 g, cholesterol 0 mg,
calcium 5 mg, sodium 350 mg
Calories 107: from protein 4%,
from carbohydrate 32% from fat 64%

# Pineapple Apricot Butter

*This luscious spread has a velvety texture*
*and rich buttery flavor—and it's fat free!*

1½ cups chopped dried apricots
⅔ cup chopped dried pineapple

1½ cups apple cider
¼ cup frozen apple juice concentrate

Place apricots, pineapple, and cider in a medium saucepan and bring to a boil. Reduce heat to low, add apple juice concentrate, and simmer, stirring frequently, for 25 minutes, or until liquid has been absorbed. Set aside for 10 minutes to cool slightly.

Purée mixture in food processor or blender. Spoon into a covered container and store in refrigerator for up to 2 weeks.

---

### NUTRITION ANALYSIS: PER 3-TABLESPOON SERVING

**Enlightened Pineapple Apricot Butter**
Protein 1 g, carbohydrate 24 g, fiber 2 g, fat 0 g,
saturated fat 0 g, cholesterol 0 mg,
calcium 17 mg, sodium 11 mg
Calories 95: from protein 2%,
from carbohydrate 98%, from fat 0%

**Traditional Pineapple Apricot Butter**
Protein 1 g, carbohydrate 30 g, fiber 2 g, fat 7 g,
saturated fat 4 g, cholesterol 18 mg,
calcium 2 mg, sodium 10 mg
Calories 177: from protein 2%,
from carbohydrate 64%, from fat 34%

# Spiced Peach Butter

*The enlightened approach to making fruit butters creates
delectable spreads that are not only fat-free but sugar-free too!*

*Makes
3 Cups*

1½ cups chopped dried peaches
3 tablespoons pure maple syrup

1⅓ cups apple cider

Place peaches, maple syrup, and cider in a medium saucepan and bring to a boil over medium-high heat. Reduce heat to low and simmer, stirring constantly, for 25 minutes, or until liquid has been absorbed. Set aside for 10 minutes to cool slightly.

Purée mixture in food processor or blender. Spoon into a covered container and store in refrigerator for up to 2 weeks.

## NUTRITION ANALYSIS: PER 2-TABLESPOON SERVING

**Enlightened Spiced Peach Butter**
Protein 1 g, carbohydrate 24 g, fiber 2 g, fat 0 g,
saturated fat 0 g, cholesterol 0 mg,
calcium 6 mg, sodium 1 mg
Calories 94: from protein 5%,
from carbohydrate 95%, from fat 0%

**Traditional Peach Butter**
Protein 2 g, carbohydrate 27 g, fiber 2 g, fat 7 g,
saturated fat 5 g, cholesterol 19 mg,
calcium 2 mg, sodium 2 mg
Calories 167: from protein 3%,
from carbohydrate 61%, from fat 36%

# Marvelous Muffins
# and Loaves

When you want to whip up a quick and delicious accompaniment to a meal, quickbreads are an easy choice. However, even simple treats such as muffins or tea breads can be the source of unwanted fat and calories. As in all of my baking, I use fruit purées to replace the fat. And I often add fiber-rich dried fruits and nutritious soynuts or sunflower seeds. Baking the Enlightened way, you can make scrumptious treats with all of the flavor and texture you expect, with a fraction of the fat and no cholesterol.

The method for making quickbreads is fairly standard. The dry and liquid ingredients are mixed in separate bowls. Any additions—such as dried fruit, nuts, or chocolate chips—are added to the dry ingredients, minimizing mixing and handling. Then the dry and liquid ingredients are combined with a wooden spoon or spatula just until the dry mixture is moistened.

The preparation time can be streamlined even more by completing the early stages in advance. Serve a basket of fragrant muffins at breakfast, fresh from the oven with a minimum of fuss, by assembling the dry and the liquid ingredients, the night before. Store each *separately,* covered, in the refrigerator. The following morning, simply combine as directed and bake. Note: Heavy-weight muffin pans will absorb and hold the heat better, and muffins baked in pans such as these will rise higher and have better color. In addition to muffins and quickbreads, there are a few bread machine loaves in this chapter. Serve these wholesome baked goods with pride, knowing that they are as good for you as they are *delicious!*

# Recipes

Awesome Apricot Muffins
Cranberry Spice Muffins
Cranberry Walnut Muffins
Blueberries, Oats, and Roses Muffins
Yam Good Muffins!
Banana Bread with Roasted Soynuts
Chocolate Chip Banana Bread
Cinnamon Raisin Bread
Cranberry Banana Bread
Hearty Whole Wheat Bread
Spiced Pineapple Zucchini Bread
Pumpkin Raisin Bread
Southern-Style Sweet Potato Bread
Cranberry Apple Coffee Cake
Blueberry Apple Pancakes

# Awesome Apricot Muffins

*Brandied apricots elevate these delicious muffins to new heights.*
*Serve with Pineapple Apricot Butter (page 221).*

olive oil cooking spray
1 cup chopped apricots
½ cup apricot brandy or water
2 cups whole wheat pastry flour
¼ cup whole-grain yellow cornmeal
¼ cup soy flour
1 teaspoon ground cinnamon
1 tablespoon nonaluminum baking
  powder

½ teaspoon sea salt
½ cup prune purée
½ cup Sucanat unrefined cane sugar
2 tablespoons liquid Fruitsource
2 tablespoons egg replacer powder
½ cup water
½ cup soymilk
1 tablespoon pure vanilla extract
½ cup Tosteds soynuts

Preheat oven to 350°. Spray muffin cups with olive oil cooking spray.

Place apricots in saucepan, add brandy, and warm over medium heat for 5 minutes, or until brandy is absorbed. Set aside. In a medium bowl, combine pastry flour with cornmeal, soy flour, cinnamon, baking powder, and salt. Set aside.

In a large bowl, blend prune purée with sugar and Fruitsource. In a small bowl, whisk egg replacer powder with water until foamy. Add to sugar mixture with soymilk and vanilla, and mix thoroughly. Quickly fold the dry ingredients into the liquid and add apricots, stirring just until blended. Top muffins with soynuts and bake for 20 to 25 minutes, or until toothpick inserted in middle comes out clean.

> THIS RECIPE makes 16 muffins. Use 2 muffin pans, filling the empty muffin cups ⅓ full with water before baking.

## NUTRITION ANALYSIS: PER MUFFIN

**Enlightened Awesome Apricot Muffins**
Protein 5 g, carbohydrate 33 g, fiber 4 g, fat 2 g,
saturated fat 0 g, cholesterol 0 mg,
calcium 94 mg, sodium 181 mg
Calories 184: from protein 12%,
from carbohydrate 78%, from fat 10%

**Traditional Apricot Muffins**
Protein 5 g, carbohydrate 36 g, fiber 2 g, fat 12 g,
saturated fat 6 g, cholesterol 58 mg,
calcium 108 mg, sodium 320 mg
Calories 291: from protein 8%,
from carbohydrate 53%, from fat 39%

# Cranberry Spice Muffins

*These muffins have a sophisticated
flavor and spicy kick.*

*12
Muffins*

olive oil cooking spray
2 cups whole wheat pastry flour
½ cup, plus 1 tablespoon whole grain
    yellow cornmeal
¼ cup soy flour
1 teaspoon nonaluminum baking
    powder
1 teaspoon baking soda
1¼ teaspoons ground cinnamon
¼ teaspoon ground nutmeg
⅛ teaspoon ground cloves

½ teaspoon sea salt
1 cup dried cranberries
½ cup prune purée
¾ cup evaporated cane sugar
2 tablespoon egg replacer powder
½ cup cold water
½ cup enriched 1 % fat vanilla
    soymilk
3 tablespoons unsalted sunflower
    seeds

Preheat oven to 350°. Spray muffin cups with oil.

In a medium bowl, combine the pastry flour with the cornmeal, soy flour, baking powder, baking soda, cinnamon, nutmeg, cloves, and salt. Stir in the cranberries and set aside.

In a large bowl, mix the prune purée with the cane sugar. In a small cup, whisk together the egg replacer powder with the water until foamy. Add to the sugar mixture, stir to blend, and add the soymilk. Quickly fold the dry ingredients into the liquid mixture. Pour into prepared muffin cups and sprinkle tops with sunflower seeds. Bake 25 minutes, or until tester comes out clean.

## NUTRITION ANALYSIS: PER MUFFIN

**Enlightened Cranberry Spice Muffins**
Protein 5 g, carbohydrate 46 g, fiber 4 g, fat 2 g,
saturated fat 0 g, cholesterol 0 mg,
calcium 54 mg, sodium 251 mg
Calories 214: from protein 8%,
from carbohydrate 83%, from fat 9%

**Traditional Cranberry Spice Muffins**
Protein 6 g, carbohydrate 44 g, fiber 2 g, fat 13 g,
saturated fat 6 g, cholesterol 60 mg,
calcium 50 mg, sodium 340 mg
Calories 312: from protein 7%,
from carbohydrate 56%, from fat 37%

# Cranberry Walnut Muffins

*Split leftover muffins and toast under
the broiler for a delightful snack.*

olive oil cooking spray
1¾ cups whole wheat pastry flour
¾ cup rolled oats
¼ cup soy flour
2 tablespoons whole grain yellow
    cornmeal
1 teaspoon nonaluminum baking
    powder
½ teaspoon baking soda
1 teaspoon ground cinnamon

½ teaspoon sea salt
1 cup dried cranberries
⅓ cup chopped walnuts
½ cup unsweetened applesauce
¾ cup evaporated cane sugar
2 tablespoons egg replacer powder
½ cup cold water
½ cup enriched 1% fat vanilla
    soymilk

Preheat oven to 350°. Spray muffin cups with olive oil.

In a medium bowl, combine pastry flour, oats, soy flour, corn-meal, baking powder, baking soda, cinnamon, and salt. Stir in cranberries and walnuts. Set aside.

In a large bowl, combine the applesauce with evaporated cane sugar. In a small cup, whisk egg replacer with water until foamy. Add to applesauce mixture with soymilk. Quickly fold the dry ingredients into the liquid mixture. Spoon into muffin cups. Bake 20 minutes, or until tester comes out clean.

FOR AN ADDED treat, spread with wholesome Pineapple Apricot Butter (page 221) or Spiced Peach Butter (page 222).

---

### NUTRITION ANALYSIS: PER MUFFIN

**Enlightened Cranberry Walnut Muffins**
Protein 5 g, carbohydrate 38 g, fiber 4 g, fat 3 g,
saturated fat 0 g, cholesterol 0 mg,
calcium 54 mg, sodium 184 mg
Calories 192: from protein 10%,
from carbohydrate 76%, from fat 14%

**Traditional Cranberry Walnut Muffins**
Protein 6 g, carbohydrate 40 g, fiber 2 g, fat 14 g,
saturated fat 6 g, cholesterol 22 mg,
calcium 49 mg, sodium 283 mg
Calories 304: from protein 8%,
from carbohydrate 51%, from fat 41%

# Blueberries, Oats, and Roses Muffins

*The great flavor and texture of these delicious muffins
are enhanced with the intoxicating aroma of roses.*

*12
Muffins*

olive oil cooking spray
1½ cups whole wheat pastry flour
¾ cup rolled oats
⅓ cup yellow cornmeal
2 tablespoons soy flour
1 teaspoon nonaluminum baking
    powder
1 teaspoon baking soda
1 teaspoon ground cinnamon
¼ teaspoon ground nutmeg
½ teaspoon sea salt

¾ cup dried blueberries
½ cup prune purée
¾ cup evaporated cane sugar
2 tablespoons egg replacer powder
½ cup cold water
½ cup plus 1 tablespoon enriched
    1 % fat vanilla soymilk
1 teaspoon rose water
¼ cup Tosteds soynuts

Preheat oven to 350°. Spray muffin cups with oil.

In a medium bowl, combine pastry flour, oats, cornmeal, soy flour, baking powder, baking soda, cinnamon, nutmeg, and salt. Stir in the blueberries and set aside.

In a large bowl, combine the prune purée with the cane sugar. In a small cup, whisk together the egg replacer powder with the water until foamy. Add to the sugar mixture, stir to blend, and add the soymilk and rose water. Quickly fold the dry ingredients into the liquid mixture. Pour into prepared muffin cups and sprinkle tops with soynuts. Bake 25 minutes, or until tester comes out clean.

## NUTRITION ANALYSIS: PER MUFFIN

**Enlightened Blueberries, Oats, and Roses Muffins**
Protein 5 g, carbohydrate 44 g, fiber 4 g, fat 2 g,
saturated fat 0 g, cholesterol 0 mg,
calcium 56 mg, sodium 255 mg
Calories 210: from protein 10%,
from carbohydrate 83%, from fat 7%

**Traditional Blueberry Oat Muffins**
Protein 6 g, carbohydrate 43 g, fiber 2 g, fat 13 g,
saturated fat 6 g, cholesterol 60 mg,
calcium 53 mg, sodium 366 mg
Calories 314: from protein 8%,
from carbohydrate 55%, from fat 37%

# Yam Good Muffins!

*Outstanding flavor, texture, and eye appeal*
*make these tasty muffins just perfect!*

olive oil cooking spray
2 cups Multi-Grain Baking Mix
   (page 195)
1 teaspoon ground allspice
1 teaspoon ground ginger
½ cup dried currants
¼ cup prune purée

¾ cup mashed cooked yams
⅔ cup evaporated cane sugar
¼ cup strong brewed coffee
¼ cup plus 2 tablespoons water
1 teaspoon pure vanilla extract
¼ cup Tosteds soynuts
nutmeg for garnish

Preheat oven to 350°. Spray muffin pan with olive oil.

In a medium bowl, combine Multi-Grain Baking Mix with allspice, ginger, and currants, and set aside.

In a large bowl, blend prune purée and yams. Add evaporated cane sugar and mix well. Add brewed coffee, water, and vanilla. Mix thoroughly. Fold the dry ingredients into the liquid, mixing just until blended. Spoon batter into prepared muffin cups. Top with soynuts, and sprinkle with nutmeg. Bake for 20 minutes, or until tester comes out clean.

THIS BEARS repeating: Tosteds are my soynut of choice for topping baked goods. A special roasting process produces a light, crunchy texture. *And,* they are not overly salty.

## NUTRITION ANALYSIS: PER MUFFIN

**Enlightened Yam Good Muffins!**
Protein 5 g, carbohydrate 31 g, fiber 3 g, fat 2 g,
saturated fat 0 g, cholesterol 0 mg,
calcium 75 mg, sodium 231 mg
Calories 151: from protein 12%,
from carbohydrate 78%, from fat 10%

**Traditional Sweet Potato Muffins**
Protein 5 g, carbohydrate 36 g, fiber 2 g, fat 16 g,
saturated fat 8 g, cholesterol 51 mg,
calcium 51 mg, sodium 230 mg
Calories 300: from protein 7%,
from carbohydrate 47%, from fat 46%

# Banana Bread with Roasted Soynuts

*This banana bread is topped with crunchy roasted soynuts that add the goodness of soy with ¹/₃ less fat than traditional nuts.*

olive oil cooking spray
2 cups whole wheat pastry flour
¼ cup soy flour
1 teaspoon nonaluminum baking
   powder
1 teaspoon baking soda
1 teaspoon ground cinnamon
⅛ teaspoon ground nutmeg
¼ teaspoon sea salt

⅓ cup prune purée
¾ cup evaporated cane sugar
1 cup mashed ripe bananas
   (2 medium)
1 tablespoons egg replacer powder
¼ cup water
1 teaspoon pure vanilla extract
¾ cup enriched vanilla soymilk
½ cup Tosteds soynuts

Preheat oven to 350°. Spray 9-by-5-inch loaf pan with olive oil.

In a medium bowl, combine whole wheat flour, soy flour, baking powder, baking soda, cinnamon, nutmeg, and salt. Set aside.

In a large bowl, blend prune purée with sugar. Add mashed bananas and blend. In a small bowl, whisk egg replacer powder with water until foamy. Add to banana mixture with vanilla and soymilk, and mix thoroughly. Fold the dry ingredients into the liquid, mixing just until blended. Pour batter into prepared pan and top with soynuts. Bake for 50 minutes, or until toothpick inserted in the middle comes out clean.

NUTRITION ANALYSIS: PER SLICE

**Enlightened Banana Bread with Roasted Soynuts**
Protein 7 g, carbohydrate 40 g, fiber 5 g, fat 2 g,
saturated fat 0 g, cholesterol 0 mg,
calcium 80 mg, sodium 240 mg
Calories 200: from protein 13%,
from carbohydrate 78%, from fat 9%

**Traditional Banana Nut Bread**
Protein 6 g, carbohydrate 38 g, fiber 2 g, fat 14 g,
saturated fat 6 g, cholesterol 64 mg,
calcium 62 mg, sodium 278 mg
Calories 293: from protein 8%,
from carbohydrate 51%, from fat 41%

# Chocolate Chip Banana Bread

*This moist quickbread, made with sweet chocolate chips and a crunchy cinnamon topping, is more like a dessert.*

olive oil cooking spray
¾ cup enriched 1% fat soymilk
1 tablespoon lemon juice
1 cup whole wheat pastry flour
1 cup rolled oats
1 teaspoon nonaluminum baking
  powder
1 teaspoon baking soda
1 teaspoon ground cinnamon
½ teaspoon sea salt

½ cup dairy-free chocolate chips
¼ cup unsweetened applesauce
1 cup mashed ripe bananas
  (2 medium)
¾ cup evaporated cane sugar
1 tablespoon egg replacer powder
¼ cup water
1 teaspoon pure vanilla extract

*Topping:*
2 tablespoons soy grits
2 tablespoons Sucanat, unrefined
  cane sugar

1 teaspoon ground cinnamon
nutmeg for garnish

Preheat oven to 350°. Spray a 9-by-5-inch loaf pan with olive oil cooking spray. Combine soymilk and lemon juice in a small glass measuring cup and set aside.

In a medium bowl, combine pastry flour, oats, baking powder, baking soda, cinnamon, and salt. Stir in chocolate chips and set aside.

In a large bowl, blend applesauce with bananas. Add evaporated cane sugar, mixing well. In a small bowl, whisk egg replacer powder with water until foamy. Add to applesauce mixture with vanilla and soymilk mixture, and mix thoroughly. Fold the dry ingredients into the liquid, stirring just until mixed. Pour batter into prepared pan.

BANANA BREAD is a very popular treat, and generally considered a healthy indulgence. However, traditional banana breads can be loaded with unhealthy fat and cholesterol.

**Chocolate Chip Banana Bread** *(continued)*

*For the topping:* In a small bowl, combine the soy grits, Sucanat, and cinnamon. Distribute evenly over batter, and sprinkle with nutmeg. Bake for 55 minutes, or until tester inserted in middle comes out clean.

---

NUTRITION ANALYSIS: PER SLICE

Enlightened Chocolate Chip Banana Bread
Protein 4 g, carbohydrate 39 g, fiber 4 g, fat 4g,
saturated fat 1 g, cholesterol 0 mg,
calcium 67 mg, sodium 285 mg
Calories 195: from protein 13%,
from carbohydrate 78%, from fat 9%

Traditional Chocolate Chip Banana Bread
Protein 5 g, carbohydrate 38 g, fiber 2 g, fat 18 g,
saturated fat 11 g, cholesterol 58 mg,
calcium 99 mg, sodium 420 mg
Calories 328: from protein 8%,
from carbohydrate 51%, from fat 41%

# Cinnamon Raisin Bread

*For this delightful bread, set the controls on your bread machine to
"Whole Grain" and "Medium Crust." Add the wholesome ingredients
according to your manufacturer's recommendations and walk away!*

### Small Loaf (about 1 pound)
- ¾ cup water
- 1 tablespoon olive oil
- 1½ tablespoons maple syrup
- 1 tablespoon vital wheat gluten
- 1½ tablespoon mashed potato flakes
- ½ teaspoon sea salt
- 1 cup whole wheat flour
- ¾ cup plus 2 tablespoons unbleached flour
- 2 tablespoons yellow cornmeal
- 1½ teaspoons ground cinnamon
- 1¼ teaspoons fast-rising yeast
- ⅓ cup golden raisins

### Large Loaf (about 2 pounds)
- 1½ cups water
- 2 tablespoons olive oil
- 3 tablespoons maple syrup
- 2 tablespoons vital wheat gluten
- 3 tablespoons mashed potato flakes
- 1 teaspoon sea salt
- 2 cups whole wheat flour
- 1¾ unbleached flour
- ¼ cup yellow cornmeal
- 1 tablespoon ground cinnamon
- 2½ teaspoons fast-rising yeast
- ⅔ cup golden raisins

Place all the ingredients, except for the raisins, in the baking
pan of the bread machine in the order presented. Or, follow the
instructions for your machine if they differ in the order presentation. In some cases, as in the DAK and Welbilt bread
machines, the manufacturer will recommended that the yeast
be added first. If that is the case, simply read the ingredient list
from bottom to top, beginning with yeast. Add raisins at the
"beep."

W HETHER YOU are a
novice who has never baked
bread before or an expert who
can't seem to find the time to
bake as often as you'd like, you
will now find homemade bread
as easy as pushing a button.

## NUTRITION ANALYSIS: PER SLICE

### Enlightened Cinnamon Raisin Bread
Protein 4 g, carbohydrate 21 g, fiber 2 g, fat 2 g,
saturated fat 0 g, cholesterol 0 mg,
calcium 13 mg, sodium122 mg
Calories 108: from protein 12%,
from carbohydrate 73%, from fat 15%

### Traditional Cinnamon Raisin Bread
Protein 3 g, carbohydrate 17 g, fiber 1 g, fat 4 g,
saturated fat 3 g, cholesterol 24 mg,
calcium 38 mg, sodium 150 mg
Calories 115: from protein 9%,
from carbohydrate 59%, from fat 32%

# Cranberry Banana Bread

*Orange blossom water enhances the flavor and
aroma of this moist quickbread.*

*10
Servings*

olive oil cooking spray
2 cups whole wheat pastry flour
⅓ cup yellow cornmeal
1 teaspoon nonaluminum baking
    powder
1 teaspoon baking soda
1 teaspoon ground cinnamon
½ teaspoon sea salt
⅔ cup dried cranberries
¼ cup prune purée

1 cup mashed ripe banana
    (2 medium)
¾ cup evaporated cane sugar
1 tablespoon egg replacer powder
¼ cup cold water
½ cup fresh orange juice
1 teaspoon pure vanilla extract
1 teaspoon orange blossom water
¼ cup unsalted sunflower seeds
cinnamon and nutmeg for garnish

DRIED FRUIT adds
flavor, texture, and color to
baked goods. Cranberries
are a great choice.

Preheat oven to 350°. Spray 9-by-5-inch loaf pan with olive oil cooking spray.

In a medium bowl, combine pastry flour, cornmeal, baking powder, baking soda, cinnamon, and salt. Stir in cranberries and set aside.

In a large bowl, combine the prune purée and banana. Add evaporated cane sugar and mix thoroughly. In a small cup, whisk egg replacer powder with water until foamy. Add to prune purée mixture with orange juice, vanilla, and orange blossom water. Quickly fold the dry ingredients into the liquid mixture. Pour batter into prepared loaf pan, and sprinkle with sunflower seeds, cinnamon, and nutmeg. Bake for 50 minutes, or until tester comes out clean.

## NUTRITION ANALYSIS: PER SLICE

**Enlightened Cranberry Banana Bread**
Protein 5 g, carbohydrate 50 g, fiber 4 g, fat 2 g,
saturated fat 0 g, cholesterol 0 mg,
calcium 48 mg, sodium 287 mg
Calories 231: from protein 8%,
from carbohydrate 83%, from fat 9%

**Traditional Cranberry Banana Bread**
Protein 5 g, carbohydrate 43 g, fiber 2 g, fat 21 g,
saturated fat 9 g, cholesterol 80 mg,
calcium 54 mg, sodium 404 mg
Calories 375: from protein 5%,
from carbohydrate 45%, from fat 50%

# Hearty Whole Wheat Bread

*Mashed potatoes or potato cooking water, when added
to any bread recipe, promotes a moist and even texture.
Convenient mashed potato flakes produce comparable results.*

### Small Loaf (about 1 pound)

¾ cup water

1 tablespoon olive oil

1½ tablespoons liquid Fruitsource

1 tablespoon vital wheat gluten

1½ tablespoons mashed potato flakes

½ teaspoon sea salt

1¾ cups plus 2 tablespoons whole
    wheat flour

2 tablespoons oat bran

1¼ teaspoons fast-rising yeast

### Large Loaf (about 2 pounds)

1½ cups water

2 tablespoons olive oil

3 tablespoons liquid Fruitsource

2 tablespoons vital wheat gluten

3 tablespoons mashed potato flakes

1 teaspoon sea salt

3¾ cups whole wheat flour

¼ cup oat bran

2½ teaspoons fast-rising yeast

Place the ingredients in the baking pan of the bread machine in the
order presented. Or, follow the instructions for your machine if
they differ in the order presentation. (In some cases, as in the DAK
and Welbilt bread machines, the manufacturer will recommended
that yeast be added first. If that is the case, simply read the ingredient list from bottom to top, beginning with yeast.)

T OAST AND serve with
Pineapple Apricot Butter
(page 221)

---

NUTRITION ANALYSIS: PER SLICE

| Enlightened Hearty Whole Grain Bread | Traditional White Bread |
|---|---|
| Protein 5 g, carbohydrate 23 g, fiber 4 g, fat 2 g, saturated fat 0 g, cholesterol 0 mg, calcium 11 mg, sodium136 mg Calories 122: from protein 15%, from carbohydrate 69%, from fat 16% | Protein 3 g, carbohydrate 23 g, fiber 1 g, fat 4 g, saturated fat 2 g, cholesterol 20 mg, calcium 7 mg, sodium 135 mg Calories 136: from protein 9%, from carbohydrate 50%, from fat 41% |

# Spiced Pineapple Zucchini Bread

*Zucchini bread is a perennial favorite. In this recipe, dried pineapple adds an unexpected flavor, and chopped almonds a delightful crunch.*

*2 Loaves,
10 Servings
Each*

olive oil cooking spray
2⅓ cups whole wheat pastry flour
⅔ cup oat bran
⅓ cup yellow cornmeal
½ teaspoon sea salt
1 teaspoon nonaluminum baking powder
2 teaspoons baking soda
1 teaspoon ground cinnamon
¼ teaspoon ground nutmeg

⅛ teaspoon ground cloves
1 cup diced dried pineapple
½ cup chopped almonds
1 12.3-ounce package lite silken tofu
½ cup unsweetened applesauce
2 cups evaporated cane sugar
½ cup enriched 1% fat soymilk
1 tablespoon pure vanilla extract
2 cups coarsely shredded zucchini

Preheat oven to 350°. Spray two 9-by-5-inch loaf pans with olive oil cooking spray.

In a large bowl, combine the flour, oat bran, cornmeal, salt, baking powder, baking soda, cinnamon, nutmeg, and cloves. Stir in the pineapple and almonds. Set aside.

Place the tofu in food processor and blend until smooth, about 1 minute. Add applesauce, evaporated cane sugar, soymilk, and vanilla. Quickly fold the tofu mixture into the dry ingredients, and add the zucchini. Do not overbeat. Divide the batter between the prepared pans. Bake on center rack of oven for 60 minutes or until tester comes out clean. Set aside to cool.

## NUTRITION ANALYSIS: PER SLICE

**Enlightened Spiced Pineapple Zucchini Bread**
Protein 4 g, carbohydrate 34 g, fiber 3 g, fat 2 g, saturated fat 0 g, cholesterol 0 mg, calcium 42 mg, sodium 188 mg
Calories 162: from protein 10%, from carbohydrate 79%, from fat 11%

**Traditional Spiced Pineapple Zucchini Bread**
Protein 4 g, carbohydrate 34 g, fiber 2 g, fat 13 g, saturated fat 2 g, cholesterol 27 mg, calcium 45 mg, sodium 232 mg
Calories 262: from protein 6%, from carbohydrate 50%, from fat 44%

# Pumpkin Raisin Bread

*I like to toast this moist and hearty raisin bread under the broiler.
Try it with Spiced Peach Butter (page 222).*

olive oil cooking spray
1 cup whole wheat flour
1 cup unbleached white flour
¼ cup yellow cornmeal
1 cup Sucanat unrefined cane sugar
1 teaspoon ground cinnamon
½ teaspoon ground nutmeg
¼ teaspoon ground cloves
1 teaspoon nonaluminum baking
  powder
1 teaspoon baking soda

¼ teaspoon sea salt
¾ cup golden raisins
⅓ cup prune purée
½ cup pumpkin purée
1 tablespoon liquid Fruitsource
1 tablespoons egg replacer powder
¼ cup water
1 tablespoon pure vanilla extract
1 cup enriched 1% fat soymilk
cinnamon and nutmeg for garnish
⅓ cup Tosteds soynuts

Preheat oven to 350°. Spray 9-by-5-inch loaf pan with olive oil cooking spray.

In a medium bowl, combine whole wheat flour, white flour, cornmeal, Sucanat, cinnamon, nutmeg, cloves, baking powder, baking soda, and salt. Add raisins and set aside.

In a large bowl, blend prune purée with pumpkin purée and Fruitsource. In a small bowl, whisk egg replacer powder with water until foamy. Add to pumpkin mixture with vanilla and soymilk. Mix thoroughly. Fold dry ingredients into the liquid, mixing just until blended. Pour batter into prepared pan and sprinkle with cinnamon and nutmeg. Top with soynuts. Bake for 50 minutes, or until tester inserted in middle comes out clean.

---

### NUTRITION ANALYSIS: PER SLICE

**Enlightened Pumpkin Raisin Bread**
Protein 5 g, carbohydrate 50 g, fiber 4 g, fat 1 g,
saturated fat 0 g, cholesterol 0 mg,
calcium 90 mg, sodium 275 mg
Calories 222: from protein 8%,
from carbohydrate 86%, from fat 6%

**Traditional Pumpkin Raisin Bread**
Protein 6 g, carbohydrate 42 g, fiber 2 g, fat 17 g,
saturated fat 8 g, cholesterol 76 mg,
calcium 78 mg, sodium 409 mg
Calories 335: from protein 6%,
from carbohydrate 48%, from fat 46%

# Southern-Style Sweet Potato Bread

*This quickbread is a tasty way to use up leftover yams.*

*10 Servings*

olive oil cooking spray
2¼ cups Multi-Grain Mix (page 195)
1¼ teaspoons ground cinnamon
¼ teaspoon ground nutmeg
⅛ teaspoon ground cloves
¼ cup prune purée

¾ cup evaporated cane sugar
1 cup mashed cooked yams
¼ cup orange juice
¼ cup water
1 teaspoon pure vanilla extract
3 tablespoons unsalted sunflower seeds

SWEET POTATOES, popular throughout the southern United States find their way into many entrées, side dishes, and desserts. Yams are sweet potatoes grown from a special strain. They are darker orange in color, and have a sweeter flavor and more moist texture than other sweet potatoes.

Preheat oven to 350°. Spray a 9-by-5-inch loaf pan with olive oil.

In a medium bowl, combine Multi-Grain Mix, cinnamon, nutmeg, and cloves. Set aside.

In a large bowl, combine prune purée with sugar. Add yams and blend with orange juice, water, and vanilla. Fold the dry ingredients into the liquid, mixing just until blended. Pour batter into prepared pan, top with sunflower seeds, and sprinkle with nutmeg. Bake for 50 minutes, or until tester inserted in middle comes out clean.

## NUTRITION ANALYSIS: PER SLICE

**Enlightened Sweet Potato Bread**
Protein 4 g, carbohydrate 35 g, fiber 2 g, fat 2 g, saturated fat 0 g, cholesterol 0 mg, calcium 84 mg, sodium 316 mg, Calories 170: from protein 10%, from carbohydrate 78%, from fat 12%

**Traditional Sweet Potato Bread**
Protein 4 g, carbohydrate 31 g, fiber 1 g, fat 18 g, saturated fat 9 g, cholesterol 59 mg, calcium 99 mg, sodium 384 mg Calories 298: from protein 6%, from carbohydrate 40%, from fat 54%

# Cranberry Apple Coffee Cake

*Having Multi-Grain Mix, on hand
makes quick work of this delicious coffee cake.*

olive oil cooking spray

*Topping*
1 Granny Smith apple, peeled and
 diced
½ cup dried cranberries
1 tablespoon lemon juice
½ cup Sucanat, unrefined cane sugar

¼ teaspoon ground cinnamon
⅛ teaspoon nutmeg, plus a little
 more for garnish
⅓ cup soynuts
¼ cup low-fat granola

*Coffee Cake*
2¼ cups Multi-Grain Mix
 (page 195)
½ cup evaporated cane sugar
1 teaspoon ground cinnamon

¾ cup plus 1 tablespoon water
¼ cup unsweetened applesauce
1 teaspoon pure vanilla extract

Preheat oven to 350°. Spray an 8-by-8-inch square baking pan with olive oil
cooking spray.

*For the topping:* In a small bowl, combine apple, cranberries, lemon juice,
Sucanat, cinnamon, and nutmeg. Set aside.

*For the cake:* In a large bowl, combine Multi-Grain Mix with evaporated
cane sugar and cinnamon. Add water, applesauce, and vanilla. Stir just until
mixed. Pour batter into prepared pan. Distribute apple mixture evenly over top,
then sprinkle with soynuts and granola. Pat topping very lightly into batter, and
sprinkle with nutmeg. Bake for 35 minutes, or until tester comes out clean.

NUTRITION ANALYSIS: PER SERVING (1 2-BY-2½-INCH SQUARE)

**Enlightened Cranberry Apple Coffee Cake**
Protein 4 g, carbohydrate 32 g, fiber 3 g, fat 2 g,
saturated fat 0 g, cholesterol 0 mg,
calcium 47 mg, sodium 145 mg
Calories 151: from protein 10%,
from carbohydrate 80%, from fat 10%

**Traditional Cranberry Apple Coffee Cake**
Protein 5 g, carbohydrate 40 g, fiber 2 g, fat 14 g,
saturated fat 7 g, cholesterol 46 mg,
calcium 47 mg, sodium 300 mg
Calories 299: from protein 7%,
from carbohydrate 52%, from fat 41%

# Blueberry Apple Pancakes

*With a wholesome quick mix on hand,*
*pancakes are not just for weekends!*

*18*
*3-Inch*
*Pancakes*

2 cups Multi-Grain Mix (page 195)
3 tablespoons evaporated cane sugar
½ cup peeled chopped apples
½ cup dried blueberries
1 cup water

¼ cup apple juice
1 tablespoon olive oil
¼ teaspoon ground cinnamon
olive oil cooking spray

You don't need a griddle to make pancakes. An electric frying pan, set to 350°, provides even, controlled heat and makes perfect pancakes.

Combine Multi-Grain Mix, sugar, apples, and blueberries in a large bowl. Stir in water, apple juice, and oil. Stir to mix and add cinnamon. Spray griddle, electric frying pan, or 10-inch frying pan with olive oil cooking spray and heat 2 minutes on medium-high heat. Drop batter onto prepared pan with a ¼ cup measure. Cook for about 3 minutes, flipping when bubbles start to appear. Cook for about 2 minutes on the other side, and serve.

NUTRITION ANALYSIS: PER SERVING (3 PANCAKES)

Enlightened Blueberry Apple Pancakes
Protein 6 g, carbohydrate 44 g, fiber 3 g, fat 4 g,
saturated fat 0 g, cholesterol 0 mg,
calcium 118 mg, sodium 438 mg
Calories 224: from protein 10%,
from carbohydrate 75%, from fat 15%

Traditional Blueberry Apple Pancakes
Protein 7 g, carbohydrate 48 g, fiber 1 g, fat 11 g,
saturated fat 6 g, cholesterol 62 mg,
calcium 171 mg, sodium 542 mg
Calories 322: from protein 9%,
from carbohydrate 61%, from fat 30%

# Sweet Sensations

This chapter is dedicated to the health-conscious dessert lover. Here you will find fabulous, over-the-top favorites, such as Strawberry Banana "Cream" Pie and Chocolate Raspberry Ganache, recreated *healthfully!* Normally, a traditional cream pie, or ganache-style cake would contain an excessive amount of fat, calories, and cholesterol. These outstanding desserts are every bit as rich-tasting as their counterparts, with just a fraction of the calories and fat, and absolutely no cholesterol.

You *can* have your cake and eat it too! Enlightened desserts are made without a drop of butter, oil, or shortening. Instead we use fruit purées, whose natural pectins replace fat in baked goods. Silken tofu, soymilk, and egg replacers stand in for traditional ingredients like eggs and and dairy products, binding baked goods and providing silky, rich texture.

Puddings prepared in the traditional fashion are high in calories and contain an unhealthy amount of fat, especially saturated fat. The luscious puddings in this chapter contain only a gram or two of fat. Brandied Peach Custard, Pineapple Mango Pudding, and Maple Walnut Pudding, are delectable baked puddings made entirely without eggs or cream—and you won't be able to tell the difference! Baking a pudding intensifies both the flavor and texture. Over-the-top desserts that have a very healthy bottom line are my specialty and a great way to complete a meal healthfully.

# Recipes

Apple Almond Bundt Cake

Mocha Java Bundt Cake with Espresso Glaze

Black Forest Bundt Cake with Cherry Blossom Sauce

Fruit Tunnel Cake with Peanut Butter Icing

Pumpkin Spice Cake

Spiced Chocolate Cake with Boiled Pineapple Icing

Boiled Pineapple Icing

Chocolate Raspberry Ganache

Strawberry Banana "Cream" Pie

Brandied Peach Custard

Mandarin–Orange Blossom Pudding

Maple Walnut Pudding

Pineapple Mango Pudding

Poached Pears with Brandied Almond "Cream"

Chocolate Raspberry Phyllo Cups

Mocha Cranberry Brownies with Orange Blossom Glaze

Chocolate Chip Okara Spice Bars

Rich and Creamy Mocha Shake

Chocolate-Covered Tosteds 'n' Fruit

# Apple Almond Bundt Cake

*This delightful cake features a rich tasting, almond-studded batter layered with spiced apples.*

olive oil cooking spray
¾ cup enriched 1% fat soymilk
1 tablespoon plus 1 teaspoon lemon
   juice
2 medium Granny Smith apples,
   peeled and diced
3 tablespoons Sucanat, unrefined
   cane sugar
1 teaspoon ground cinnamon
¼ teaspoon ground nutmeg
2½ cups whole wheat pastry flour

⅓ cup whole grain yellow cornmeal
1 teaspoon nonaluminum baking
   powder
1 teaspoon baking soda
½ teaspoon sea salt
½ cup chopped almonds
1 12.3-ounce package lite silken tofu
⅓ cup prune purée
1½ cups evaporated cane sugar
¼ teaspoon almond extract

Preheat oven to 350°. Spray a 12-cup Bundt pan with olive oil.

In a small glass liquid measuring cup, combine soymilk and 1 teaspoon lemon juice and set aside. Place the apples in a medium bowl and drizzle with 1 tablespoon lemon juice. Add Sucanat, cinnamon, and nutmeg. Set aside. In a large bowl, combine flour, cornmeal, baking powder, baking soda, salt, and almonds. Set aside.

Place the tofu in a food processor and process until smooth. Add prune purée and sugar and blend. Add soymilk mixture and almond extract. Blend. Fold the tofu mixture into the dry ingredients, mixing just until blended. Spoon ⅓ of the batter into prepared pan and, using a slotted spoon, top with half of the apple mixture. Alternate layers of batter and apples, ending with batter. Bake for 45 minutes, or until tester comes out clean.

## NUTRITION ANALYSIS: PER SLICE

### Enlightened Apple Almond Bundt Cake
Protein 7 g, carbohydrate 49 g, fiber 4 g, fat 4 g,
saturated fat 0 g, cholesterol 0 mg,
calcium 83 mg, sodium 272 mg
Calories 249: from protein 11%,
from carbohydrate 75%, from fat 14%

### Traditional Apple Almond Bundt Cake
Protein 7 g, carbohydrate 66 g, fiber 3 g, fat 25 g,
saturated fat 2 g, cholesterol 36 mg,
calcium 64 mg, sodium 336 mg
Calories 505: from protein 5%,
from carbohydrate 51%, from fat 44%

# Mocha Java Bundt Cake with Espresso Glaze

*This could be called the "disappearing" cake! Not only does the zucchini "disappear" into the cake, this cake is so delicious, you won't be able to keep it around for long.*

olive oil cooking spray
1½ cups unbleached white flour
½ cup cocoa powder
½ cup oat bran
¼ cup whole grain yellow cornmeal
1 teaspoon ground cinnamon
¼ teaspoon ground nutmeg
1 teaspoon nonaluminum baking powder
1 teaspoon baking soda
½ teaspoon sea salt
½ cup chopped walnuts

½ cup prune purée
1¼ cups evaporated cane sugar
1 tablespoon egg replacer powder
¼ cup water
⅔ cup strong brewed coffee
½ tablespoon pure vanilla extract
1 medium zucchini, coarsely shredded (about 1¼ cups)

*Glaze*
½ cup powdered sugar
2 teaspoons strong brewed coffee

Preheat oven to 350°. Spray a 12-cup Bundt pan with olive oil cooking spray.

In a medium bowl, combine flour, cocoa, oat bran, cornmeal, cinnamon, nutmeg, baking powder, baking soda, and salt. Add walnuts and set aside.

In a large bowl, blend prune purée with evaporated cane sugar. In a small bowl, whisk egg replacer powder with water until foamy. Add to sugar mixture with coffee and vanilla. Fold dry ingredients into the liquid alternately with the zucchini. Mix just until blended. Pour into prepared pan and bake for 40 minutes, or until tester inserted comes out clean.

*For the glaze:* Sift the powdered sugar into a medium bowl. Add the coffee, stirring until blended. Drizzle onto cooled cake.

---

## NUTRITION ANALYSIS: PER SLICE

### Enlightened Mocha Java Bundt with Espresso Glaze
Protein 4 g, carbohydrate 33 g, fiber 3 g, fat 4 g,
saturated fat 1 g, cholesterol 0 mg,
calcium 37 mg, sodium 241 mg
Calories 165: from protein 9%,
from carbohydrate 72%, from fat 19%

### Traditional Mocha Java Bundt with Espresso Glaze
Protein 5 g, carbohydrate 36 g, fiber 1 g, fat 22 g,
saturated fat 11 g, cholesterol 71 mg,
calcium 41 mg, sodium 307 mg
Calories 350: from protein 6%,
from carbohydrate 40%, from fat 54%

# Black Forest Bundt Cake with Cherry Blossom Sauce

*This rendition of the classic dessert is made healthy because of the Enlightened approach to baking—virtually no added fat!*

olive oil cooking spray
2 cups whole wheat pastry flour
½ cup cocoa powder
¼ cup oat bran
1 teaspoon nonaluminum baking powder
1 teaspoon baking soda
1 teaspoon ground cinnamon

½ teaspoon sea salt
1 cup dried cherries
1 12.3-ounce package lite silken tofu
⅓ cup prune purée
1¼ cups evaporated cane sugar
½ cup fresh orange juice
1 teaspoon pure vanilla extract
1 teaspoon orange blossom water

### Cherry Blossom Sauce

¾ cup orange juice
3½ tablespoons agar flakes
1 12.3-ounce package lite silken tofu
1 cup evaporated cane sugar

1½ tablespoon kirsch (cherry brandy)
1 teaspoon orange blossom water
1 10-ounce jar dark cherry preserves

Preheat oven to 350°. Spray a 12-cup Bundt pan with olive oil cooking spray.

In a medium bowl, combine flour, cocoa, oat bran, baking powder, baking soda, cinnamon, and salt. Add dried cherries and set aside.

Place tofu in food processor and process until smooth. Add prune purée, evaporated cane sugar, orange juice, vanilla, and orange blossom water. Blend. Fold tofu mixture into the dry ingredients, mixing just until blended. Pour batter into prepared pan. Bake for 40 minutes, or until tester comes out clean.

*For the Cherry Blossom Sauce:* Combine orange juice with agar flakes and heat in microwave for 45 seconds, or on stovetop for 2 minutes. Set aside.

Place tofu in food processor and process. Add evaporated cane sugar and blend. Add orange juice mixture, kirsch, and orange blossom water. Blend until

**Black Forest Bundt Cake with Cherry Blossom Sauce** *(continued)*

smooth. Set aside, covered, in refrigerator. Once the cake has cooled, split it crosswise, and spread cherry preserves on the bottom half. Replace the top. Slice, and drizzle Cherry Blossom Sauce over each slice.

---

NUTRITION ANALYSIS: PER SERVING (1 SLICE CAKE WITH $1/3$ CUP SAUCE)

| Enlightened Black Forest Bundt Cake with Cherry Blossom Sauce | Traditional Black Forest Bundt Cake with Cherry Sauce |
|---|---|
| Protein 6 g, carbohydrate 44 g, fiber 3 g, fat 1 g, saturated fat 0 g, cholesterol 0 mg, calcium 52 mg, sodium 221 mg Calories 204: from protein 14%, from carbohydrate 81%, from fat 5% | Protein 4 g, carbohydrate 52 g, fiber 3 g, fat 16 g, saturated fat 10 g, cholesterol 58 mg, calcium 39 mg, sodium 261 mg Calories 422: from protein 4%, from carbohydrate 56%, from fat 40% |

# Fruit Tunnel Cake
## with Peanut Butter Icing

*Filled with spiced figs and cranberries, and topped
with a lush peanut butter icing, this festive cake is scrumptious.*

olive oil cooking spray

### Filling

1 cup chopped dried Calimyrna figs

¼ cup dried cranberries

2 tablespoons Sucanat, unrefined
cane sugar

½ teaspoon ground cinnamon

dash ground nutmeg

### Cake

2⅓ cups whole wheat pastry flour

½ cup whole grain yellow cornmeal

2 tablespoons oat bran

1 teaspoon nonaluminum baking
powder

1 teaspoon baking soda

1 teaspoon ground cinnamon

½ cup unsalted soynut pieces

½ teaspoon sea salt

1 12.3-ounce package lite silken tofu

⅓ cup prune purée

1½ cups evaporated cane sugar

¾ cup fresh orange juice

1 tablespoon pure vanilla extract

### Icing

1 12.3-ounce package lite silken tofu

1 cup evaporated cane sugar

½ cup low-fat peanut butter

⅔ cup fresh orange juice

3 rounded tablespoons agar flakes

1 tablespoon pure vanilla extract

Preheat oven to 350°. Spray a tube pan with olive oil cooking
spray.

*For the filling:* Combine figs, cranberries, Sucanat, cinnamon,
and nutmeg. Set aside.

*For the cake:* In a large bowl, combine the flour, cornmeal, oat
bran, baking powder, baking soda, cinnamon, soynuts, and salt. Set
aside.

Place tofu in food processor and blend. Add prune purée and
process. Add sugar, juice, and vanilla, and process to blend thoroughly. Fold the tofu mixture into the dry ingredients quickly, just

Figs are high in
fiber—more dietary fiber
per serving than any other
common dried or fresh
fruit. About ¼ cup pro-
vides 20 percent of the
RDA for fiber.

**Fruit Tunnel Cake with Peanut Butter Icing** *(continued)*

until mixed. Do not overmix. Pour half the batter into prepared pan and cover with fig filling. Cover with remaining batter and place on the middle rack of oven. Bake 45 minutes or until tester comes out clean.

*For the icing:* Place tofu in food processor and process. Add evaporated cane sugar and peanut butter, and blend. Combine orange juice with agar flakes and heat for 1 minute in microwave on 100% power or on stovetop for 2 minutes over medium heat. Add to tofu with vanilla, and process to blend. Spread generously over cooled cake. Chill to set.

---

NUTRITION ANALYSIS: PER 1 SLICE

Enlightened Fruit Tunnel Cake
with Peanut Butter Icing
Protein 9 g, carbohydrate 43 g, fiber 4 g, fat 3 g,
saturated fat 0 g, cholesterol 0 mg,
calcium 72 mg, sodium 231 mg
Calories 225: from protein 15%,
from carbohydrate 73%, from fat 12%

Traditional Fruit Tunnel Cake
with Peanut Butter Icing
Protein 7 g, carbohydrate 71 g, fiber 3 g, fat 17 g,
saturated fat 7 g, cholesterol 66 mg,
calcium 52 mg, sodium 297 mg
Calories 454: from protein 6%,
from carbohydrate 61%, from fat 33%

# Pumpkin Spice Cake

*Old-fashioned pumpkin spice cake is easy to prepare, enticing, and delicious. Low in fat and high in fiber, this rendition is not only moist but perfumed with fragrant orange blossom water.*

olive oil cooking spray
1 cup rolled oats
2 cups whole wheat pastry flour
⅓ cup whole grain yellow cornmeal
1½ teaspoons ground cinnamon
¾ teaspoon ground ginger
½ teaspoon ground nutmeg
¼ teaspoon ground cloves
1 teaspoon nonaluminum baking powder

1 teaspoon baking soda
½ teaspoon sea salt
1 12.3-ounce package lite silken tofu
¼ cup prune purée
1 cup pumpkin purée
1½ cups evaporated cane sugar
1 teaspoon orange blossom water
⅔ cup fresh orange juice

Preheat oven to 350°. Spray a tube pan with olive oil cooking spray.

Place oats in food processor and blend for a minute, until reduced to flour. Place in a large bowl and add pastry flour, cornmeal, cinnamon, ginger, nutmeg, cloves, baking powder, baking soda, and salt. Set aside.

Place tofu in food processor and process until smooth, scraping down halfway. Add prune purée and pumpkin purée and blend. Add evaporated cane sugar, orange blossom water, and orange juice. Blend until smooth. Fold tofu mixture into dry ingredients, just until mixed. Pour into prepared pan and bake for 50 minutes, or until tester comes out clean.

SERVE THIS wonderful cake with a dusting of powdered sugar.

## NUTRITION ANALYSIS: PER SLICE

**Enlightened Pumpkin Spice Cake**
Protein 7 g, carbohydrate 45 g, fiber 4 g, fat 1 g,
saturated fat 0 g, cholesterol 0 mg,
calcium 59 mg, sodium 267 mg
Calories 209: from protein 12%,
from carbohydrate 82%, from fat 6%

**Traditional Pumpkin Spice Cake**
Protein 5 g, carbohydrate 48 g, fiber 2 g, fat 17 g,
saturated fat 10 g, cholesterol 95 mg,
calcium 49 mg, sodium 343 mg
Calories 363: from protein 6%,
from carbohydrate 52%, from fat 42%

*12
Servings*

# Spiced Chocolate Cake with Boiled Pineapple Icing

*You can have your cake and eat it too—healthfully!*

olive oil cooking spray
2 cups whole wheat pastry flour
½ cup cocoa powder
¼ cup soy flour
¼ cup oat bran
1½ teaspoons ground cinnamon
½ teaspoon ground nutmeg
¼ teaspoon ground cloves
1 teaspoon nonaluminum baking
    powder

1 teaspoon baking soda
½ teaspoon sea salt
½ cup nondairy chocolate chips
1 12.3-ounce package lite silken tofu
½ cup prune purée
1½ cups evaporated cane sugar
1 tablespoon pure vanilla extract
½ cup enriched 1% fat soymilk
1 recipe Boiled Pineapple Icing
    (recipe follows)

Preheat oven to 350°. Spray tube pan with olive oil cooking spray.

In a large bowl, combine pastry flour, cocoa powder, soy flour, oat bran, cinnamon, nutmeg, cloves, baking powder, baking soda, and salt. Stir in chocolate chips and set aside.

Place tofu in food processor and blend until smooth, scraping down halfway. Add prune purée and blend. Add sugar, vanilla, and soymilk. Blend until smooth. Fold tofu mixture into dry ingredients, just until mixed. Pour into prepared pan and bake for 40 minutes, or until tester comes out clean.

Prepare icing, cool, and spread on cooled cake.

---

## NUTRITION ANALYSIS: PER SLICE

**Enlightened Spiced Chocolate Cake
with Boiled Pineapple Icing**
Protein 9 g, carbohydrate 57 g, fiber 5 g, fat 4 g,
saturated fat 1 g, cholesterol 0 mg,
calcium 84 mg, sodium 299 mg
Calories 284: from protein 12%,
from carbohydrate 77%, from fat 11%

**Traditional Spiced Chocolate Cake
with Boiled Pineapple Icing**
Protein 7 g, carbohydrate 70 g, fiber 3 g, fat 19 g,
saturated fat 11 g, cholesterol 62 mg,
calcium 61 mg, sodium 342 mg
Calories 480: from protein 5%,
from carbohydrate 61%, from fat 34%

# Boiled Pineapple Icing

*This is an especially delicious icing
with heightened flavor and unique texture.*

---

1 12.3-ounce package lite silken tofu
1 cup canned pineapple chunks,
    drained, reserving juice
¾ cup evaporated cane sugar

2 tablespoons arrowroot
½ tablespoon pure vanilla extract
⅓ cup chopped dried pineapple

Place tofu in food processor and process until smooth. Add pineapple chunks, evaporated cane sugar, and ¼ cup reserved pineapple juice. Blend. Add arrowroot and vanilla. Blend. Scrape into medium saucepan and heat over medium-low heat for 5 minutes, stirring frequently. Set aside to cool. Spread over cake and top with chopped dried pineapple.

THIS DAIRY-FREE icing achieves the fluffy texture of the traditional version, without the use of beaten egg whites.

---

NUTRITION ANALYSIS: PER ¼-CUP SERVING

**Enlightened Boiled Pineapple Icing**
Protein 2 g, carbohydrate 13 g, fiber 0 g, fat 0 g,
saturated fat 0 g, cholesterol 0 mg,
calcium 15 mg, sodium 30 mg
Calories 63: from protein 14%,
from carbohydrate 82%, from fat 4%

**Boiled Pineapple Icing**
Protein 1 g, carbohydrate 39 g, fiber 0 g, fat 4 g,
saturated fat 2 g, cholesterol 10 mg,
calcium 35 mg, sodium 277 mg
Calories 190: from protein 3%,
from carbohydrate 80%, from fat 17%

*16
Servings*

# Chocolate Raspberry Ganache

*Traditional ganache cakes are rich with whipped cream and melted chocolate. Our version is elegant, rich-tasting, and much healthier!*

olive oil cooking spray

### Cake
¾ cup enriched 1% fat soymilk
2 tablespoons lemon juice
2¼ cups whole wheat pastry flour
¾ cup cocoa powder
1½ teaspoons nonaluminum
   baking powder
1½ teaspoons baking soda

2 teaspoon ground cinnamon
½ teaspoon sea salt
1 12.3-ounce package lite silken tofu
½ cup Lighter Bake or prune purée
1¾ cups evaporated cane sugar
1 teaspoon pure vanilla extract

### Raspberry Maple Filling
1 12-ounce package unsweetened
   frozen raspberries
⅔ cup frozen apple juice
   concentrate, thawed

⅓ cup pure maple syrup
2 teaspoons pure vanilla extract
2 tablespoons cornstarch
2 tablespoons cold water

### Ganache Topping
1 12.3-ounce package lite silken tofu
½ cup cocoa powder

6 tablespoons liquid Fruitsource
1 tablespoon pure vanilla extract

THIS IS A terrific cake for an intimate Valentines' Day dinner. The filling and topping for this scrumptious dessert can be made a day in advance, and will profit from refrigerating overnight.

Preheat oven to 350°. Spray three 8- or 9-inch round cake pans with olive oil cooking spray.

*For the cake:* Combine soymilk and lemon juice in a glass measuring cup and set aside. In a large bowl, combine the flour, cocoa, baking powder, baking soda, cinnamon, and salt. Mix thoroughly and set aside.

Place tofu in food processor and blend until smooth, about a minute. Add Lighter Bake, evaporated cane sugar, soymilk, and vanilla. Fold the tofu mixture into the dry ingredients and divide the batter between the prepared pans. Bake on center rack of oven for 30 minutes or until tester inserted comes out clean. Set aside to cool.

*For the filling:* Place raspberries in a medium saucepan, add juice concentrate and cook over medium heat, stirring frequently, until raspberries have softened. Suspend a wire mesh colander over a bowl. Pour raspberries into the colander and mash pulp with the back of a spoon. Discard the seeds and return the liquid to the saucepan. Add maple syrup and vanilla. Simmer over low heat for 3 minutes. Blend cornstarch with water in a small bowl and add to the raspberry mixture. Stir to blend and continue to simmer until the mixture begins to thicken. Set aside to cool.

*For the topping:* Place tofu in food processor and blend. Place the cocoa powder in a small bowl and set aside. Heat the liquid Fruitsource in a small glass measuring cup in the microwave on 100% power for 20 seconds. Whisk the hot Fruitsource into the cocoa powder to form a chocolate syrup. Add to the tofu with the vanilla and blend until smooth. Set aside.

*To assemble:* Place one cake layer on a cake dish, spread with half the raspberry filling, and add the second cake layer. Spread with the remaining filling and position the last layer on top. With a spatula, spread the chocolate ganache over the cake. Refrigerate until ready to serve.

---

NUTRITION ANALYSIS: PER SLICE

Enlightened Chocolate Raspberry Ganache
Protein 7 g, carbohydrate 45 g, fiber 5 g, fat 2 g,
saturated fat 0 g, cholesterol 0 mg,
calcium 86 mg, sodium 274 mg
Calories 225: from protein 12%,
from carbohydrate 82%, from fat 6%

Traditional Chocolate Raspberry Ganache
Protein 6 g, carbohydrate 61 g, fiber 4 g, fat 38 g,
saturated fat 23 g, cholesterol 119 mg,
calcium 50 mg, sodium 383 mg
Calories 578: from protein 4%,
from carbohydrate 40%, from fat 56%

# Strawberry Banana "Cream" Pie

*This pie is so rich-tasting that everyone
will be amazed that it is dairy- and egg-free!*

olive oil cooking spray

1 recipe Deep-Dish Whole Wheat
Pie Crust (page 194)

### Filling
¾ cup enriched 1% fat soymilk
3 rounded tablespoons agar flakes
1 12.3-ounce package lite silken tofu,
plus remainder of tofu from crust
1 medium banana, broken into
pieces

1 tablespoon lemon juice
1¼ cups evaporated cane sugar
1 tablespoon pure vanilla extract
1 quart fresh strawberries

### Glaze
1 cup reserved strawberries
¼ cup apple juice concentrate,
thawed
5 tablespoons evaporated cane sugar

1 teaspoon pure vanilla extract
1 tablespoon cornstarch
1 tablespoon cold water

Preheat oven to 400°. Lightly spray a deep-dish pie pan with oil.

Make Deep-Dish Whole Wheat Pie Crust using ⅓ cup of a 12.3-ounce package of lite silken tofu, setting aside the remainder for the filling. Bake pastry "blind," (without filling). Prick pastry several times with a fork, and bake for 15 minutes in the center of preheated oven. Set aside to cool.

*For the filling:* Combine the soymilk and agar flakes in a medium glass measuring cup and set aside. Place the tofu (you will have one package plus ⅔ package remaining from the crust recipe) in a food processor. Blend until smooth. Add the banana and lemon juice and pulse to blend. Add evaporated cane sugar, soymilk mixture, and vanilla, and process.

THIS FIVE-STAR dessert makes a beautiful presentation. As with any fresh fruit dessert, use up within 36 hours.

Scrape the tofu mixture into a medium saucepan and bring to a boil over medium heat, stirring frequently. Reduce heat to low and simmer for 5 minutes. Set aside to cool, about 20 minutes. Pour into baked crust.

Set aside 1 cup of strawberries. Slice the remaining strawberries and arrange in an overlapping circular pattern on top of the filling. Refrigerate the pie while preparing the glaze.

*For the glaze:* Slice the reserved strawberries and place them in a medium saucepan with the juice concentrate. Bring to a boil over medium-high heat, and simmer for 3 minutes. Place a wire mesh colander over a bowl, and press the berry mixture through the mesh with the back of a large spoon. Return the seedless berry mixture to the saucepan, over medium heat, and stir in the evaporated cane sugar and vanilla. In a small bowl, blend the cornstarch with the water, and add to the berry mixture. Reduce heat to low and simmer for 5 minutes. Cool slightly, then pour over pie. Return to refrigerator and chill for several hours.

---

NUTRITION ANALYSIS: PER SLICE

**Enlightened Strawberry Banana "Cream" Pie**
Protein 9 g, carbohydrate 51 g, fiber 4 g, fat 4 g,
saturated fat 0 g, cholesterol 0 mg,
calcium 78 mg, sodium 126 mg
Calories 273: from protein 13%,
from carbohydrate 73%, from fat 14%

**Traditional Strawberry Banana Cream Pie**
Protein 5 g, carbohydrate 56 g, fiber 2 g, fat 22 g,
saturated fat 9 g, cholesterol 123 mg,
calcium 83 mg, sodium 283 mg
Calories 434: from protein 5%,
from carbohydrate 51%, from fat 44%

# Brandied Peach Custard

*In a word? Luscious!*

4 fresh peaches, peeled and diced
⅓ cup apricot brandy
1 cup enriched 1% fat soymilk
3 rounded tablespoons agar flakes
1 12.3-ounce package lite silken tofu

¾ cup chopped dried apricots
1 cup fresh orange juice
1¼ cups evaporated cane sugar
1 tablespoon pure vanilla extract

*Topping*
2 tablespoons low-fat granola
¼ teaspoon ground cinnamon
⅛ teaspoon ground nutmeg

1½ teaspoons Sucanat, unrefined
cane sugar

Preheat oven to 350°.

Combine peaches and brandy in a medium saucepan over medium-high heat. Bring mixture to a boil, reduce heat to medium low, and cook for 10 minutes, or until liquid is thickened and has the consistency of a syrup. Set aside. Combine the soymilk and agar and heat in microwave on 100% power for 1 minute, or on stovetop for 3 minutes. Set aside.

Place tofu in food processor and blend. Add apricots and process. Add orange juice, thickened soymilk, sugar, and vanilla. Blend until smooth. Pour into a 2-quart oven-safe casserole dish and fold in peaches.

*For the topping:* Combine granola, cinnamon, nutmeg, and Sucanat and sprinkle over custard. Bake for 30 minutes or until lightly browned. Serve warm or cold. Refrigerate covered.

---

NUTRITION ANALYSIS: PER 1-CUP SERVING

**Enlightened Brandied Peach Custard**
Protein 6 g, carbohydrate 27 g, fiber 4 g, fat 1 g,
saturated fat 0 g, cholesterol 0 mg,
calcium 93 mg, sodium 65 mg
Calories 168: from protein 20%,
from carbohydrate 74%, from fat 6%

**Traditional Brandied Peach Custard**
Protein 5 g, carbohydrate 28 g, fiber 3 g, fat 33 g,
saturated fat 20 g, cholesterol 183 mg,
calcium 86 mg, sodium 239 mg
Calories 453: from protein 5%,
from carbohydrate 26%, from fat 69%

# Mandarin–Orange Blossom Pudding

*The scent of orange blossoms fill the kitchen as this pudding bakes.*

1 cup enriched 1% fat soymilk
3 rounded tablespoons agar flakes
1 12.3-ounce package lite silken tofu
2 medium bananas, broken into
  pieces
¾ cup liquid Fruitsource
1½ tablespoons lemon juice

1¼ teaspoons orange blossom water
1 tablespoon pure vanilla extract
1 11-ounce can mandarin oranges,
  drained
½ teaspoon ground cinnamon
freshly ground nutmeg

Preheat oven to 350°.

Combine soymilk and agar and heat in microwave on 100% power for 45 seconds, or on stovetop over medium-low heat for 2 minutes. Set aside.

Place tofu in food processor and blend. Add banana and process. Add Fruitsource, lemon juice, orange blossom water, and vanilla. Blend until smooth. Pour into 2-quart baking dish and fold in mandarin oranges. Sprinkle cinnamon and nutmeg over pudding. Run a butter knife through the pudding, using swirling motions. Bake for 30 minutes or until lightly browned. Serve warm or cold. Refrigerate covered.

THIS AROMATIC baked pudding is a terrific party pleaser.

---

NUTRITION ANALYSIS: PER 1-CUP SERVING

Enlightened Mandarin–Orange
Blossom Pudding
Protein 5 g, carbohydrate 36 g, fiber 2 g, fat 1 g,
saturated fat 0 g, cholesterol 0 mg,
calcium 61 mg, sodium 46 mg
Calories 168: from protein 10%,
from carbohydrate 85%, from fat 5%

Traditional Mandarin–Orange
Blossom Pudding
Protein 3 g, carbohydrate 40 g, fiber 1 g, fat 16 g,
saturated fat 9 g, cholesterol 104 mg,
calcium 65 mg, sodium 161 mg
Calories 307: from protein 4%,
from carbohydrate 51%, from fat 45%

# Maple Walnut Pudding

*This pudding features a crunchy
topping of cinnamon spiced walnuts. Scrumptious!*

2 12.3-ounce packages lite silken tofu
1 medium banana, broken into
    pieces
⅔ cup liquid Fruitsource

½ cup maple syrup
1½ tablespoons lemon juice
1 tablespoon pure vanilla extract

### Topping

⅓ cup chopped walnuts
½ teaspoon ground cinnamon
⅛ teaspoon ground nutmeg

1½ teaspoons Sucanat, unrefined
    cane sugar

Preheat oven to 350°.

Place tofu in food processor and blend. Add banana and process. Add Fruitsource, maple syrup, lemon juice, and vanilla. Blend until smooth. Pour into a 2-quart oven-safe casserole dish and set aside.

Combine walnuts, cinnamon, nutmeg, and Sucanat. Sprinkle over pudding. Bake, uncovered, for 30 minutes, or until lightly browned. Serve warm or cold. Refrigerate covered.

## NUTRITION ANALYSIS: PER 1-CUP SERVING

**Enlightened Maple Walnut Pudding**
Protein 10 g, carbohydrate 45 g, fiber 1 g, fat 5 g,
saturated fat 0 g, cholesterol 0 mg,
calcium 77 mg, sodium 118 mg
Calories 261: from protein 15%,
from carbohydrate 68%, from fat 17%

**Traditional Maple Walnut Pudding**
Protein 8 g, carbohydrate 53 g, fiber 1 g, fat 28 g,
saturated fat 13 g, cholesterol 183 mg,
calcium 109 mg, sodium 176 mg
Calories 480: from protein 6%,
from carbohydrate 43%, from fat 51%

# Pineapple Mango Pudding

*Garnish this pudding with fresh mint leaves to make a lovely presentation.*

1 cup orange juice
3 rounded tablespoons agar flakes
1 12.3-ounce package lite silken tofu
1 medium banana, broken into
     pieces
1 tablespoon lemon juice
1 24-ounce package frozen mango
     chunks, thawed

1 8-ounce can crushed pineapple,
     drained
1½ cups evaporated cane sugar
½ teaspoon ground cinnamon
¼ teaspoon ground nutmeg

Preheat oven to 350°.

Combine orange juice and agar flakes and set aside. Place tofu in food processor and process until smooth. Add banana and lemon juice and blend. Add mango, pineapple, and evaporated cane sugar. Blend until smooth. Pour into a 2-quart oven-safe casserole dish. Sprinkle cinnamon and nutmeg over pudding. Run a butter knife, through pudding, using swirling motions. Bake, uncovered, for 35 minutes, or until lightly browned. Serve warm or cold. Refrigerate covered.

MAKE SURE you choose agar *flakes.* Agar powder is far more concentrated and will not produce the same result.

## NUTRITION ANALYSIS: PER 1-CUP SERVING

**Enlightened Pineapple Mango Pudding**
Protein 4 g, carbohydrate 43 g, fiber 3 g, fat 1 g,
saturated fat 0 g, cholesterol 0 mg,
calcium 36 mg, sodium 49 mg
Calories 202: from protein 8%,
from carbohydrate 88%, from fat 4%

**Traditional Pineapple Mango Pudding**
Protein 2 g, carbohydrate 46 g, fiber 3 g, fat 18 g,
saturated fat 11 g, cholesterol 114 mg,
calcium 49 mg, sodium 157 mg
Calories 360: from protein 3%,
from carbohydrate 52%, from fat 45%

# Poached Pears with Brandied Almond "Cream"

*Easy, elegant, and healthful,
this dessert is a heavenly finish to any meal.*

---

*8
Servings*

4 firm, ripe Bosc pears, peeled,
    halved vertically, and cored
juice of 1 lemon

*Brandied Almond "Cream"*
1 12.3-ounce package extra-firm
    silken tofu, drained
⅓ cup pure maple syrup
2 tablespoons apricot brandy or
    frozen apple juice concentrate

1 cup white wine or apple juice
½ cup pure maple syrup
¼ teaspoon almond extract

¼ teaspoon almond extract
¼ cup sliced almonds for garnish
    (optional)

Place pears in a large bowl, drizzle with lemon juice, and set aside.

Combine wine, maple syrup, and almond extract in a large saucepan, and warm over medium-high heat for 2 minutes. Reduce heat to medium-low, and add pears. Cover and simmer for 15 minutes, or until pears are tender when pierced gently with a fork. Using a slotted spoon, gently remove pears to a large bowl. Raise heat to medium high, and bring the poaching liquid to a boil. Cook, stirring frequently, for about 5 minutes, or until liquid is reduced by about a third and is the consistency of thin syrup. Pour over the pears. Cover and refrigerate for up to 4 hours.

*For the "Cream":* Place tofu in food processor. Blend until smooth, about a minute or so, scraping down once with a spatula. Add the maple syrup, brandy, and almond extract. Process for 3

RATHER THAN the lite that I usually prefer, this dish calls for regular Mori Nu silken tofu, because of its denser texture, which mimics the mouthfeel of heavy cream.

minutes, until fluffy and mixed thoroughly. Refrigerate for at least an hour. For a lovely presentation, cut the poached pear halves lengthwise into thin slices, leaving the slices *attached* at the stem end. Transfer pear to a plate, using a metal spatula. Press pear gently at the base to fan out slices. Spoon syrup over fanned pear and place a dollop of almond "Cream" alongside. Sprinkle with sliced almonds if desired.

---

NUTRITION ANALYSIS: PER SERVING (ONE HALF PEAR WITH $1/2$ CUP "CREAM" TOPPING)

| Enlightened Poached Pears with Brandied Almond "Cream" | Traditional Poached Pears with Brandied Almond Cream |
|---|---|
| Protein 4 g, carbohydrate 49 g, fiber 4 g, fat 2 g, saturated fat 0 g, cholesterol 0 mg, calcium 60 mg, sodium 20 mg Calories 241: from protein 7%, from carbohydrate 87%, from fat 6% | Protein 2 g, carbohydrate 53 g, fiber 4 g, fat 16 g, saturated fat 10 g, cholesterol 54 mg, calcium 53 mg, sodium 55 mg Calories 372: from protein 3%, from carbohydrate 58%, from fat 39% |

# Chocolate Raspberry Phyllo Cups

*This lovely dessert makes an elegant presentation.*

olive oil cooking spray
24 large Fillo Factory pastry shells

½ cup Cookie Crumb Topping
  (page 197)

### Chocolate Layer

1 12.3-ounce package lite silken tofu
1 ripe banana, broken into pieces
⅓ cup cocoa powder
1 cup liquid Fruitsource

1 tablespoon pure vanilla extract
¾ cup enriched 1% fat vanilla
  soymilk
3 tablespoons agar flakes

### Raspberry Layer

1 12-ounce package frozen
  raspberries
3 tablespoons cold water
½ cup maple syrup

¼ cup Sucanat, unrefined cane sugar
2 tablespoons kirsch
2 tablespoons cornstarch
2 tablespoons cold water

Preheat oven to 375°. Lightly spray two baking pans with olive oil cooking spray.

*For the chocolate layer:* Place tofu in food processor and process. Add banana and blend. Place cocoa in a medium bowl and set aside. Heat Fruitsource in microwave for 45 seconds, or on stovetop for 1 minute over medium-low heat until hot. Add Fruitsource to cocoa and, using a small wire whisk, mix into a smooth syrup. Add chocolate syrup to tofu mixture along with vanilla. Combine soymilk and agar flakes and heat in microwave for a minute (almost to a boil), stirring halfway, or on stovetop for 2 minutes over medium heat. Blend into tofu mixture. Fill pastry shells ⅔ full with chocolate filling. Top each with 1 teaspoon of Cookie Crumb Topping. Bake for 20 minutes or until firm at the center. Cool on wire racks.

CONVENIENT and widely available, Fillo Factory pastry shells are low in fat and shelf-stable!

*For the raspberry layer:* Place frozen raspberries with 3 tablespoons of water in a medium saucepan over medium-high heat. Cook, stirring occasionally, for 5 minutes, or until thawed. Pour raspberries into wire mesh colander placed over a medium bowl. Press berries against colander using the back of a table-spoon. Return the raspberry purée to the saucepan, and place over medium-high heat. Add maple syrup, Sucanat, and kirsch brandy and bring to a boil. In a small bowl, combine cornstarch and cold water, add to the raspberry mixture, and reduce heat to medium. Cook for 5 minutes, stirring frequently. Cool slightly.

Add to chocolate-filled shells, and top each with 1 teaspoon of cookie crumbs. Refrigerate for at least 1 hour before serving.

NUTRITION ANALYSIS: PER SERVING (1 PHYLLO CUP)

**Enlightened Chocolate Raspberry Phyllo Cups**
Protein 5 g, carbohydrate 39 g, fiber 1 g, fat 4 g,
saturated fat 1 g, cholesterol 0 mg,
calcium 33 mg, sodium 158 mg
Calories 211: from protein 9%,
from carbohydrate 75%, from fat 16%

**Traditional Chocolate Raspberry Phyllo Cups**
Protein 3 g, carbohydrate 35 g, fiber 1 g, fat 16 g,
saturated fat 10 g, cholesterol 41 mg,
calcium 29 mg, sodium 210 mg
Calories 296: from protein 4%,
from carbohydrate 47%, from fat 49%

# Mocha Cranberry Brownies with Orange Blossom Glaze

*Each of my books features an exceptional brownie recipe.
Here is a scrumptious frosted brownie.*

*30
Brownies*

olive oil cooking spray
1¾ cups unbleached white flour
¾ cup cocoa powder
¼ cup oat bran
¼ cup whole grain yellow cornmeal
1 teaspoon ground cinnamon
¼ teaspoon ground nutmeg
1 teaspoon nonaluminum baking
   powder

1 teaspoon baking soda
½ teaspoon sea salt
1 cup dried cranberries
1 12.3-ounce package lite silken tofu
½ cup prune purée
1½ cups evaporated cane sugar
½ cup strong brewed coffee
½ tablespoon pure vanilla extract

*Glaze*

1 cup powdered sugar
2 tablespoons orange juice

½ teaspoon orange blossom water

Preheat oven to 350°. Spray a 9-by-13-inch baking pan with olive oil.

In a large bowl, combine flour, cocoa, oat bran, cornmeal, cinnamon, nutmeg, baking powder, baking soda, and salt. Stir in cranberries and set aside.

Place tofu in food processor and process until smooth. Add prune purée and blend. Add evaporated cane sugar, coffee, and vanilla. Blend until smooth, scraping down mixture halfway. Fold tofu mixture into dry ingredients, just until mixed. Do not overmix. Pour into pan. Bake for 45 minutes, or until tester comes out clean. Set aside on cooling rack to cool, then cut into 2-inch squares.

*For the glaze:* Sift the powdered sugar into a medium bowl. Add juice and orange blossom water and mix well. Drizzle over cooled brownies.

---

### NUTRITION ANALYSIS: PER BROWNIE

**Enlightened Mocha Cranberry Brownies with
Orange Blossom Glaze**
Protein 2 g, carbohydrate 20 g, fiber 1 g, fat 1 g,
saturated fat 0 g, cholesterol 0 mg,
calcium 18 mg, sodium 108 mg
Calories 85: from protein 8%,
from carbohydrate 87%, from fat 5%

**Traditional Mocha Cranberry Brownies with
Orange Blossom Glaze**
Protein 2 g, carbohydrate 26 g, fiber 2 g, fat 11 g,
saturated fat 7 g, cholesterol 39 mg,
calcium 26 mg, sodium 138 mg
Calories 203: from protein 4%,
from carbohydrate 48%, from fat 48%

# Chocolate Chip Okara Spice Bars

*Rich in nutrients, these bars are
as good to eat as they are good for you.*

olive oil cooking spray
1 cup rolled oats
2 cups whole wheat pastry flour
¼ cup soy flour
1 teaspoon nonaluminum baking
    powder
1 teaspoon baking soda
1 teaspoon ground cinnamon
¼ teaspoon ground nutmeg
½ teaspoon sea salt

1 cup dried cranberries
½ cup dairy-free chocolate chips
⅔ cup prune purée
1¼ cups evaporated cane sugar
2 tablespoons liquid Fruitsource
¾ cup dry roasted okara
    (see box)
2 tablespoons egg replacer powder
¼ cup cold water
¾ cup soymilk

Preheat oven to 350°. Spray a 9-by-13-inch baking pan with olive oil cooking spray.

Place oats in food processor or blender and process to a coarse flour, about 20 seconds. Place in a medium bowl, and combine with pastry flour, soy flour, baking powder, baking soda, cinnamon, nutmeg, and salt. Mix in cranberries and chocolate chips, and set aside.

In a large bowl, blend prune purée with evaporated cane sugar, Fruitsource, and okara. In a small bowl, whisk egg replacer powder with water until foamy. Add to sugar mixture with soymilk and mix thoroughly. Quickly fold the dry ingredients into the liquid and pour into prepared pan. Bake for 50 minutes, or until tester comes out clean. Cool, then cut into bars.

Drying okara will increase its shelf-life, and make it a more useful baking ingredient, To dry okara, drain it, then spread on a baking pan. Bake at 300 degrees for about 20 minutes, stirring occasionally. Store, covered, in the refrigerator.

---

## NUTRITION ANALYSIS: PER SERVING (1 SPICE BAR)

### Chocolate Chip Okara Spice Bars
Protein 4 g, carbohydrate 43 g, fiber 3 g, fat 2 g,
saturated fat 1 g, cholesterol 0 mg,
calcium 48 mg, sodium 191 mg
Calories 203: from protein 7%,
from carbohydrate 83%, from fat 10%

### Traditional Chocolate Chip Spice Bars
Protein 4 g, carbohydrate 38 g, fiber 1 g, fat 16 g,
saturated fat 5 g, cholesterol 28 mg,
calcium 58 mg, sodium 238 mg
Calories 305: from protein 5%,
from carbohydrate 49%, from fat 46%

*3
Servings*

# Rich and Creamy Mocha Shake

*Love those rich milkshakes, but not all the fat, calories, and cholesterol?*
*Here is a healthier approach to this summer favorite.*

¼ cup cocoa powder
⅓ cup liquid Fruitsource
1 cup Silk enriched vanilla soymilk
3 tablespoon dry vanilla soymilk

1 cup Sweet Nothings fat-free vanilla
   soy ice cream
3 tablespoons strong brewed coffee

Place cocoa powder in a small bowl and set aside. Microwave Fruitsource on 100% power for 30 seconds, or simmer on stovetop for 2 minutes. Whisk hot Fruitsource into cocoa until smooth. Place soymilk in food processor or blender with the chocolate mixture and the soymilk powder. Blend. Add the soy ice cream and coffee and blend. Chill and serve.

## NUTRITION ANALYSIS: PER 1-CUP SERVING

### Enlightened Mocha Shake
Protein 6 g, carbohydrate 49 g, fiber 0 g, fat 2 g,
saturated fat 0 g, cholesterol 0 mg,
calcium 163 mg, sodium 83 mg
Calories 239: from protein 10%,
from carbohydrate 83%, from fat 7%

### Traditional Mocha Shake
Protein 6 g, carbohydrate 37 g, fiber 0 g, fat 23 g,
saturated fat 14 g, cholesterol 81 mg,
calcium 178 mg, sodium 107 mg
Calories 357: from protein 6%,
from carbohydrate 39%, from fat 55%

# Chocolate-Covered Tosteds 'n' Fruit

*Quick and easy to prepare,*
*these treats are bound to become a family favorite!*

olive oil cooking spray
2 cups Tosteds soynuts
1½ cups mixed dried fruit, such as
blueberries, strawberries, and
cherries

⅓ cup cocoa powder
2 tablespoons arrowroot
¾ cup liquid Fruitsource
1½ tablespoons pure vanilla extract
¼ teaspoon almond extract

Spray a cookie sheet with olive oil cooking spray.

Combine soynuts and fruit in a large bowl and set aside. Combine cocoa and arrowroot in a small bowl and set aside. Microwave Fruitsource for 25 seconds, or heat on stovetop over low heat for 1 minute. Using a wire whisk, blend the hot Fruitsource into the cocoa mixture until a chocolate syrup is formed. Add vanilla and almond extracts, and pour over fruit and soynuts. Combine thoroughly with a rubber spatula. Place rounded tablespoonfuls of mixture on prepared cookie sheet and place in the freezer for 10 to 15 minutes. Serve immediately. Store remaining candies in freezer, as they will become soft when left at room temperature.

THESE *delectable* chocolate candies are ready-to-eat right out of the freezer.

## NUTRITION ANALYSIS: PER CANDY

**Enlightened Chocolate-Covered Tosteds 'n' Fruit**
Protein 3 g, carbohydrate 10 g, fiber 2 g, fat 1 g,
saturated fat 2 g, cholesterol 0 mg,
calcium 15 mg, sodium 10 mg
Calories 63: from protein 18%,
from carbohydrate 63%, from fat 19%

**Traditional Chocolate-Covered Peanuts 'n' Fruit**
Protein 3 g, carbohydrate 13 g, fiber 1 g, fat 6 g,
saturated fat 2 g, cholesterol 2 mg,
calcium 22 mg, sodium 41 mg
Calories 110: from protein 10%,
from carbohydrate 44%, from fat 46%

# RESOURCE GUIDE

**Advanced Ingredients, Inc.**
331 Capitola Avenue, Suite F
Capitola, CA 95010
(888) 238-4647
www.advancedingredients.com
*Fruitsource liquid sweetener.*

**Arrowhead Mills**
110 South Lawton
Hereford, TX 79045
(806) 364-0730
(806) 364-8242 (Fax)
*A variety of flours and grain products.*

**Boca Foods Co.**
P.O. Box 8995
Madison, WI 53708
www.bocaburger.com
*Boca Burgers and Boca Burger Crumbles.*

**Bob's Red Mill Natural Foods, Inc.**
Milwaukie, OR 97222
www.bobsredmill.com
*Variety of specialty stone-ground flours, baking mixes, dried beans, and more.*

**Dixie USA, Inc.**
Dixie Diner's Club (DDC)
P.O. Box 1969
15555 FM 2920
Tomball, TX 77377
(800) 233-3668
www.dixiediner.com
*Over 150 plant-based whole soy products. Fillo Factory shelf-stable phyllo shells, snacks, beverages, egg and dairy substitutes, quick-fix mixes, Textured Vegetable Protein, and more.*

**EnerG Foods, Inc.**
5960 First Avenue S.
Seattle, WA 98108
(800) 331-5222
www.ener-g.com
*EnerG Egg Replacer, tapioca flour, and allergy-free products.*

**Fairview Farms of Iowa**
2304 150th Street
Corwith, IA 50430
(888) 526-9296
www.fairviewfarms.com
*Laura Beans (soybeans), Tosteds (roasted soynuts), and Laura soy flour. Also nigari and everything you need for soymilk and tofu making.*

**Florida Crystals, Inc.**
Palm Beach, FL 33480
www.floridacrystals.com
*Florida Crystals organic and conventional evaporated cane sugar.*

269

**Follow Your Heart**
Earth Island
7848 Alabama Avenue
Canoga Park, CA 91305
(818) 347-9946
www.followyourheart.com/
    Vegenaise.html
*Vegenaise and Follow Your Heart salad
dressings.*

**The Grain and Salt Society**
273 Fairway Drive
Asheville, NC 28805
(800) TOP-SALT (867-7258)
www.celtic-seasalt.com
*The source of Celtic Sea Salt and many
wholesome foods and accessories.*

**The Hain Celestial Group**
50 Charles Lindbergh Boulevard
Uniondale, NY 11553
(516) 237-6200
(516) 237-6240 (Fax)
www.thehainfoodgroup.com
*Hain Pure Foods has acquired a
number of natural foods companies
including Westsoy, Arrowhead Mills,
HealthValley, Garden of Eatin', and
others.*

**Health Valley**
16100 Foothill Boulevard
Irwindale, CA 91706
(626) 334-3241
*Fat free cookies, granola, and more.*

**Imagine Foods, Inc.**
1245 San Carlos Avenue
San Carlos, CA 94070
(800) 333-6339
www.imaginefoods.com
*Nondairy rice and soy beverages,
puddings, frozen desserts, stuffed
sandwiches, and soups.*

**Lightlife Foods, Inc.**
153 Industrial Boulevard
Turners Falls, MA 01376
(800) SOY-EASY (769-3279)
www.lightlife.com
*Wide variety of soy analogs, tempeh,
Gimme Lean, Smart Ground, hot
dogs, sausages, burgers, shrink-wrapped
seitan, and more.*

**Live Food Products**
Box 7
Santa Barbara, CA 93102
(805) 968-1028
www.bragg.com
*Bragg Liquid Aminos*

**The Mail Order Catalog**
413 Farm Road
P.O. Box 180
Summertown, TN 38483
(800) 695-2241
www.healthy-eating.com
*Wide variety of vegetarian foods, dairy
and egg substitutes, soyfoods such as
Textured Vegetable Protein, cookbooks,
and more.*

Melissa's/World Variety
Produce, Inc.
P.O. Box 21127
Los Angeles, CA 90021
www.melissas.com
(800) 588-0151
*The largest distributor of specialty
produce in the United States with
over 1,000 items. Exotic fruits and
vegetables, soyfoods, dried fruits,
chiles, mushrooms, jarred items,
and more.*

Miyako Oriental Foods, Inc.
4287 Puente Avenue
Baldwin Park, CA 91706
(626) 962-9633
*Cold Mountain Miso: organic mellow
white, light yellow, and red miso.*

Morinaga Nutritional Foods, Inc.
2050 West 190th Street, Suite 110
Torrance, CA 90504
(800) 669-8638
www.morinu.com
*Mori Nu Silken Tofu and Silken Tofu
Lite, Tofu Hero, and Mori Nu soups.*

Nasoya Foods, Inc.
One New England Way
Ayer, MA 01432
(800) 229-TOFU (8638)
www.nasoya.com
*Tofu, baked tofu, Nayonaise, salad
dressings, puddings.*

nSpire Natural Foods
14855 Wicks Boulevard
San Leandro, CA 94577
(510) 686-0116
www.nspiredfoods.com
*A variety of wholesome snack foods,
including Cloud Nine and Tropical
Source gourmet chocolates and Sunspire chocolate chips.*

Pacific Foods of Oregon, Inc.
Tualatin, OR 97062
(503) 692-9666
www.pacificfoods.com
*Nondairy soy, rice, and almond
beverages, broth, and soups.*

Quong Hop & Co.
171 Beacon Street
South San Francisco, CA 94080
(650) 553-9900
www.quonghop.com
*The Soy Deli: baked tofu, firm nigari
tofu, tempeh, burgers, and more.*

San Gennaro Foods, Inc.
9620 ML King Way
South Seattle, WA 98118
(800) 462-1916
www.sangennarofoods.com
*Variety of precooked and ready-to-use,
shelf-stable polenta.*

San Miguel Produce, Inc.
444 Navalair Road
Oxnard, CA 93033

www.sanmiguelgreens.com
*Cut 'n Clean Greens in convenient ready to use packages. The variety of greens include kale, collards, chard, spinach, and blends such as European Blend and Country Mix.*

**Sanlinx Inc.**
4755 Fowler Drive
Morristown, TN 37814
(888) 228-3082
www.soymilkmaker.com
*Soyajoy Soymilk Maker, automatic machine with stainless steel construction. Also, nigari and accessories for making tofu.*

**Simply Delicious, Inc.**
8411 Highway 86 North
Cedar Grove, NC 27231
(919) 732-5294
www.simplydelicious.com
*Variety of organic soy-based salad dressings and The Wizards vegetarian Worcestershire sauce.*

**Sokol and Co.**
5315 Dansher Road
Countryside, IL 60525
(708) 482-8250
www.solofoods.com
*Solo Prune Filling and Simon Fischer Prune Butter/Lekvar (prune purée)*

**Soyco Foods**
2441 Viscount Row
Orlando, FL 32809

www.galaxyfoods.com
*Soymage Parmesan cheese.*

**Sunsweet Growers, Inc.**
Yuba City, CA 95993
(800) 417-2253
www.sunsweet.com
*Lighter Bake fat replacer and a variety of dried fruits, such as prunes, apricots, raisins, and more.*

**Tree of Life**
P.O. Box 410
St. Augustine, FL 32085
(800) 260-2424
www.treeoflife.com
*Tofu, baked tofu, dairy-free rice and soy beverages, frozen vegetables, fruits, and more.*

**Vegi-Deli**
P.O. Box 881781
San Francisco, CA 94188
(888) 473-3667
www.vegideli.com
*Seitan-based meat substitutes and snack foods.*

**White Wave, Inc.**
1990 N 57th Court
Boulder, CO 80301
www.whitewave.com
*Tofu, baked tofu, seitan packed in broth, tempeh, Silk soymilk, soy yogurt, and more.*

**Wholesome Sweeteners**
8016 Highway 90A
Sugarland, TX 77478
(281) 490-9582
(281) 275-3170 (Fax)
www.wholesomefoods.com
*Organic Sucanat and organic evaporated cane sugar.*

**Wildwood Natural Foods**
135 Bolinas Road
Fairfax, CA 94930
(800) 499-TOFU (8638)
www.wildwoodnaturalfoods.com

*Firm nigari and calcium-fortified tofu; baked, braised, and smoked tofu; soymilk; and more.*

**Yves Veggie Cuisine**
1138 East Georgia Street
Vancouver, BC V6A 2A8 Canada
(800) 667-9837
www.yvesveggie.com
*Variety of soyfoods, veggie Canadian bacon, deli slices, ground round, burgers, hot dogs, soy cheese, and more.*

# INTERNET RESOURCES

www.vegsource.com
This terrific resource for the health-conscious Web surfer features an online magazine with cutting-edge articles, recipes, interactive discussion boards, and many of the top experts in the field of health and nutrition. VegSource is the home of *Soy Talk with Marie Oser.*

www.vegtv.com
An all-video site promoting a healthy, plant-based lifestyle with entertaining and informative videos. Recipes, links, and an online column, *Recipe of the Week,* with Marie Oser.

www.pcrm.com
Physicians Committee for Responsible Medicine (PCRM) is a nonprofit organization with 5,000 physicians and 100,000 lay members. Founded in 1985, PCRM promotes preventive medicine through innovative programs, and encourages higher standards for ethics and effectiveness in research. PCRM publishes *Good Medicine,* a quarterly newsletter.

www.earthsave.org
Founded by John Robbins, Earthsave International promotes food choices that are healthy for people and for the planet, providing information, support, and practical programs. EarthSave publishes a quarterly newsletter.

www.drmcdougall.com
Books, videos, articles, and more from Dr. John McDougall, founder of the McDougall Plan for Healthy Living. Information about how the plant-based diet can promote dramatic and lasting health benefits.

www.vrg.org
The Vegetarian Resource Group (VRG), a nonprofit organization of health
professionals, provides information regarding issues of health and nutrition.
The Vegetarian Resource group publishes a bimonthly magazine, *The Vegetarian Journal.*

www.farmsanctuary.org
Farm Sanctuary is a nonprofit organization dedicated to ending the exploitation of animals used for food production and providing refuge for animals
rescued from factory farms.

www.farmusa.org
FARM (Farm Animal Reform Movement) is a nonprofit organization advocating a plant-based diet and the humane treatment of farm animals.

www.worldwatch.org
The Worldwatch Institute analyzes environmental data from around the
world, and publishes the monthly magazine, *WorldWatch.*

www.earthisland.org
Earth Island Institute fosters the development of projects for the conservation, preservation, and restoration of the global environment.

www.ran.org
The Rainforest Action Network has been working to protect tropical rainforests and the human rights of those living in and around those forests
through education, grassroots organizing, and nonviolent direct action.

www.yvesveggie.com
Home of Yves Veggie Cuisine, an extensive line of quality soyfoods. Health
tips, recipes, and product information.

www.morinu.com
Morinaga maker of Mori Nu products, offers recipes, books, and health information.

www.newcenturynutrition.com
NewCenturyNutrition is a web site that provides a forum where renowned researchers, teachers, and physicians from the East and West can discuss their philosophies, research findings, or health advice to enrich readers.

heart.kumu.org/nshome.html
Healing Heart Foundation founded by Dr. Neal Pinckney. Practical advice for preventing and reversing heart disease, an extensive glossary, plant-based recipes, and more.

www.yesworld.org
Youth for Environmental Sanity (YES!) founded by Ocean Robbins in 1990, YES! is a nonprofit organization that educates, and inspires young people to become environmental advocates.

www.melissas.com
Gourmet recipes, online catalog, and information regarding hundreds of items, including exotic fruits, vegetables, and soyfoods.

www.lightlife.com
Producers of many innovative products offers health information, newsletter, recipes, and links.

# RECOMMENDED READING

Attwood, Charles. *Dr. Attwood's Low-Fat Prescription for Kids.* Viking/ Penguin, 1995.

Barnard, Neal D. *Food for Life.* Crown Publishing, 1994.

———. *Eat Right, Live Longer.* Crown Publishing, 1995.

———. *The Power of Your Plate.* Crown Publishing, 1999.

———. *Turn off the Fat Genes.* Harmony Books, 2001.

Fouts, Roger. *Next of Kin.* William Morrow and Company, 1997.

Harris, William. *The Scientific Basis of Vegetarianism.* Hawaii Health Publishers, 1995.

Havala, Suzanne. *Good Foods, Bad Foods: What's Left to Eat?* John Wiley & Sons, 1998.

———. *The Natural Kitchen,* Berkley, 2000.

———. *Being Vegetarian for Dummies.* HungryMinds, 2001.

———. *Vegetarian Cooking for Dummies.* HungryMinds, 2001.

Lyman, Howard. *Mad Cowboy.* Scribner, 1998.

Masson, Jeffrey Moussaieff, and Susan McCarthy. *When Elephants Weep.* Bantam Doubleday, 1995.

McDougall, John. *The McDougall Program for Women.* Dutton, 1999.

McDougall, John, and Mary McDougall. *The McDougall Program.* Penguin Books, 1990.

———. *The McDougall Program for Maximum Weight Loss.* Plume, 1995.

———. *The McDougall Quick and Easy Cookbook.* Plume, 1999.

Messina, Mark, and Virginia Messina. *The Simple Soybean and Your Health.* Avery, 1994.

———. *The Vegetarian Way.* Crown, 1996.

Ornish, Dean. *Dr. Dean Ornish's Program for Reversing Heart Disease.* Random House, 1990.

————. *Eat More, Weigh Less.* HarperCollins, 1993.

————. *Everyday Cooking With Dr. Dean Ornish.* HarperCollins, 1997.

Oski, Frank. *Don't Drink Your Milk.* Tech Services, 1992.

Physicians Committee for Responsible Medicine, Amy Lanou, Ph.D. *Healthy Eating for Life for Children,* John Wiley & Sons, Inc., 2002.

Physicians Committee for Responsible Medicine, Kristine Kieswer. *Healthy Eating for Life for Women,* John Wiley & Sons, Inc., 2002.

Physicians Committee for Responsible Medicine, Vesanto Melina, M.S., R.D. *Healthy Eating for Life to Prevent and Treat Cancer,* John Wiley & Sons, Inc., 2002.

Physicians Committee for Responsible Medicine, Patricia Bertron, R.D. *Healthy Eating for Life to Prevent and Treat Diabetes,* John Wiley & Sons, Inc., 2002.

Pinckney, Neal. *Healthy Heart Handbook.* Health Communications, 1996.

Rhoads, Richard. *Deadly Feasts.* Simon & Schuster, 1997.

Rifkin, Jeremy. *Beyond Beef.* Dutton, 1992.

Robbins, John. *Diet for a New America.* Stillpoint, 1987.

————. *May All Be Fed.* William Morrow and Company, Inc., 1992.

————. *Reclaiming Our Health.* H.J. Kramer, 1996.

————. *The Food Revolution.* Conari Press, 2001.

Shurtleff, William, and Akiko Aoyagi. *The Book of Tofu.* Ten Speed Press, 1983.

Stepaniak, Joanne. *Compassionate Living for Healing, Wholeness & Harmony.* Keats, 2001.

# BIBLIOGRAPHY

American Cancer Society. "Cancer Facts and Figures"—1997. Atlanta: 1999.

Anderson, J. "The dependence of the effects of cholesterol and degree of saturation of the fat in the diet on serum cholesterol in man." *American Journal of Clinical Nutrition* 29:1784, 1976.

Armstrong B., and R. Doll. "Environmental factors and cancer incidence and mortality in different countries, with special reference to dietary practices." *International Journal of Cancer* 1975; 15:617-31.

Attwood, Charles R. "Milk, a Catch-22 Calcium Without the Cow." www.vegsource.com/attwood/milk.htm.

Behar, Richard, and Michael Kramer. "Something Smells Fowl." *Time,* Oct 17, 1994, p. 42.

Block, G., B. Patterson, and A. Subar. "Fruit, vegetables and cancer prevention: a review of evidence." *Nutrition and Cancer.* 1992; 18(1): 1-29.

Braitman, L. S., E. Adlin, and J. L. Stanton. "Obesity and caloric intake: the National Health and Nutrition" Examination Survey of 1971–75 (HANES 1). *Journal of Chronic Disease* 1985; 38:727–32.

Brenner, B. M., T. W. Meyer, and T. H. Histettler. "Dietary protein intake and the progressive nature of kidney disease." *New England Journal of Medicine* 1982; 307:652-59.

Brody, Jane. "Huge Study of Diet Indicts Fat and Meat." *The New York Times,* May 8, 1990.

Cadogan, J., et al. "Milk intake and bone mineral acquisition in adolescent girls: randomised, controlled intervention trial." *British Medical Journal* 1997; 315:1255-60.

Campbell, T. C., B. Parpia, and J. Chen. "Diet, lifestyle, and the etiology of coronary heart disease: The Cornell Study." *American Journal of Cardiology* 82 (10B):18T-21T (November 26, 1998).

Castelli ,W. P. "Epidemiology of coronary heart disease." *American Journal of Medicine* 1984; 76(2A):4-12.

Chen, J., et al. "Diet, Life-Style and Mortality in China. A Study of the Characteristics of 65 Chinese Counties." Oxford, UK; Ithaca, NY; Beijing, PRC; Oxford University Press; Cornell University Press; People's Medical Publishing House, 1990. 894 pp.

Cohen, P. "Serum insulin-like growth factor-I levels and prostate cancer risk—interpreting the evidence." *Journal of the National Cancer Institute* 1998; 90:876-9.

Committee on Diet, Nutrition and Cancer: Assembly of Life Sciences, National Research Council. *Diet, Lifestyle, and the Risk of Type 2 Diabetes Mellitus in Women.* Washington, D.C.: National Academy Press, 1982.

Cumming R. G., and R. J. Klineberg. "Case-control study of risk factors for hip fractures in the elderly." *American Journal of Epidemiology* 1994; 139:493-505.

———. "Calcium intake and bone mass: a quantitative review of the evidence." *Calcified Tissue International* 1990; 47(4):194-201.

Cummings, J. H, and S. A. Bingham. "Diet and the prevention of cancer." *British Medical Journal* 1998; 317:1636-1640.

Cummings, S. R., et al. "Risk factors for hip fracture in white women." *New England Journal of Medicine* 1995; 332:767-73.

Dreon, D. M., et al. "Dietary fat: carbohydrate ratio and obesity in middle-aged men." *American Journal of Clinical Nutrition* 1988; 47:995-1000.

Drewnowski, A. and C. Gomez-Carneros. "Bitter taste, Phytonutrients, and the Consumer: A Review." *American Journal of Clinical Nutrition* 2000 Dec.; 72(6):1424-35.

Feskanich, D.,et al. "Milk, dietary calcium, and bone fractures in women: a 12-year prospective study." *American Journal of Public Health* 1997; 87:992-7.

Flatt, J. P. "Energetics of intermediary metabolism." Found in: Gatrow, J. S. and D. Halliday, eds. *Substrate and energy metabolism in man.* London: John Libbey and Co., 1985.

Food and Nutrition Board, National Research Council. *Recommended Dietary Allowances,* 10th ed. Washington, D.C.: National Academy Press, 1989.

Fuster, V., et al. "The pathogenesis of coronary artery disease and the acute coronary syndromes." (1) *New England Journal of Medicine* 326:242, 1992.

Garrow, J. S. *Energy Balance and Obesity in Man.* New York: Elsevier, 1974.

Giovannucci, E., et al. "Intake of fat, meat, and fiber in relation to risk of colon cancer in men." *Cancer Research.* 1994; 54: 2390-2397.

Glassman, Peter, and David Leaf. *The Oxidative Balance: How to Lead the Antioxidant Lifestyle.* EMIS Medical Publishers, 2000.

Hatherill, J. Robert. *Eat to Beat Cancer.* Los Angeles: Renaissance Books, 1999.

Heaney, R. P., and C. M. Weaver. "Calcium absorption from kale." *American Journal of Clinical Nutrition* 1990; 51:656-7.

Heaney, R. P., et al. "Dietary changes favorably affect bone remodeling in older adults." *Journal of the American Dietetic Association* 1999; 99:1228-33.

Hill, J. D., et al. "Neuropathological Manifestations of Cardiac Surgery." *Annals of Thoracic Surgery* 1969; 7:409-419.

Hu, F. B., et al. "Diet, Lifestyle, and the Risk of Diabetes Mellitus in Women." *New England Journal of Medicine* 345:790-797, Sep. 13, 2001.

Huang, Z., J. H. Himes, and P. G. McGovern. "Nutrition and subsequent hip fracture risk among a national cohort of white women." *American Journal of Epidemiology* 1996; 144:124-34.

Jackson, R. "Influence of polyunsaturated and saturated fats on plasma lipids and lipoproteins in man." *American Journal of Clinical Nutrition* 39:589, 1984.

Kieswer, Kristine. "There's No Room for Chicken in a Healthy Diet." *Good Medicine,* 2000; 9(2):8-94.

Lipid Research Clinics Program. "The Lipid Research Clinic's Coronary Primary Prevention Trial Results, II." *Journal of the American Medical Association* 1984: 251(3):365-74.

Malone, W. F. "Studies evaluating antioxidants and beta-carotene as chemopreventives." *American Journal of Clinical Nutrition* 1991; 53(suppl): 305S-313S.

McDonald, C. J., and J. F. Fitzgerald. "CABG surgical mortality in different centers." *Journal of the American Medical Association.* 1992 Feb 19; 267(7):932-3.

McDougall, John. *The McDougall Program.* New York: Plume Books, 1991.

Minamoto, T., M. Mai, and Z. Ronai. "Environmental factors as regulators and effectors of multistep carcinogenesis." *Carcinogenesis* 1999; 20(4):519-27.

Murkin, J. M. "Anesthesia, the brain, and cardiopulmonary bypass." *Annals of Thoracic Surgery* 1993; 56: 1461-1463.

National Cancer Institute. "Cancer Rates and Risks." Washington, D.C., 1985.

National Research Council. "Diet, nutrition, and cancer." Washington, D.C.: National Academy Press, 1982.

Nestel, P. "Lowering of Plasma Cholesterol...With Consumption of Polyunsaturated Fats." *New England Journal of Medicine* 288:379, 1973.

Nicholson, A. "Diet and the Prevention and Treatment of Breast Cancer." *Alternative Therapies in Health and Medicine* 1996; 2:32-38.

Nordin, C. B. E. "Calcium and osteoporosis." *Journal of Nutrition* 1997; 3(7/8):664-86.

O'Connor, G. T., et al. "A regional prospective study of in-hospital mortality associated with coronary artery bypass grafting." *Journal of the American Medical Association* 1991 Aug 14; 266(6):803-9.

Ornish, D., et al. "Can lifestyle changes reverse coronary heart disease?" *Lancet* 1990; 336:129-33.

Pennington, J. A. T. *Bowes and Church's Food Values of Portions Commonly Used.* New York: Harper and Row, 1989.

Physicians Committee for Responsible Medicine. *Calcium in Plant Based Diets.* www.pcrm.org.

———. *Food Choices for Health.* www.pcrm.org.

———. *The Protein Myth.* www.pcrm.org.

———. *The Role of Calcium.* www.pcrm.org.

Position of the American Dietetic Association: "Phytochemicals and functional foods." *Journal of the American Dietetic Association* 1995; 95:493.

Position of the American Dietetic Association: "Vegetarian diets." *Journal of the American Dietetic Association* 1997; 97(11):1317-21.

Reddy, B. "Metabolic Epidemiology of Large Bowel Cancer." *Cancer* 42:2832, 1978.

Remer, T., and F. Manz. "Estimation of the renal net acid excretion by adults consuming diets containing variable amounts of protein." *American Journal of Clinical Nutrition* 1994; 59:1356-61.

Robbins, John. *The Food Revolution.* Berkeley, CA: Conari Press, 2001.

Salonen, J. T, et al. "Iron sufficiency is associated with hypertension and excess risk of myocardial infarction" The Kuopio Ischaemic Heart Disease Risk Factor Study (KIHD). *Circulation* 1992; 85:759-64.

Schnall, P. L., et al. "The relationship between 'job strain,' workplace diastolic blood pressure, and left ventricular mass index." *Journal of the American Medical Association* 1990; 263:1929-35.

Sellmeyer, D. E., et al. "A High Ratio of Dietary Animal to Vegetable Protein Increases the Rate of Bone Loss and the Risk of Fracture in Post-menopausal Women." *American Journal of Clinical Nutrition* 2001; 73:118-122

Singh, V. N., and S. Gaby. "Premalignant lesions: role of antioxidant vitamins and beta-carotene in reduction and prevention of malignant transformation." *American Journal of Clinical Nutrition* 1991; 53(suppl): 385S-390S.

Skog, K. I., et al. "Carcinogenic heterocyclic amines in model systems and cooked foods: a review on formation, occurrence, and intake." *Food and Chemical Toxicology* 1998; 36:879-96.

Slavin, J., et al. "The Role of Whole Grains in Disease Prevention." *Journal of the American Dietetic Association* 2001; 101(7):780-785.

Steinbrook, R. "Hospital Death Rates for Five Surgeries Vary," *Los Angeles Times,* March 27, 1988.

Steinmetz, K., and J. Potter. "Vegetables, fruit and cancer." *International Journal of Epidemiology.* Cancer Causes Control. 1991; 2 (suppl): 325-357.

Trout, D. L. "Vitamin C and cardiovascular risk factors." *American Journal of Clinical Nutrition* 1991; 53:322S-5S.

Tymchuk, C. N., et al. "Evidence of an inhibitory effect of diet and exercise on prostate cancer cell growth." Departments of Physiological Science, Medicine and Urology, University of California-Los Angeles, *The Journal of Urology* 2001; 166:1185-1189.

Ulbricht, T. "Coronary heart disease:seven dietary factors." *Lancet* 338:985,1991.

Weaver, C. M., and K. L. Plawecki. "Dietary calcium: adequacy of a vegetarian diet." *American Journal of Clinical Nutrition* 1994; 59(suppl):1238S-41S.

Weisberger, J. "Nutrition and Cancer—On the Mechanisms bearing on Causes of Cancer of the Colon, Breast, Prostate, and Stomach," *Bulletin of the New York Academy of Medicine,* 56:673, 1980.

Weisburger, J. H. "Nutritional approach to cancer prevention with emphasis on vitamins, antioxidants, and carotenoids." *American Journal of Clinical Nutrition* 1991; 53(suppl): 226S-237S.

Williams, S. V., et al. "Differences in mortality from coronary artery bypass graft surgery at five teaching hospitals." *Journal of the American Medical Association* 1991 Aug 14; 266(6):810-5.

Willitt, W. C., et al. "Relation of meat, fat, and fiber intake to colon cancer in a prospective study among women. " *New England Journal of Medicine* 1990; 323:1664-72.

World Cancer Research Fund and American Institute for Cancer Research. "Food, Nutrition and the Prevention of Cancer: a Gobal Perspective." 1997.

Wynder, E. "Dietary Fat and Colon Cancer." *Journal of the National Cancer Institute* 54:7, 1975.

———. "The Dietary Environment and Cancer." *Journal of the American Dieticians Association* 71:385, 1977.

Wynder, E. L., et al. "Diet and breast cancer in causation and therapy." *Cancer* 1986; 58:1804-13.

Ziegler, R. G. "Vegetables, fruits, and carotenoids and the risk of cancer." *American Journal of Clinical Nutrition* 1991; 53(suppl):251S-259S.

# INDEX

Acorn squash:
    Gingered, Soup, 105–106
    Hearty Stuffed Squash, 124
Advanced Ingredients, Inc., 269
Agar flakes, 259
Allergies, milk, 12
Alzheimer's disease, 2
American diet, 5–6, 16
American Institute for Cancer Research
    (AICR), 8
*American Journal of Clinical Nutrition,*
    11, 13
Amino acids, 15–16, 22
Anderson, James, Dr., 21
Angina, 6
Angioplasty, 6
Angostura, 49
Animal products:
    characteristics of, 2, 5–8, 25
    high-protein, 16
Anthocyanins, 27
Antioxidants, 5, 25–26
Appetizers, *see* Dips
    Black Bean Cakes with Creamy Dijon
        Sauce, 91–92
    Chilled Asparagus with Creamy Dill
        Dressing, 93
    Creamy "Cheese" Bites, 63
    Garlic and Thyme Pita Crisps, 74
    Mushroom-Okara Pâté, 83
    "Sausage" in a Blanket, 75
    "Sausage" Turnovers, 76–77
    Sun-Dried Tomato Quiche Bites,
        57–58
Apples:
    applesauce, 42
    Granny Smith, 45
Apricot(s):
    dried, 44

    Muffins, 225
    Pineapple Butter, 221, 227
Arrowhead Mills, 40, 45, 269
Arrowroot, 42
Arthritis, 18
Artichoke hearts, 42
Asparagus:
    "Beef" and, Oriental, 158
    Chilled with Creamy Dill Dressing,
        93
    Dilled, 85
    Dilled, and Wild Mushrooms, 161
    Hearty "Chicken" and, 127, 212
        and "Sausage" Fajitas, 138
Attwood, Charles, Dr., 13
Avocado, 42

Bacon, *see* Veggie Canadian Bacon (Yves)
Bacterial growth, 9
Baking:
    Awesome Apricot Muffins, 225
    Banana Bread with Roasted Soynuts,
        230
    Blueberries, Oats, and Roses Muffins,
        228
    Blueberry Apple Pancakes, 240
    Chocolate Chip Banana Bread,
        231–232
    Chocolate Chip Okara Spice Bars, 265
    Cinnamon Raisin Bread, 233
    Cranberry Apple Coffee Cake, 239
    Cranberry Banana Bread, 234
    Cranberry Spice Muffins, 226
    Cranberry Walnut Muffins, 227
    Hearty Whole Wheat Bread, 235
    preparation time, 223
    Pumpkin Raisin Bread, 237
    Pumpkin Spice Cake, 249
    recipes list, 224

Baking *(continued)*
    Southern-Style Sweet Potato Bread,
      238
    Spiced Chocolate Cake with Boiled
      Pineapple Icing, 250
    Spiced Pineapple Zucchini Bread, 236
    Yam Good Muffins!, 229
Baking mixes:
    Cookie Crumb Topping, 197
    Deep-Dish Whole Wheat Pie Crust,
      194
    Multi-Grain Baking Mix, 195, 239
Baking powder, 42
Balsamic vinegar, 42, 147, 209
Bananas:
    Bread with Roasted Soynuts, 230
    Chocolate Chip Banana Bread,
      231–232
    Strawberry Banana "Cream" Pie,
      254–255
Barbara's Bakery, 42
Barbara's Mashed Potato Flakes, 42
Barbecue sauce, 33
Barilla lasagna noodles, 42
Barley:
    and Chicken Soup, 101–102
    pearl, quick cooking, 48
    miso, 38
Barnard, Neal, Dr., 3, 12, 16
Basmati rice, 43
Beans:
    Black Bean Cakes with Creamy Dijon
      Sauce, 91–92
    canned, 31
    garbanzo, 45, 107–108
    dried, 31
    Great Northern, 45
    Hawaiian Unbaked, 181
    nutritional characteristics of, 22
    Red, with Rice and "Sausage," 161,
      186
    sweet, 159
Beef, disadvantages of, 7
"Beef":
    and Asparagus Oriental, 158
    Balsamic, and Broccoli, 152
    Chunky Vegetable Soup, 103
    Vindaloo, 160

Beef Not!, 37, 41
Bell peppers, Crumbled Tofu with Peas,
    Tomatoes and, 161, 185
Beta-carotene, 25
Beverages:
    red wine, 27
    Rich and Creamy Mocha Shake, 266
Bile acids, 9
Binge eating, 18
Black Bean Cakes with Creamy Dijon
    Sauce, 91–92
Blood pressure, soyfoods and, 21
Blueberries:
    dried, 44
    Muffins, 228
    Roasted Garlic Couscous with Walnuts
      and, 184
Bob's Red Mill Natural Foods, Inc., 40,
    45, 269
Boca Foods Co., 269
Bok choy, 130
Bovine growth hormone (rBGH), 12
Bragg Liquid Aminos, 33, 37
Bread machines, 223, 233
Breads:
    Banana Bread with Roasted Soynuts,
      230
    Chocolate Chip Banana, 231–232
    Cinnamon Raisin, 233
    nutritional characteristics of, 19
    Pumpkin Raisin, 237
    Spiced Pineapple Zucchini, 236
    Sweet Potato, Southern-Style, 238
    whole grain, 146
    Whole Wheat, Hearty, 235
Breast cancer, 2, 7, 9, 11, 27
Brewer's Yeast, 32, 47
Broccoli:
    Balsamic "Beef" and, 152
    with Brown Rice and Pine Nuts, 177
    "Cream" of, 89, 100
    Individual Quiche, 69–70
    nutritional characteristics of, 13
    and Potato Curry, 156
Broth powder:
    characteristics of, 32
    defined, 37
    onion, 153

vegetarian, 34
vegetarian chicken-/beef-flavored, 49
Broth powders, vegetarian, 34
Brown rice:
    with Broccoli and Pine Nuts, 177
    and Tomato Pilaf, 173
Brownies, Mocha Cranberry, with Orange
        Blossom Glaze, 264
Brussels Sprouts, Curried, and Baby
        Carrots, 161, 164
Burgers:
    A-Maize-ing Okara, 154
    Onion Okara, 153
    Quick Soy, 155
Butter/spreads:
    margarine, 19
    Pineapple Apricot Butter, 221, 227
    Spiced Peach Butter, 222, 227, 237
Butternut squash, 121
Bypass surgery, 6

Cakes:
    Apple Almond Bundt Cake, 243
    Black Forest Bundt Cake with Cherry
        Blossom Sauce, 245–246
    Chocolate Raspberry Ganache,
        252–253
    Fruit Tunnel Cake with Peanut Butter
        Icing, 247–248
    Mocha Java Bundt Cake with Espresso
        Glaze, 244
    Pumpkin Spice, 249
    Spiced Chocolate Cake with Boiled
        Pineapple Icing, 250
Calcium:
    plant sources of, 13–15
    recommended daily allowance (RDA),
        12–13
    in soyfoods, 21, 23
    sources of, generally, 11, 21, 23, 48,
        161
Campbell, T. Colin, Dr., 3, 8
Canadian bacon, 41
Cancer, see specific types of cancer
    animal protein and, 16
    antioxidants and, 26
    dairy product intake and, 11–12
    dietary sources of, 2, 7–8
    disease prevention, 8–9
    hormone-stimulated, 27
    prevalence of, 7
Canthaxanthin, 28
Capers, 43
Capsaicin, 28
Carbohydrates:
    characteristics of, 19
    restrictions, 18
Cardiovascular disease:
    antioxidants and, 27
    dietary causes of, 8, 25
Carotenoids, 27–28
Carrots:
    Baby, Curried Brussel Sprouts and,
        161, 164
    baby-cut, 42
    julienne baby–cut, 129
Casseroles:
    Broken Pasta, 172
    Cassoulet, 118
    Creamy Mushroom Cauliflower Bake,
        182
    Gratin Topping, 196
    Hearty Tempeh and Potato Roast, 150
    Roasted Corn and Potato, 187, 196
Cassoulet, 118
Cataracts, dietary causes of, 12, 26
Cauliflower:
    in "Cheese" Sauce, 161, 163
    Creamy Mushroom Bake, 182
    nutritional benefits of, 22
Cellu baking powder, 42
Cheese/"Cheese":
    "Cheesy" Fondue Pot, 54, 59
    Creamy "Cheese" Bites, 63
    Homemade Dairy-Free, 202
    nutritional characteristics of, 13, 18
    Open-Faced Grilled Triangles, 146,
        202
    Parmesan alternatives, 40
    Sauce, 161, 163
    soy, 40
Chick'n Strips, 143
"Chicken":
    and Barley Soup, 101–102
    Hearty, with Asparagus, 127, 212
    Kung Pao, 115

"Chicken" (continued)
    Moroccan Tagine, 116–117
    Pineapple, 143
    Roasted, and Vegetables, 111, 126
Chicken consumption, increase in, 7
Chicken Not!, 37, 41, 116, 126
Chile:
    beans, with chopotle peppers, 43
    Tempeh, 82
China-Cornell-Oxford Project, 8
Chinese food:
    Balsamic "Beef" and Broccoli, 152
    "Beef" and Asparagus Oriental, 158
    Kung Pao "Chicken," 115
    Sesame Noodles, Cold, 89, 109, 201
Chlorophyll, 28
Chocolate:
    chips, dairy-free, 43
    Chocolate Chip Okara Spice Bars, 265
    Chocolate-Covered Tosteds 'n' Fruit,
        267
    Chocolate Raspberry Ganache,
        252–253
    Chocolate Raspberry Phyllo Cups,
        262–263
    Spiced Chocolate Cake with Boiled
        Pineapple Icing, 250
    Richly Chocolate Fondue, 54, 87
Cholesterol:
    antioxidants and, 27
    blockage and, 6
    dietary, 7
    high-protein animal products and, 16
    levels, 2, 5
    in milk, 11
    sources of, 5–7
    soyfoods and, 21
Cloud Nine, 43
Cocoa butter, 5
Coconut milk, 46
Coconut oil, 5
Coffee cake, Cranberry Apple, 239
Cold Mountain, 38
Colon cancer, 2, 7–9
Corn:
    nutritional characteristics of, 22
    Roasted, and Potato Gratin, 187
    roasted sweet, 48

    Savory Medallions, 171
Cornstarch, 42–43
Coronary bypass surgery, 6
Coronary heart disease, 2, 6–8, 10, 19
Courmarin, 28
Couscous:
    Golden Raisin, Soynut Pilaf and, 183
    nutritional characteristics of, 43
    Roasted Garlic, with Blueberries and
        Walnuts, 184
Cow's milk, see Milk
Cranberries:
    dried, 44
    Fruit Tunnel Cake with Peanut Butter
        Icing, 247–248
    Mocha Cranberry Brownies with
        Orange Blossom Glaze, 264
    muffins, 226–227
Creams, see Sauces
    Brandied Almond, 260–261
    Ginger, 149
    Tomato-Basil, 114
Crème It!, 37
Crème of Mushroom Soup, Sauce and
    Gravy Mix (DDC), 46
Crepes:
    Dilled Asparagus and Wild
        Mushrooms, 161
    Just Peachy Dessert, 86
    Light and Lovely, 85
    nutritional characteristics of, 53
Crock-Pots, 131
Curcumin, 28
Currants, dried, 44
Curry:
    Burmese, 148
    Coconut Sauce, 198
    Potato, 156
    Vegetable, 145
Curry powder, 43
Cut 'n Clean Greens, 128

Daidzein, 27
Dairy products:
    calcium intake, 11–13
    cow's milk 11
    "Got Milk?" ad campaign, 10–11
    high intake of, 11–12

nutritional characteristics of, 7
osteoporosis and, 11
Dates, 44
DDC (Dixie Diners Club), 34, 37, 39–41, 46–47
Degenerative diseases, 8
Desserts:
 Apple Almond Bundt Cake, 243
 Black Forest Bundt Cake with Cherry Blossom Sauce, 245–246
 Boiled Pineapple Icing, 251
 Brandied Peach Custard, 241, 256
 Chocolate Chip Okara Spice Bars, 265
 Chocolate-Covered Tosteds 'n' Fruit, 267
 Chocolate Raspberry Ganache, 252–253
 Chocolate Raspberry Phyllo Cups, 262–263
 Fruit Tunnel Cake with Peanut Butter Icing, 247–248
 healthy, characteristics of, 241
 Just Peachy Crepes, 86
 Mandarin-Orange Blossom Pudding, 257–258
 Maple Walnut Pudding, 241
 Mocha Cranberry Brownies with Orange Blossom Glaze, 264
 Mocha Java Bundt Cake with Espresso Glaze, 244
 Pineapple Mango Pudding, 241, 259
 Poached Pears with Brandied Almond "Cream," 260–261
 Pumpkin Spice Cake, 249
 recipes list, 242
 Rich and Creamy Mocha Shake, 266
 Richly Chocolate Fondue, 54, 87
 Spiced Chocolate Cake with Boiled Pineapple Icing, 250
 Strawberry Banana "Cream" Pie, 254–255
Diabetes, 2, 8, 18, 21
Diet for a Small Planet (Lappe), 1
Dips:
 "Bacon" and Chive, 73
 "Cheesy" Fondue Pot, 59
 Spinach-Artichoke, 72
Disease prevention strategies, 8

Dixie USA, Inc., 269
Dressings:
 Creamy Dill, 93, 122
 Creamy Dilled, 89
 Creamy Italian, 95

Earth Island Institute, 276
Earthsave International, 275
Eat, Drink, and Be Healthy (Willett), 11
Eat to Beat Cancer (Hatherill), 1
Edamame:
 balsamic marinade, 209
 Chilled Pasta Salad with, 97
 Easy Salad, 98
 marinated, 53
 nutritional characteristics of, 37
 Savory Sesame Marinade, 218
 Shelled, and Mushrooms in Spring Onion Marinade, 60
 Shelled, in Balsamic Marinade, 62
 Shelled, in Sesame Marinade, 61
 Succotash, 161, 166
 Tempeh and Sweet Beans, 159
 Vegetable Medley with, 188
Eden brand, 31
Egg alternatives:
 Egg Not!, 37
 EnerG egg replacer powder, 44
Eggplant, Japanese, 46
Eggs, nutritional characteristics of, 7. See also Egg alternatives
EnerG Foods, Inc., 269
Energy foods, 19
Enterolactone, 27
Entertaining:
 meal preparation tips, 53
 recipes for, 55–88
Entrees:
 A-Maize-ing Okara Burgers, 154
 Balsamic "Beef" and Broccoli, 152
 Balsamic "Chicken," 147
 Basque Stew, 131
 "Beef" and Asparagus Oriental, 158
 "Beef" Vindaloo, 160
 "Beefy" Polenta Bake, 141–142
 Braised Tempeh with Mushrooms and Tomatoes, 157
 Broccoli and Potato Curry, 156

Entrees (continued)
  Burmese Curry, 148
  Caribbean Mobay, 111, 132
  Cassoulet, 118
  Creamed Penne and "Ham," 140
  Five-Spice Tofu and Snow Peas in
      Ginger "Cream," 149
  Ginger Tempeh Wrap, 122
  Grilled Marinated Tofu and Vegetables,
      120
  Grilled Polenta with Tomato-Basil
      Cream, 111–112
  Harvest Medley, 121
  Hearty "Chicken" with Asparagus,
      127, 212
  Hearty Stuffed Squash, 124
  Hearty Tempeh and Potato Roast, 150
  Kung Pao "Chicken," 115
  Linguine al Pesto, 111, 136
  Marinated Tofu and Baby Bok Choy,
      130
  Mexican Polenta, 123
  Moroccan "Chicken" Tagine, 116–117
  Neopolitan Pasta and Lentils, 111, 125
  North African Stew (Sikbadj), 151
  Onion Okara Burgers, 153
  Open-Faced Grilled "Cheese"
      Triangles, 146, 202
  Penne with Tofu Tomato Sauce, 144
  Pineapple "Chicken," 143
  Quick Soy Burgers, 155
  recipe list, 112–113
  Roasted "Chicken" and Vegetables,
      111, 126
  "Sausage" and Asparagus Fajitas, 138
  Sauteed Polenta with Sweet Italian
      "Sausage," 134
  Sloppy Joes, 111, 137
  Southern Greens and "Sausage," 128
  South of the Border Tofu, 133
  Tempeh and Sweet Beans, 159
  Tempeh Kebabs, 135
  Thai Tofu and Peanut Sauce, 129
  Tofu and Snow Peas, 119
  Vegetable Curry with Tofu, 145
  Yam Patties with Curry Sauce, 139
Equol, 27
Esophagus, cancer of the, 7

Estrogen level, significance of, 9, 27
Exercise:
  in disease prevention, 8, 10
  weight control and, 20

Fairview Farms of Iowa, 38, 41, 88, 205,
      269
FARM (Farm Animal Reform
      Movement), 276
Farm Sanctuary, 276
Fat(s):
  applesauce replacement, 42
  as energy source, 19
  nutritional characteristics, 2, 6, 11
Featherweight baking powder, 42
Federal Trade Commission, 10
Fiber-rich foods, 2
Figs, 247–258
Fish, 18
Flavonoids, 27–28
Flesh foods, 2, 7, 9
Florida Crystals, Inc., 33, 44, 269
Flour:
  corn, 43
  gluten, 50
  oat, 44
  oat bran, 44
  purchase guidelines, 32
  soy, 40
  tapioca, 42
  whole grain yellow cornmeal, 45
  whole wheat, 45
  whole wheat pastry, 45
Folic acid, sources of, 22, 25, 161
Follow Your Heart, 49, 270
Fondues:
  "Cheesy," 54, 59
  Richly Chocolate, 54, 87
Food and Agriculture Organization
      (United Nations), 8
Food and Drug Administration (FDA),
      21–22
Food for Life (Barnard), 16
Food, Nutrition and the Prevention of
      Cancer: a Global Perspective
      (AICR), 8
Food Revolution, The (Robbins), 6
Framingham Heart Study, 6–7

Free radicals, 25
Fruit, *see specific types of fruit*
    disease prevention and, 3, 8
    dried, 43–44, 234
    phytochemicals, 27
Fruitsource, 45

Gall-bladder disease, 18
Garbanzo beans:
    nutritional characteristics of, 45
    Tomato Vegetable Soup with, 107–108
Garlic:
    dried minced, 44
    granulated, 45
Gimme Lean sausage (Lightlife), 38, 111,
    138
Gingerol, 28
Gingerroot, 46
Glazes/Icing:
    Boiled Pineapple Icing, 250
    Cherry Blossom Sauce, 245–246
    Espresso Glaze, 244
    Orange Blossom Glaze, 264
    Peanut Butter Icing, 247–248
"Got Milk?" ad campaign, 10
Gourmet cooking:
    Asian Marinade, 208
    Balsamic Marinade, 209
    Barbecue Baked Tofu, homemade, 207,
    220
    "Cheese," Homemade Dairy-Free, 202
    Coconut Curry Sauce, 198
    Cookie Crumb Topping, 197
    Creamy Dijon Sauce, 199
    Deep-Dish Whole Wheat Pie Crust,
    194
    Fragrant Soy Marinade, 211
    Ginger Baked Tofu, homemade, 206
    Gratin Topping, 196
    Lively, 212
    Multi-Grain Baking Mix, 191, 195
    Orient Express Marinade, 213
    Pacific Blend Marinade, 214
    Pineapple Apricot Butter, 221
    Pungent Ginger Marinade, 215
    recipe list, 193
    Red Miso Marinade, 216
    Roasted Chile Marinade, 217
    Savory Sesame Marinade, 218
    Soymilk, homemade, 203-204
    Spiced Peach Butter, 222, 237
    Spicy Peanut Sauce, 200
    Spring Onion Marinade, 219
    Sweet 'n' Sassy Marinade, 210
    Szechuan Sesame Sauce, 201
    tips for, 191-192
    Tofu, homemade, 205
    Zesty Barbecue Marinade, 220
Grain and Salt Society, The, 270
Grains:
    protein intake, 16
    soyfoods, 22
Grapes Leaves, Stuffed, 80–81
Greens:
    assorted, 42
    Southern, and "Sausage," 128
Grilled foods:
    Open-Faced "Cheese" Triangles, 146,
    202
    Polenta, with Tomato-Basil Cream, 114
    Tofu, Marinated, with Vegetables, 120
Grits, soy, 40
Ground beef alternatives, 22, 38, 111
Ground Round, ground beef alternatives,
    22, 38

Hain Celestial Group, The, 270
"Ham":
    Creamed Penne and, 140
    Kale, White Beans, and, 161
Harris, William, Dr., 10
Harvard Nurses' Health Study, 11
Harvard School of Public Health, 11–12
Haterill, Robert, Dr., 12
Healing Heart Foundation, The, 13, 277
Health food stores, as resource, 22–24,
    37, 44, 120, 218
Health Valley, 197, 270
Heart attack:
    causes of, 6
    prevention strategies, 7, 10
Heart disease, 18. *See also* Cardiovascular
    disease; Coronary heart disease
Herbs:
    phytochemicals in, 27
    purchase guidelines, 32

High-fat diets, 9
High-fiber diets, 5, 9–10
High-protein animal foods, 16
Holiday meal planning, Festive Roast,
    78–79
Hoppin' John, 84
Hormone levels, significance of, 9–10
Hydrogenation, 19

Imagine Foods, Inc., 270
Imagine No-Chicken Broth, 32
Indoles, 28
Information resources:
    food resource guide, 269–273
    Internet sites, 275–277
    reading suggestions, 279–280
Insulin-like growth factor (IGF-1), 11–12
International Agency on Research in
    Cancer, 8
Internet resources, 275–277
Iron, sources of, 22, 48
Ischemia, 6
Isoflavones, 28
Isothiocyanates, 27–28
Italian food, see Pasta
    Linguine al Pesto, 111, 136
    Sauteed Polenta with Sweet Italian
        "Sausage," 134
    Savory "Sausage" Lasagna, 67–68
    Spinach-Stuffed Shells, 65–66

Journal of the National Institutes of Health,
    11
Juice, Florida Crystals evaporated cane, 45

Kale:
    Mexicali Kale, 161
    nutritional characteristics of, 46, 161
    Pineapple Basmati Pilaf, 176
    with Toasted Pine Nuts and Raisins,
        161
    White Beans and "Ham" and, 161
    Whole Wheat Couscous Pilaf, 175
KAL Nutritional Yeast, 32, 47
Ketchup, fruit-sweetened, 33, 45
Kidney(s):
    damage/disease, 16, 21
    stones, 18

Kosher foods, 48
Kradjian, Robert, Dr., 16

Lacto-ovo vegetarian, defined, 1–2
Lappe, Frances Moore, 1
Large intestine, function of, 9
Larynx, cancer of the, 7
Lasagna:
    Barilla noodles, 42
    Savory "Sausage," 67–68
    tofu in, 111
Laura Beans, 37–38
LDL, 5
Lean Links Italian (Lightlife), 111
Leeks, 47
Legumes:
    in disease prevention, 8
    phytochemicals in, 27
    protein intake, 16
    soyfoods, 22
Lentils:
    Hearty Yams and, 178
    Neopolitan Pasta and, 125
    nutritional characteristics of, 22
Lifestyle, generally:
    changes, 2, 21, 24
    degenerative diseases and, 8
    disease prevention and, 8
    free radicals and, 25
    plant-based, 18
    sedentary, 18
    vegan, 23
Lighter Bake, 46
Lightlife Foods, Inc., 38, 40 41, 49, 111,
    270, 277
Lignans, 28
Liquid Fruitsource, 33, 45, 69
Live Food Products, 270
Liver cancer, 7
Low-fat diets, benefits of, 5, 9–10
Low-fat, high-fiber diets, in disease
    prevention, 9–10
Lung cancer, 7
Lycopenes, 29, 31

McDougall, John, Dr., 3, 16, 18–19, 275
McDougall Plan for Healthy Living,
    18–19, 275

*McDougall Program, The* (McDougall), 16
Magnesium, 13
Mail Order Catalog, The, 41, 270
Main courses, *see* Entrees
Mainstream Vegan, 23–24
Mammograms, 9
Margarine, 19
Marinades:
  Asian, 208
  Balsamic, 62, 209
  Fragrant Soy, 211
  Lively, 212
  Orient Express, 213
  Pacific Blend, 214
  Pungent Ginger, 215
  Red Miso, 216
  Roasted Chile, 217
  Savory Sesame, 218
  sesame, 61
  Spring Onion, 60, 219
  Sweet 'n' Sassy, 210
  Zesty Barbecue, 220
Mayonnaise, 33, 38–39
Meat(s), generally:
  alternatives, 22–24. *See also* Ground
    beef alternatives
  -centered diets, 5
  protein-rich, 18
  red, 1
Meatballs, ground beef alternatives
  Gimme Lean, 38
  soy, 22
Melissa's/World Variety Produce, Inc., 44,
    271, 277
Mexican dishes:
  Ginger Tempeh Wrap, 122
  Hearty Tortilla Wraps, 71
  Mexicali Kale, 161
  Mexican Polenta, 123
  Potato Quesadillas, 56
  "Sausage" and Asparagus Fajitas,
    138
Middle Eastern foods, Stuffed Grape
    Leaves, 80–81
Milk, *see* Soymilk
  allergies to, 12
  lite coconut, 46
  nonfat, 12

nutritional characteristics, 7, 11–12, 23
  skim, 12
Mirin, 46
Miso:
  country barley, 38
  Easy and Delicious Soup, 104
  Red, Marinade, 216
  mellow white, 38
Miyako Oriental Foods, Inc., 271
Monounsaturated fats, 19
Mori Nu:
  products, generally, 276
  silken tofu, 39, 260
  soups, 32, 34, 38, 161, 199, 201
Morinaga Nutritional Foods, Inc., 271,
    276
Mouth cancer, 7
Muffins:
  Apricot, Awesome, 225
  Blueberries, Oats, and Roses, 228
  Cranberry Spice, 226
  Cranberry Walnut, 227
  Yam Good!, 229
Muir Glen, 33, 45
Multi-Grain Baking Mix, 191, 239
Mushroom(s):
  baby portabellos, 46
  Braised Tempeh with Tomatoes and,
    157
  broth powder, 46
  button, 46
  Creamy Cauliflower Bake, 182
  cremini, 46
  Dilled Asparagus and, 161
  dried medley, 44
  Shitake, 46
  wild, 46, 85
Mustard, dijon, 43, 91–92, 199

Nasoya Foods, Inc., 38, 271
National Dairy Council, 11
Nayonaise, 38–39
NewCenturyNutrition, 277
*New England Journal of Medicine,* 21
nSpire Natural Foods, 271
Nutmeats, 47
Nuts, phytochemicals in, 27. *See also* Pine
    nuts; Soynuts; Tosteds; Walnuts

Oat flour, purchase guidelines, 32
Oats, muffins, 228
Obesity, 9, 18
Oils, use of, 19–20
Okara:
  A-Maize-ing Burgers, 154
  Braised Veggies with Baked Tofu and,
    189
  Chocolate Chip Spice Bars, 265
  dry roasted, 39
  nutritional characteristics of, 39
  Onion Burgers, 153
Olive oil:
  cooking spray, 47
  nutritional characteristics of, 19–20
Onions:
  Bermuda, 47
  broth powder, 153
  Okara Burgers, 153
  red, 47
  Spanish, 47
  Spring Onion Marinade, 60, 219
  sweet, 47
  white, 47
  yellow, 47
Oranges, 22
Organosulfurs, 29
Ornish, Dean, Dr., 3, 19
Orzo, 48
Osteoporosis, 10, 18, 21–22

Pacific Foods of Oregon, Inc., 41, 271
Paella, 64
Palm oil, 5
Pancakes, Blueberry Apple, 240
Pancreatic cancer, 7
Pantry suggestions:
  baking needs, 35
  canned/jarred goods, 33–34
  cereals, 35
  condiments, 36
  dry foods, 34
  flours, 35
  ingredient notes, 36–41
  miscellaneous, 35–36
  pasta, 34
  sauces, prepared, 36
  soups, 34

sweeteners, 35
Pasta:
  Barilla lasagna noodles, 42
  Broken, Casserole, 172
  Chilled Salad with Edamame, 97
  Cold Sesame Noodles, 109, 201
  Creamed Penne and "Ham," 140
  Lasagna, Savory "Sausage," 67–68
  Linguine al Pesto, 111, 136
  Neopolitan, and Lentils, 111, 125
  nutritional characteristics of, 19
  panette, 97
  Penne, Creamed and "Ham," 140
  Penne with Tofu Tomato Sauce, 144
  Salad, Caribbean, 96, 214
  Shells, Spinach-Stuffed, 65–66
Pastry:
  Fillo pastry shells, 44
  whole wheat flour, 45
Pâté, Mushroom-Okara, 83
Peach(es):
  Brandied Custard, 241, 256
  dried, 44
  Just Peachy Dessert Crepes, 86
  Spiced Butter, 222, 227, 237
Pears:
  Poached, with Brandied Almond
    "Cream," 260–261
  Yams with "Bacon," Raisins and, 179
Peas, see Snow peas
  Crumbled Tofu with Tomatoes, Bell
    Peppers and, 161, 185
  nutritional characteristics of, 22
Penne:
  Creamed, and Ham, 140
  with Tofu Tomato Sauce, 144
  Pepper, chopotle, 43
  Pepperoni:
  veggie, 22, 41, 111
Potatoes, 161, 180
Pharynx, cancer of the, 7
Phenolic acid, 29
Phyllo cups, chocolate raspberry, 262–263
Physicians Committee for Responsible
    Medicine (PCRM), 9–10, 12, 275
Phytochemicals:
  characteristics of, 5, 9–10, 26–29
  sources of, generally, 161

Phytoestrogens, 9–10, 27
Pie, Strawberry Banana "Cream,"
    254–255
Pilaf:
    Basmatic, Pineapple, 176
    Kasha, 174
    Soynut, Couscous with Golden Raisins
        and,183
    Tomato, Brown Rice and, 173
Pinckney, Neal, Dr., 13, 277
Pineapple(s):
    Apricot Butter, 221, 227
    Boiled Icing, 250
    dried chunks, 44
    Pineapple Mango Pudding, 241, 259
    Spiced Pineapple Zucchini Bread, 236
Pine nuts:
    Brown Rice with Broccoli and, 177
    toasted, 161
Pita crisps, Garlic and Thyme, 74
Plant-based diet:
    benefits of, 2–3, 25
    cancer prevention and, 8–9
    characteristics of, 5
    defined, 2
    for disease prevention, 9
    protein intake, 16–17
Plaque, development of, 6
Polenta:
    "Beefy" Bake, 141–142
    Grilled, Tomato-Basil Cream, 114
    Mexican, 123
    San Gennaro (Food Merchants), 45,
        114
    Sauteed with Sweet Italian "Sausage,"
        134
Polyunsaturated fats, 19–20
Pork products, 7
Potato(es):
    Curry, Broccoli and, 156
    Gratin, Roasted Corn and, 187
    Harvest Medley, 121
    Hearty Tempeh and Potato Roast, 150
    mashed, 42
    nutritional characteristics of, 19, 22
    "Pepperoni," 161, 180
    Quesadillas, 53, 56
Poultry, 18. See also Chicken

Pressure cooker, use of, 31
Preventive Medicine Research Institute,
    19
Prostate cancer, 2, 7, 9, 11–12, 27
Protease inhibitors, 29
Protein(s):
    amino acids, 15–16
    calculation of, 16
    characteristics of, 2
    kidney damage and, 16
    plant sources, 15–18
    sources of, 48
    soy, 22
Prune purée, 48
Puddings/custards:
    Brandied Peach Custard, 241, 256
    Mandarin-Orange Blossom, 257–258
    Pineapple Mango Pudding, 241, 259
Pumpkin:
    Raisin Bread, 237
    Spice Cake, 249

Quercetin, 29
Quiche:
    Individual Broccoli, 69–70
    tofu in, 111
Quinoa, 48
Quong Hop & Co., 271

Rainforest Action Network, 276
Raisins:
    Cinnamon Raisin Bread, 233
    Golden, with Couscous and Soynut
        Pilaf, 183
    Pumpkin Raisin Bread, 237
    Yams with "Bacon," Pears, and, 179
Raspberries:
    Chocolate Raspberry Ganache,
        252–253
    Chocolate Raspberry Phyllo Cups,
        262–263
Recommended daily allowance
    (RDA), 12
Rectal cancer, 7
Red pepper, crushed, 32
Red Star Nutritional Yeast, 32, 47
Resource Guide, 269–273
Resveratrol, 27

Rice, *see* Pilaf
    basmati, 43
    Brown, with Broccoli and Pine Nuts,
      177
    Brown, and Tomato Pilaf, 173
    Hearty Summer Salad, 99
    nutritional characteristics of, 19
    Red Beans with "Sausage," 161, 186
    Stuffed Grape Leaves, 80–81
Rice cookers, 173
Roasted Chicken Not!, 39
Robbie's Foods, 49
Robbins, John, 6, 275
Rosmarinic acid, 29
Rumford baking powder, 42

Saffron, 48
Salad dressings, 39. *See also* Dressings
Salads:
    California Chef's, 89, 94
    Caribbean Pasta, 89, 96, 214
    Easy Edamame, 98
    Hearty Summer Rice, 89, 99
Salsa, 33
Salt:
    Celtic sea, 43, 191
    sea, 48
S & W Foods, 43, 49
San Gennaro Foods, Inc., 271
Sanlinx Inc., 272
San Miguel Produce, Inc., 271–272
Saponins, 29
Saturated fats, 2, 5–6, 11, 20–21
Sauces:
    barbecue, 33
    Brandied Almond "Cream," 260–261
    "Cheese," 161, 163
    Creamy Dijon, 91–92, 199
    Curry, 139
    Peanut, 129
    Pesto, 136
    Spicy Peanut, 200
    Szechuan Sesame, 109, 201
    Tofu Tomato, 144
    "Sausage":
    and Asparagus Fajitas, 138
    in a Blanket, 75
    Red Beans and Rice with, 161, 186

Savory Lasagne, 67–68
Smart Links Italian, 39
soy, 2
Southern Greens and, 128
Sweet Italian, Sauteed Polenta with, 134
Turnovers, 76–77
Save Yourself from Breast Cancer
    (Kradjian), 16
Scallions, 47
*Scientific Basis of Vegetarianism, The*
    (Harris), 10
Sea salt, 43, 48, 191
Seafood, 7
Sea vegetables, 31, 157
Seeds, 27
Seitan, 49, 127, 213–214, 220
Selenium, 25
Shallots, 4
Shopping guidelines, 31–33. *See also*
    Pantry suggestions
Shortening, 19
Shoyu, 39
Side dishes:
    Braised Veggies with Baked Tofu and
      Okara, 189
    Broken Pasta Casserole, 172
    Brown Rice and Tomato Pilaf, 173
    Brown Rice with Broccoli and Pine
      Nuts, 177
    Cauliflower in "Cheese" Sauce, 161,
      163
    Couscous, Golden Raisin, and Soynut
      Pilaf, 183
    Creamy Mushroom Cauliflower Bake,
      182
    Crumbled Tofu with Peas, Tomatoes,
      and Bell Pepper, 161, 185
    Curried Brussels Sprouts and Baby
      Carrots, 161, 164
    Dilled Asparagus and Wild
      Mushrooms, 161, 165
    Edamame Succotash, 161, 166
    Hawaiian Unbaked Beans, 181
    Hearty Yams and Lentils, 178
    Kale with Toasted Pine Nuts and
      Raisins, 161, 167
    Kale, White Beans, and "Ham," 161,
      169

Kasha Pilaf, 174
Mexicali Kale, 161, 168
Oven Roasted Balsamic Veggies, 170
"Pepperoni" Potatoes, 161, 180
recipe list, 162
Red Beans and Rice with "Sausage,"
    161, 186
Roasted Corn and Potato Gratin, 187,
    196
Roasted Garlic Couscous with
    Blueberries and Walnuts, 184
Savory Corn Medallions, 171
Vegetable Medley with Edamame, 188
Yams, "Bacon," Pears, and Raisins, 179
Sikbadj, 151
Simply Delicious, Inc., 39, 272
Skaff, Ned and Rose, 80
Sloppy Joes, 111, 137
Smart Chick'n Strips, 40
Smart Ground, 38
Smart Links Italian Sausage, 39
Smart Steak-Style Strips, 40
Snacks, Trail Mix, Tosteds, 88
Snow peas:
    Five-Spice Tofu and Snow Peas in
        Ginger Sauce, 149
    Tofu and, 119
Sokol and, Co., 48, 272
Solo Levkar, 48
Sonoma Foods, 49
Soups/stews:
    Basque Stew, 131
    "Beef" Vindaloo, 160
    "Beefy" Polenta Bake, 141–142
    "Chicken" and Barley, 101–102
    Chunky Vegetable "Beef", 103
    "Cream" of Broccoli, 89, 100
    Easy and Delicious Miso, 104
    Gingered Acorn Squash, 89, 105–106
    North African Stew (Sikbadj), 151
    prepared, 32
    Tomato Vegetable, with Garbanzos,
        107–108
Soybeans, 22, 27
Soy burgers, quick, 155
Soyco Foods, 272
Soy Deli, The, 37–38
Soy flour, 40

Soyfoods,:
    description of, 37–41
    health benefits of, 21–22
Soy grits, 40
Soymage, 40
Soymilk:
    homemade, 191, 203–204
    Mexican Polenta, 123
    nutritional characteristics of, 22–23, 40
    Rich and Creamy Mocha Shake, 266
Soy Power, 41
Soy products, benefits of, 9–10
Soy seasoning, 33
Soymage, 40
Soynuts:
    Creamy Mushroom Cauliflower Bake,
        182
    nutritional characteristics of, 40,
    roasted, 41
    Roasted, Banana Bread with, 230
    tosteds, 115
Soyrizo, 168
Soyrizo vegetarian chorizo, 40
Spanish foods, Paella, 64. See also Mexican
    dishes
Spices:
    phytochemicals in, 27
    purchase guidelines, 32
Spinach:
    -Artichoke Dip, 72
    -Stuffed Shells, 65–66
Spock, Benjamin, Dr., 3
Squash, Hearty Stuffed, 124. See also
    specific types of squash
Starchy foods, 19
Stomach cancer, 7
Strawberries, Banana "Cream" Pie,
    254–255
Stroke, 6, 18
Stuffed shells:
    Spinach-Stuffed, 65–66
    tofu, 111
Sucanat, 33, 49
Succotash, Edamame, 161, 166
Sugar, see Sweeteners
    brown, 49
    evaporated cane, 44
    Sucanat evaporated cane, 49

Sulforaphane, 27, 29
Sun–dried tomatoes, Quiche Bits, 53, 57–58
Sunspire, 43
Sunsweet Growers, Inc., 272
Sweet potato(es):
    Bread, Southern–Style, 238
    yams compared with, 178

Tamari, 40
Tea, green, 27
Tempeh:
    Braised, with Mushrooms and Tomatoes, 157
    Chili, 82
    Ginger Wrap, 122
    Harvest Medley, 121
    Hearty, and Potato Roast, 150
    Kebabs, 135, 217
    nutritional characteristics of, 23, 40–41, 111
    Pacific Blend Marinade, 214
    Pungent Ginger Marinade, 215
    Red Miso Marinade, 216
    Roasted Chile Marinade, 217
    Spicy Peanut Sauce, 200
    and Sweet Beans, 159
    Sweet 'n' Sassy Marinade, 210
    Zesty Barbecue Marinade, 220
Terpenes, 29
Textured Vegetable Protein (TVP), 32, 41, 111, 116, 147, 155
Thai Kitchen, 46
Tofu:
    baked, 37
    Baked, with Braised Veggies and Okara, 189
    Barbecue Baked, homemade, 207
    Chinese–style, 111, 119, 133, 191
    Crumbled, with Peas, Tomatoes, and Bell Pepper, 161, 185
    description of, 41
    Festive Holiday Roast, 78–79
    firm nigari, 37–38
    Five-Spice, and Snow Peas in Ginger "Cream," 149
    Fragrant Soy Marinade, 211
    Ginger Baked, homemade, 206

Grilled Marinated and Vegetables, 120
Hero, 49
homemade, 191, 205
Japanese-style, 111
Marinated, and Baby Bok Choy, 130
nutritional characteristics of, 23
Pacific Blend Marinade, 214
Pungent Ginger Marinade, 215
Red Miso Marinade, 216
Savory "Sausage" Lasagna, 67–68
silken, 39, 111
and Snow Peas, 119
South of the Border, 133
Sweet 'n' Sassy Marinade, 210
Thai, and Peanut Sauce, 129
Tomato Sauce, 144
Vegetable Curry with, 145
Zesty Barbecue Marinade, 220
Tomatoes:
    Braised Tempeh with Mushrooms and, 157
    Crumbled Tofu with Peas, Bell Peppers and, 161, 185
    diced, 43
    nutritional characteristics of, 31
    Pilaf, Brown Rice and, 173
    stewed, 32, 49
    sun-dried, 49
    sun-dried, quiche bites, 57–58
    Tofu Tomato Sauce, 144
    Vegetable Soup with Garbanzos, 107–108
Tortillas:
    Hearty Wraps, 71
    whole wheat, 50
Tosteds:
    Chocolate-Covered, with Fruit, 267
    nutritional characteristics of, 37, 4
    Trail Mix, 88
Trail Mix, Tosteds, 88
Trans-fats, 19–20
Tree of Life, 37, 272
Tropical oils, 5
Tropical Source, 43
Tumors, 27
Turtle Island Foods, 41

U.S. Department of Agriculture (USDA), 7, 10
U.S. National Cancer Institute, 8
Uterine cancer, 7, 9

Vanilla extract, pure, 48
Vegan, defined, 23
Vegan diet, *see* Plant-based diet
Vegenaise, 33, 49
Vegetable(s), generally:
    Braised, with Baked Tofu and Okara, 189
    disease prevention and, 3, 8
    increased consumption of, 1
    as magnesium source, 13
    Medley with Edamame, 188
    microwaved, 177
    Oven Roasted Balsamic, 170
    phytochemicals in, 27
    protein in, 22
    protein intake and, 16
    Spicy Peanut Sauce, 200
    Spring Onion Marinade, 219
Vegetable oil, 19
Vegetarian diet, *see* Plant-based diet
Vegetarian Resource Group (VRG), 276
Vegetarian Support Formula, 32, 47
Veggie Canadian Bacon (Yves):
    nutritional benefits, 22, 41, 111
    Yams with Pears, Raisins, and, 179
Veggie Cuisine (Yves), 273, 276
Veggie Dogs, 22
Veggie Pepperoni (Yves), 22, 41, 111
Vegi-Deli, 272
Vegsource.com, 275
vegtv.com, 191, 203, 275
Very-low-calorie diets, 18
Vitamin A, 161
Vitamin $B_{12}$, 23, 32, 47
Vitamin C, 25, 46, 161
Vitamin E, 25
Vitamin K, 46

Walnuts:
    Cranberry Muffins, 227
    Roasted Garlic Couscous with Blueberries and, 184
Water:
    orange blossom, 48
    rose, 48
Weight control/maintenance, 2, 8, 18–20
Weight-lifting, 20
Westbrae Foods, 38, 45
Western diet, 2, 7–8, 16
Wheat gluten, vital, 49–50
White Wave, Inc., 37, 41, 49, 272
Whole grains:
    in disease prevention, 3, 8
    magnesium source, 13
    phytochemicals in, 27
    purchase guidelines, 32
Wholesome Sweeteners, 33, 44, 49, 273
Wildwood Natural Foods, 37, 273
Willett, Walter, Dr., 11
Wine, red, 27
Wizard, The, 49
Worchestershire sauce, vegetarian, 49
World Cancer Research Fund, 8
World Health Organization, 8, 12
Worldwatch Institute, 276

Yams:
    with "Bacon," Pears, and Raisins, 179
    Hearty, and Lentils, 178
    muffins, 229
    Patties with Curry Sauce, 139
Yeast:
    active dry, 42
    nutritional, 32, 47
Youth for Environmental Sanity (YES!), 277

Zone-type diets, 18
Zucchini:
    Mocha Java Bundt Cake with Espresso Glaze, 244
    Spiced Pineapple Zucchini Bread, 236

# About the Author

Marie Oser, the best-selling author of *Soy of Cooking* and *More Soy Cooking,* is a newspaper columnist whose work focuses on health, nutrition, and the plant-based diet. She specializes in developing original gourmet recipes that are low in fat, high in fiber, and rich in phytochemicals. Her work has been endorsed by prominent medical and nutrition professionals such as Drs. Dean Ornish, John McDougall, and Neal Barnard. Her column, *The Enlightened Kitchen,* is distributed nationally on the Scripps Howard Wire Service.

A soyfoods expert, Marie hosts a popular discussion board, *Soy Talk* at *VegSource.com,* a site with well over one million unique visitors every month. Marie is co-host and on-camera chef at *VegTv.com,* where she and VegTv founder Jane Velez-Mitchell, an award-winning television journalist, produce streaming videos with a focus on food and health. Jane and Marie have just completed a one-hour special, *VegTv News Presents: Fun Food California Style,* and have several other television projects in development.

Marie has appeared on networks such as CNN, ABC, National Public Radio, QVC The Fine Living Channel, and Discovery. Marie lives in Southern California, where her live talk radio feature, *The Enlightened Kitchen,* airs weekly on KVTA-AM 1520. Marie teaches classes in healthy gourmet cooking at cooking schools and at Cedars Sinai Medical Center in Los Angeles and conducts seminars at universities such as Pepperdine in Malibu.

The book that started it all!

Now you can create elegant meals that are as healthy as they are delicious. *Soy of Cooking* is a gourmet guide to preparing savory meatless dishes that incorporate nutrient-rich soyfoods into your diet. Create meals that are high in antioxidants and phytochemicals, as well as fiber and vitamins. With more than 170 enticing recipes, this innovative cookbook shows how to combine creative techniques and easy-to-find soyfoods to make healthy starters, main dishes, desserts, and more.

## SOY OF COOKING
### *Easy-to-Make Vegetarian, Low-Fat, Fat-Free, and Antioxidant-Rich Gourmet Recipes*

By Marie Oser

Published by John Wiley & Sons, Inc.   $16.95   ISBN 0-471-34705-1
Available wherever books are sold

"In the *Soy of Cooking,* Marie Oser shows the myriad ways to make soy delicious and nutritious."
—Dean Ornish, M.D., author of *Everyday Cooking with Dean Ornish*

"Full of excellent recipes that taste superb."
—John Robbins, author of *The Food Revolution* and *Diet for a New America*

"The recipes are familiar enough to become instant successes in your home, yet sensational enough to be served in 5-star restaurants."
—John McDougall, M.D., Director of the McDougall Program, St. Helena Hospital; and Mary McDougall, author of *The New McDougall Cookbook*

Want to create 170 *more* rich-tasting, scrumptious, *healthful* dishes?

In *More Soy Cooking: Healthful Renditions of Classic Traditional Meals*, Marie Oser again shares her secrets to creating delicious dishes—healthfully! From hearty soups to succulent salads and dressings, from to-die-for desserts to elegant, easy-to-make entrees, Oser gives our favorite recipes a healthy makeover by introducing alternative ingredients and techniques to replace high-fat, cholesterol-laden fare. From Sweet Italian "Sausage" with Peppers to Stuffed Mushrooms Florentine, each recipe is low in fat, high in fiber, rich in phytochemicals, and 100% cholesterol- and dairy-free.

## MORE SOY COOKING
*Healthful Renditions of Classic Traditional Meals*

By Marie Oser

Published by John Wiley & Sons, Inc.   $16.95   ISBN 0-471-37761-9
Available wherever books are sold

"A wonderful follow-up to *Soy of Cooking*—a beautifully written treasure chest of terrific recipes."

—Neal Barnard, M.D., President, Physicians Committee for Responsible Medicine

"When it comes to creating traditional-style meals using healthy ingredients—and making it all come out fantastic—*More Soy Cooking* is the answer."

—John Robbins, author of *Diet for a New America* and founder, EarthSave International

"A cornucopia of traditional recipes that have been made healthier and lower in fat as well as many original taste treats to nourish and comfort just about everyone."

— Neal Pinckney, Ph.D., Director of the Healing Heart Foundation and author of *Healthy Heart Handbook*